Q... Sexual Assault

For Healthcare, Social Service, and Law Enforcement Professionals

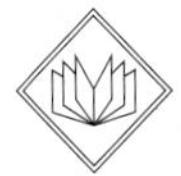

G.W. Medical Publishing, Inc.
St. Louis

Contents in Brief

Quick-Reference
Sexual Assault

For Healthcare, Social Service, and Law Enforcement Professionals

Angelo P. Giardino, MD, PhD
Associate Chair - Pediatrics
Associate Physician-in-Chief
St. Christopher's Hospital for Children
Associate Professor in Pediatrics
Drexel University College of Medicine
Philadelphia, Pennsylvania

Elizabeth M. Datner, MD
Assistant Professor
University of Pennsylvania School of Medicine
Department of Emergency Medicine
Assistant Professor of Emergency Medicine in Pediatrics
Children's Hospital of Philadelphia
Philadelphia, Pennsylvania

Janice B. Asher, MD
Assistant Clinical Professor
Obstetrics and Gynecology
University of Pennsylvania Medical Center
Director
Women's Health Division of Student Health Service
University of Pennsylvania
Philadelphia, Pennsylvania

Barbara W. Girardin, RN, PhD
Forensic Health Care
Palomar Pomerado Health
Escondido, California

Diana K. Faugno, RN, BSN, CPN, FAAFS, SANE-A
District Director
Pediatrics/Nicu
Forensic Health Service
Palomar Pomerado Health
Escondido, California

Mary J. Spencer, MD
Clinical Professor of Pediatrics
University of California San Diego School of Medicine
Medical Director
Child Abuse Prevention and Sexual Assault Response Team
Palomar Pomerado Health
Escondido, California

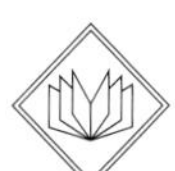

G.W. Medical Publishing, Inc.
St. Louis

Publishers: Glenn E. Whaley and Marianne V. Whaley
Design Director: Glenn E. Whaley
Managing Editors: Ann Przyzycki
Kristine Feeherty
Associate Editors: Grant Armstrong
Christine Bauer
Book Design/Page Layout: G.W. Graphics
Vicky Ho
Print/Production Coordinator: Charles J. Seibel, III
Cover Design: G.W. Graphics
Color Prepress Specialist: Terry L. Williams
Developmental Editor: Elaine Steinborn
Indexer: Nelle Garrecht

Printed in Canada

Publisher:
G.W. Medical Publishing, Inc.
77 Westport Plaza, Suite 366, St. Louis, Missouri 63146-3124 USA
Phone: (314)542-4213 Fax: (314)542-4239 Toll Free: (800)600-0330
http://www.gwmedical.com

Library of Congress Cataloging-in-Publication Data

Quick-reference sexual assault : for healthcare professionals, social services, and law enforcement / Angelo P. Giardino . . . [et al.].
p. ; cm.
Includes bibliographical references and index.
ISBN 1-878060-38-4 (pbk. : alk. paper)
1. Rape.
[DNLM: 1. Forensic Medicine--methods. 2. Sex Offenses.
3. Patient Care Team. 4. Physical Examination--methods.
W 795 Q6 2003] I. Giardino, Angelo P.
RA1141.Q53 2003
616.85'8--dc21

2003009538

Contributors

Joyce A. Adams, MD
Clinical Professor of Pediatrics
Division of General Academic Pediatrics and Adolescent Medicine
University of California, San Diego Medical Center
San Diego, California

Randell Alexander, MD, PhD
Associate Professor
Clinical Pediatrics
Morehouse School of Medicine
Forensic Pediatrician
Department of Pediatrics
Morehouse School of Medicine
Atlanta, Georgia

Eileen Allen, RN, BSN, DABFN
SANE Program Coordinator
Monmouth County Prosecutor's Office
Freehold, New Jersey

Sarah Anderson, RN, MSN
University of Virginia
Department of Emergency Medicine (Registered Nurse)
School of Nursing (Doctoral Student)
Charlottesville, Virginia

Joanne Archambault
Training Director
Sexual Assault Training and Investigations (SATI, Inc.)
Retired Sergeant
San Diego Police Department
Sex Crimes Unit

Janice B. Asher, MD
Assistant Clinical Professor
Obstetrics and Gynecology
University of Pennsylvania Medical Center
Director
Women's Health Division of Student Health Service
University of Pennsylvania
Philadelphia, Pennsylvania

Tracy Bahm, JD
Senior Attorney
Violence Against Women Program
American Prosecutors Research Institute (APRI)
Alexandria, Virginia

Kathy Bell, RN
Forensic Nurse Examiner
Tulsa Police Department
Tulsa, Oklahoma

Patrick E. Besant-Matthews, MD
Forensic Pathology and Forensic Medicine
Legal and Law Enforcement Consultations
Private Practice
Dallas, Texas

Sandra L. Bloom, MD
CEO, Community Works
Philadelphia, Pennsylvania

Duncan T. Brown, JD
Staff Attorney
National Center for Prosecution of Child Abuse
American Prosecutors Research Institute (APRI)
Alexandria, Virginia

Mary-Ann Burkhart, JD
Senior Attorney
National Center for Prosecution of Child Abuse
American Prosecutors Research Institute (APRI)
Alexandria, Virginia

Susan Chasson, MSN, CNM, JD
Lecturer
College of Nursing
Brigham Young University
Provo, Utah

Michael Clark, MSN, CRNP
Nurse Practitioner
Department of Emergency Medicine
Hospital of the University of Pennsylvania
Clinical Lecturer
University of Pennsylvania School of Nursing
Philadelphia, Pennsylvania

Sharon W. Cooper, MD, FAAP
Adjunct Associate Professor of Pediatrics
University of North Carolina School of Medicine
Chapel Hill, North Carolina
Clinical Assistant Professor of Pediatrics
Uniformed Services University of Health Sciences
Bethesda, Maryland
Chief
Developmental Pediatric Service
Womack Army Medical Center
Fort Bragg, North Carolina

Elizabeth M. Datner, MD
Assistant Professor
University of Pennsylvania School of Medicine
Department of Emergency Medicine
Assistant Professor of Emergency Medicine in Pediatrics
Children's Hospital of Philadelphia
Philadelphia, Pennsylvania

Sue Dickinson, RN, BSN, PHN, CEDN, SANE-A
Forensic Nurse Examiner
Palomar Pomerado Health
Escondido, California

Colette M. Eastman, DO
Obstetrics, Gynecology, and Reproductive Medicine
Physician Consultant/Instructor, Sexual Assault Response Team
Poway, California

Thomas Ervin, RNC, FN, BSc †
Reception and Release Coordinator
California State Prison at Corcoran
Department of Corrections
State of California

†Deceased

Diana K. Faugno, RN, BSN, CPN, FAAFS, SANE-A
District Director
Pediatrics/Nicu
Forensic Health Service
Palomar Pomerado Health
Escondido, California

Anne B. Finigan, RN, MScN, ACNP
Forensic Clinical Nurse Specialist/Nurse Practitioner
Regional Sexual Assault and Domestic Violence Treatment Centre
St. Joseph's Health Care London
London, Ontario
Canada

Martin A. Finkel, DO, FACOP, FAAP
Professor of Pediatrics
Medical Director
Center for Children's Support
School of Osteopathic Medicine
University of Medicine and Dentistry of New Jersey
Stratford, New Jersey

Marla J. Friedman, DO
Fellow, Pediatric Emergency Medicine
Emergency Medicine
Alfred I. duPont Hospital for Children
Wilmington, Delaware

Donna Gaffney, RN, DNSc, FAAN
Associate Professor, Acute Care Nurse Practitioner Program
College of Nursing
Seton Hall University
South Orange, New Jersey

Ann E. Gaulin, MS, MFT
Director of Counseling Services
Women Organized Against Rape
Philadelphia, Pennsylvania

Angelo P. Giardino, MD, PhD
Associate Chair - Pediatrics
Associate Physician-in-Chief
St. Christopher's Hospital for Children
Associate Professor in Pediatrics
Drexel University College of Medicine
Philadelphia, Pennsylvania

Eileen R. Giardino, PhD, RN, CRNP
Associate Professor
LaSalle University, School of Nursing
Nurse Practitioner
LaSalle University, Student Health Center
Philadelphia, Pennsylvania

Barbara W. Girardin, RN, PhD
Forensic Health Care
Palomar Pomerado Health
Escondido, California

Holly M. Harner, CRNP, PhD, MPH, SANE
Assistant Professor
William F. Connell School of Nursing
Boston College
Chestnut Hill, Massachusetts

Caren Harp, JD
Senior Attorney/Director
National Juvenile Justice Prosecution Center
American Prosecutors Research Institute (APRI)
Alexandria, Virginia

William C. Holmes, MD, MSCE
Assistant Professor of Medicine and Epidemiology
Philadelphia Veterans Affairs Medical Center
Center for Clinical Epidemiology and Biostatistics
University of Pennsylvania School of Medicine
Philadelphia, Pennsylvania

Jeffrey R. Jaeger, MD
Assistant Professor of Medicine
University of Pennsylvania Health System
Clinical Faculty, Institute for Safe Families
Philadelphia, Pennsylvania

Susan Bieber Kennedy, RN, JD
Senior Attorney
Violence Against Women Program
American Prosecutors Research Institute (APRI)
Alexandria, Virginia

Lisa Kreeger, JD
Senior Attorney
Violence Against Women Program Manager
DNA Forensics Program Manager
American Prosecutors Research Institute (APRI)
Alexandria, Virginia

Susan Kreston, JD
Deputy Director
National Center for Prosecution of Child Abuse
American Prosecutors Research Institute (APRI)
Alexandria, Virginia

Linda E. Ledray, RN, PhD, SANE-A, FAAN
Director
Sexual Assault Resource Service
Hennepin County Medical Center
Minneapolis, Minnesota

Carolyn J. Levitt, MD
Assistant Professor of Pediatrics
Department of Pediatrics
University of Minnesota
Director
Midwest Children's Resource Center
Children's Hospitals and Clinics
St. Paul, Minnesota

Patsy Rauton Lightle
Supervisory Special Agent
Lieutenant, Department of Child Fatalities
South Carolina Law Enforcement Division
Columbia, South Carolina

Judith A. Linden, MD, FACEP, SANE
Assistant Professor
Emergency Medicine
Boston University School of Medicine
Associate Residency Director
Boston University School of Medicine
Boston Medical Center
Boston, Massachusetts

John Loiselle, MD
Associate Professor of Pediatrics
Jefferson Medical College
Assistant Director, Emergency Medicine
Alfred I. duPont Hospital for Children
Wilmington, Delaware

Kathi Makoroff, MD
Mayerson Center for Safe and Healthy Children
Cincinnati Children's Hospital Medical Center
Cincinnati, Ohio

Jeanne Marrazzo, MD, MPH
Assistant Professor
Department of Medicine
Division of Allergy and Infectious Diseases
University of Washington
Seattle, Washington
Medical Director
Seattle STD/HIV Prevention Training Center
Seattle, Washington

Claire Nelli, RN, SANE-A
Manager—SART Department
Villa View Community Hospital
San Diego, California

Patrick O'Donnell, PhD
Supervising Criminalist, DNA Laboratory
San Diego Police Department
San Diego, California

Jason Payne-James, LLM, FRCS (Edin & Eng)**, DFM, RNutr**
Forensic Physician
Forensic Medical Examiner - Metropolitan Police Service and City of London Police
Director - Forensic Healthcare Services, Ltd.
Editor-in-Chief, *Journal of Clinical Forensic Medicine*
London, England
United Kingdom

Christine M. Peterson, MD
Director of Gynecology
Department of Student Health
Assistant Professor of Clinical Obstetrics and Gynecology
University of Virginia School of Medicine
Charlottesville, Virginia

Millicent Shaw Phipps, JD
Staff Attorney
Violence Against Women Program
American Prosecutors Research Institute (APRI)
Alexandria, Virginia

Hannah Ufberg Rabinowitz, MSN, ARNP, FNA, NCGNP
Clinical Education
Aventura Hospital
Aventura, Florida

William J. Reed, MD, FAAP
Assistant Professor of Pediatrics
Texas A&M College of Medicine
Behavioral and Adolescent Medicine
Driscoll Children's Hospital
Corpus Christi, Texas

Iris Reyes, MD, FACEP
Assistant Professor
Emergency Medicine
Hospital of the University of Pennsylvania
Assistant Medical Director
Emergency Medicine
Hospital of the University of Pennsylvania
Philadelphia, Pennsylvania

Dawn Rice, RN, BSN, FNE
Executive Director
Fort Wayne Sexual Assault Treatment Center
President
Indiana Chapter of the IAFN
Fort Wayne, Indiana

Laura L. Rogers, JD
Senior Attorney
National Center for Prosecution of Child Abuse
American Prosecutors Research Institute (APRI)
Alexandria, Virginia

Mimi Rose, JD
Chief Assistant District Attorney
Family Violence and Sexual Assault Unit
Philadelphia District Attorney Office
Philadelphia, Pennsylvania

Pamela Ross, MD
Assistant Professor of Emergency Medicine & Pediatrics
University of Virginia Health System
Charlottesville, Virginia

Rena Rovere, MS, FNP
Sexual Assault Program Director
Clinical Nurse Specialist
Department of Emergency Medicine
Albany Medical Center
Albany, New York

Bruce D. Rubin, MD
Clinical Instructor
Department of Emergency Medicine
Hospital of the University of Pennsylvania
Philadelphia, Pennsylvania

Maureen S. Rush, MS
Vice President for Public Safety
University of Pennsylvania
Division of Public Safety
Philadelphia, Pennsylvania

Charles J. Schubert, MD
Associate Professor of Pediatrics
Division of Emergency Medicine
Cincinnati Children's Hospital Medical Center
Cincinnati, Ohio

Diana Schunn, RN, BSN, SANE-A
SANE/SART Manager
Via Christi Regional Medical Center
Wichita, Kansas

Margot Schwartz, MD
Virginia Mason Medical Center
Infectious Diseases Section
Seattle, Washington
Clinical Instructor
Department of Medicine
University of Washington
Seattle, Washington

Deborah K. Scott, RN-C, BSN, ARNP, FNS
Child Protection Team
Howard Phillips Center for Children and Families
Orlando, Florida

Philip Scribano, DO, MSCE
Assistant Professor
Pediatrics and Emergency Medicine
University of Connecticut School of Medicine
Director, Child Protection Program
Connecticut Children's Medical Center
Hartford, Connecticut

Christina Shaw, JD
Staff Attorney
National Center for Prosecution of Child Abuse
American Prosecutors Research Institute (APRI)
Alexandria, Virginia

Patricia M. Speck, APRN, MSN, BC
Coordinator of Nursing Services and Interim Manager
City of Memphis Sexual Assault Resource Center
Division of Public Services and Neighborhoods
Memphis, Tennessee

Mary J. Spencer, MD
Clinical Professor of Pediatrics
University of California San Diego
School of Medicine
Medical Director
Child Abuse Prevention and Sexual Assault Response Team
Palomar Pomerado Health
Escondido, California

Norman D. Sperber, DDS
Chief Forensic Dentist, San Diego and Imperial County
Diplomate, American Board of Forensic Odontology
Distinguished Fellow, American Academy of Forensic Sciences
San Diego, California

Jeanne L. Stanley, PhD
Executive Director of Academic Services
Graduate School of Education
University of Pennsylvania
Philadelphia, Pennsylvania

Cari Michele Steele, JD
Staff Attorney
National Center for Prosecution of Child Abuse
American Prosecutors Research Institute (APRI)
Alexandria, Virginia

Jacqueline M. Sugarman, MD
Assistant Professor of Pediatrics
Department of Pediatrics
College of Medicine
University of Kentucky
Lexington, Kentucky

Kathryn M. Turman
Program Director
Office of Victim Assistance
Federal Bureau of Investigation
Washington, DC

Victor I. Vieth, JD
Director
National Center for Prosecution of Child Abuse
American Prosecutors Research Institute (APRI)
Alexandria, Virginia

Malinda Waddell, RN, MN, FNP
Director-Forensic Nurse Specialists
Long Beach, California

J. M. Whitworth, MD
Professor of Pediatrics
University of Florida
State Medical Director
Child Protection Team Program
Children's Medical Services
Department of Health
State of Florida

Dawn Doran Wilsey, JD
Senior Attorney
National Center for Prosecution of Child Abuse
American Prosecutors Research Institute (APRI)
Alexandria, Virginia

Janet S. Young, MD
Assistant Professor
University of North Carolina-Chapel Hill
Department of Emergency Medicine
Chapel Hill, North Carolina

Foreword

Sexual assault is broadly defined as unwanted sexual contact of any kind. Among the acts included are rape, incest, molestation, fondling or grabbing, and forced viewing of or involvement in pornography. Drug-facilitated behavior was recently added in response to the recognition that pharmacologic agents can be used to make the victim more malleable. When sexual activity occurs between a significantly older person and a child, it is referred to as molestation or child sexual abuse rather than sexual assault. In children, there is often a "grooming" period where the perpetrator gradually escalates the type of sexual contact with the child and often does not use the force implied in the term sexual assault. But it is assault, both physically and emotionally, whether the victim is a child, an adolescent, or an adult.

The reported statistics are only an estimate of the problem's scope, with the actual reporting rate a mere fraction of the true incidence. The financial costs of sexual assault are enormous; intangible costs, such as emotional suffering and risk of death from being victimized, are beyond measurement. Short-term and long-term consequences reach far into all emotional and physical aspects of a victim's life.

Trained professionals work every day to combat sexual assault in all its forms as well as the adverse aftereffects. This book offers information for all who deal with sexual assault—the crisis hotline staff, law enforcement personnel, prehospital providers, specialized detectives, medical and mental health staff, specialized sexual assault examiners, and counselors. The information is as current, accurate, and specific as it can be in a rapidly evolving field. This book seeks to provide this information in a most accessible manner for professionals needing an immediate resource; it will fill a need in many venues where sexual victimization is seen and care is given to victims.

Robert M. Reece, MD
Director, MSPCC Institute for Professional Education
Clinical Professor of Pediatrics, Tufts University School of Medicine
Executive Editor, the *Quarterly Child Abuse Medical Update*

Foreword

Healthcare, social service, and law enforcement professionals have the unique opportunity to make a difference in how victims of sexual assault will incorporate that event into the rest of their lives. The well-prepared professional is aware of the patient's needs and sensitive to the victim's response to the examination process. This attentiveness will go a long way in beginning the emotional healing process necessary to integrate the events. Giving control back to the victim of rape is therapeutic and should be a priority throughout the examination.

The primary purpose of the sexual assault examination by the healthcare professional is to provide for medical diagnosis and treatment. The examiner needs to keep in mind that observations may be the result of normal development, a result of trauma caused by accident or abuse, or the result of a disease condition. Treatment may be of a clinical, psychological, or emotional nature.

The evidence collection portion of the examination assists in linking the victim, the suspect, the crime scene, and the evidence. Documentation of this portion of the examination is just as important as documenting the history and physical assessment. This text provides easy-to-access information outlining forensic, biologic, and technologic evidence collection within the discussion of the many unique situations in which a sexual assault may occur.

Necessary for any professional who deals with sexual assault, this quick reference provides a base of details essential to accomplish a thorough medical forensic examination.

Kathy Bell, RN
Forensic Nurse Examiner
Tulsa Police Department
Tulsa, Oklahoma

Preface

Sex crimes are now recognized as the precipitating event for various physical, emotional, and psychological disorders. Individuals, families, and the society as a whole suffer. Professionals are charged with working to identify and document the presence of physical injury to corroborate the victim's history, which contributes to the investigation of possible sexual abuse or assault and holds offenders accountable for their crime. Aids in this process include photographic, colposcopic, video, and narrative documentation, and the quality of these media continues to improve. Secure computer programs are being used to transmit photographs so that various professionals can consult on injuries. Research investigating assault injuries continues to support the position that the presence of injury does not prove assault, nor does the absence of injury prove consent. The interdisciplinary sexual assault response team (SART) approach, in which an expert nurse examiner or physician, a sex crimes detective, an advocate, and an experienced, specialized prosecutor work in tandem, has streamlined the process for the victim. Emotional care offered from the time of the examination has softened the impact of the process and helped the victim toward recovery. More efficient and better funded DNA profiling at the local, state, and national levels allows for more timely identification of offenders.

In this text, we see the problem of sexual assault and abuse through the eyes of many professionals: physicians, paramedics, law enforcement personnel, the judicial system, social workers, and people who work with children. The knowledge shared by these concerned and caring individuals supplies the power to intervene. This book offers current, accurate, and specific data concerning the problem of sexual assault in an easy-to-access format. With this information, we become empowered participants whose effective interventions help prevent sexual assault as well as care for its victims.

Angelo P. Giardino, MD, PhD
Elizabeth M. Datner, MD
Janice B. Asher, MD
Barbara W. Girardin, RN, PhD
Diana K. Faugno, RN, BSN, CNP, FAAFS, SANE-A
Mary J. Spencer, MD

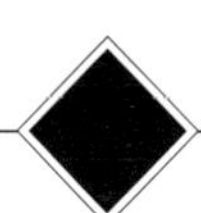

DETAILED TABLE OF CONTENTS

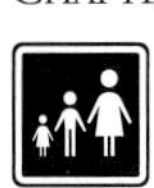

Quick-Reference

Sexual Assault

For Healthcare, Social Service, and Law Enforcement Professionals

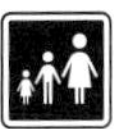

Chapter 1

Principles of Sexual Assault at Any Age

John Loiselle, MD
Marla J. Friedman, DO
Judith A. Linden, MD, FACEP, SANE
Janet S. Young, MD

Child Sexual Abuse

Child sexual abuse is not a new problem but has only been accepted as a bona fide entity that deserves professional attention since the 1970s. Its definition is subject to interpretation on multiple levels. Institutional, societal, medical, and legal terminology all differ in either definition or emphasis. A broad range of developmentally inappropriate sexual behaviors is included, covering both contact and noncontact activities. The Child Abuse Prevention and Treatment Act (CAPTA) of 1974 provided a federal legal standard that all states were mandated to follow to be eligible for funds for child abuse programs. This act defined sexual abuse as "the employment, use, persuasion, inducement, enticement, or coercion of any child to engage in, or assist any other person to engage in, any sexually explicit conduct or simulation of such conduct for the purpose of producing a visual depiction of such conduct." Principles that mark most legal definitions include the following:

- A child is defined as a person under age 18 years, with some exceptions.
- Most statutes emphasize the discrepancy between the perpetrator's and victim's ages.
- The developmental level of the child is considered.

- Laws generally distinguish who is considered a caretaker or guardian for the child.
- When the caretaker is involved in the abuse, involvement of the local child protective services (CPS) agency and law enforcement personnel is usually mandated.
- When the alleged perpetrator is also considered a child, intervention may be limited to child protective services only.
- When the perpetrator is unknown, unrelated, or not considered a caretaker or involved in the child's care, the abuse may be treated as a purely criminal case.

The generally recognized forms of sexual abuse are genital fondling, oral-genital, genital-genital, and anal-genital contact, but the perpetrator does not need to have direct physical contact with the child for sexual abuse to occur, with exhibitionism, voyeurism, and viewing, producing, or distributing pornography also included in most definitions. The use of computers and the Internet to produce, compile, possess, or disseminate child pornography as well as to seduce or attract children with the intent of sexual misuse is a recent addition to legislation. In addition, failure to protect a child is an important component of many definitions of child sexual abuse. Incest is a special category in that a different level of psychosocial problems, prognosis, and family dysfunction is involved, but the cases are handled the same with respect to reporting and meeting the legal definition of sexual abuse.

Sexual play occurs between young children of similar developmental levels and frequently involves viewing or touching, but it is considered a normal part of childhood development and curiosity.

The distinction between sexual play and sexual abuse is generally predicated on the discrepancy in age between the 2 participants, the level of control or authority the older child holds over the younger one, the degree of coercion, and the actual activity involved.

Persons who are mandatory reporters, having a responsibility for the welfare of children, should be familiar with their own state statutes.

Scope

- True magnitude is unknown.
- Rates are generally considered underestimates and are based on substantial underreporting.
- Cases may never be disclosed or may be disclosed by victims but not reported to authorities.
- Estimate for 1993 was 217 700 cases, a rate of 3.2 cases/1000 children, which is nearly double the figures for 1986.
- In 1998, 48 states reported 99 000 cases of child sexual abuse, with an overall rate of 1.6 cases/1000 children.
- Prevalence studies report much higher rates of child sexual abuse, with one third of victimized women and 40% of victimized men never disclosing the incident to anyone.
- Physicians and other mandated reporters also often fail to report all cases of sexual abuse, with a perceived lack of sufficient evidence, concern for disrupting the patient-physician relationship, fear of harming the family, and distrust of local CPS agencies cited as the most common reasons for not reporting.

• Recall bias may affect the prevalence data reported, with false childhood memories overestimating the true prevalence and denial, repressed memories, and a continuing unwillingness to disclose traumatic events generating an underestimate.

Victims

• There is no classic profile of a sexually abused child.

• Female victims account for more than 3 times the number of male victims in reported cases of child sexual abuse. Data also show that girls are 2.5 times more likely to be victims of sexual abuse than boys.

• The risk for sexual abuse is highest during preadolescence, with a smaller peak in the early school-age years.

• Sexually abused boys tend to be younger than their female counterparts.

• Race, ethnicity, and socioeconomic factors do not differ from nonabused populations.

• Children who become victims of abuse tend to be easily controlled and may have physical or mental disabilities.

• These children also often have needs for love and belonging that are not being met at home.

• Children living without one or both of their natural parents are at an increased risk of being abused. Females who live apart from their mothers or are not emotionally close to their mothers are at increased risk of sexual abuse. Abused males are more likely to live with their mothers and have no father figure at home.

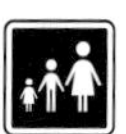

• The single most important risk factor for both males and females is the presence of a stepfather in the household.

• Other risk factors include having a mother who is ill, disabled, or extensively out of the home; substance abuse; parental conflict; violence in the home; having adolescent parents, foster parents, or parents who were sexually abused themselves; and being a sibling of an abused child.

OFFENDERS

• There is no classic profile of an abuser.

• Child sex abusers tend to be older men, but one fourth to one third of male perpetrators are adolescents.

• Women are offenders in up to 5% of cases involving female children and 20% of cases involving male children.

• The perpetrator is usually well known to the child, with male family members (father, stepfather, and uncle) the most common offenders.

• Stepfathers molest girls more often than boys, while biologic fathers molest similar numbers of girls and boys.

• Incest victims are most likely to be female children who are molested by their fathers or stepfathers.

• The typical family in which incest occurs is involved with multiple stressors, with parental conflict leading to an absence of sexual relations between the parents and that leading to the father looking to his daughter for comfort and love. The daughter may be depressed and withdrawn and have a poor self-image; she yearns for attention and affection and may be happy to fill the need in her father's life. The mother, feeling completely dependent on her husband, sees herself as powerless. She abandons her husband and daughter emotionally and physically, allowing her daughter to assume her role as wife.

• Extrafamilial abuse is more common among boys, especially those over age 12 years. Boys under age 6 years are more likely to be abused by family and friends.

• The duration of molestation is shorter on average for male victims, but the acts themselves tend to be more severe.

• While fewer than 50% of child sex offenders are mentally ill, most have an emotional disorder that prevents them from forming intimate relationships with partners their own age. They experience emotional and sexual gratification when the abuse of a child is complete. They often view their abuse as proof to themselves that they have the power to control at least that aspect of their lives.

• The victim-to-victimizer cycle is especially true for adolescent perpetrators and most often involves male victims of male offenders. The characteristics of the victim and the characteristics of the abuse often closely parallel the offender's own memory of abuse.

• Four preconditions must exist before the victimization of a child can occur:

1. Arousal: the abuser has sexual desires surrounding children.
2. Internal inhibitions: overcoming internal inhibitions related to the abuse of children; this

step is facilitated if the perpetrator experienced a traumatic childhood sexual event of his own.

3. Repeated physical contact: perpetrators are generally people on whom the child depends for emotional, physical, financial, educational, or religious support.
4. Child's resistance: overcoming the child's resistance to the sexual interaction.

• Strategies to gain the child's trust involve many forms of manipulation and are termed "engagement."

1. Abuser targets the child and they begin to share nonsexual activities.
2. Abuser uses bribery, including gifts, favors, or privileges to entice the child.
3. Abuser may shower the child with encouragement and compliments.
4. Abuser may use persuasion to deceive the child into believing that they have a special friendship.
5. Over time, activity escalates, with each interaction becoming more sexual in nature.
6. Once sexual intimacy occurs, the perpetrator focuses on maintaining the secret, now using a different form of manipulation to intimidate the child.
7. Abuser may play on the child's guilt and threaten to stop loving the child; the abuser may threaten physical violence to the child or a family member, or may actually use force or violence.

• The child becomes confused, alone, and feels betrayed, perpetuating the secret.

Indicators of Sexual Abuse

• Children may not reveal a history of sexual abuse because they fear no one will believe them, they feel guilty or ashamed and worry about being blamed, they do not want to get the perpetrator into trouble, or they fear retaliation if they tell.

• The disclosure may be offered at any time and to any number of people.

1. May occur in a place that reminds the child of the event or where the child feels safe.
2. May be to a parent at bath time or bedtime.
3. May be to a sibling or playmate.
4. May be to a teacher or guidance counselor after a sexual abuse prevention program in school.
5. May be to a physician during a routine health examination.

• A common early warning sign is the use of broad general statements, which the child uses to gauge the response of a trusted listener. These subtle suggestions should alert the listener to the possibility of sexual abuse.

• The most consistent indicator of sexual abuse in all age groups is the demonstration of sexualized behavior, defined as age-inappropriate knowledge of sexual language and behaviors. Issues to consider include family sexuality, life stress, domestic violence, and sexual abuse when confronted with this indicator.

• Other broad, nonspecific indicators of child sexual abuse can be divided into 3 categories:

1. Physical signs and symptoms: presence of a sexually transmitted disease (STD) in a young

child, presence of sperm in or on the body, discovery of childhood/teen pregnancy are obvious signs but seldom found; more likely findings are chronic abdominal pain, enuresis or encopresis, constipation secondary to anal discomfort, recurrent urinary tract infections, vaginal discharge, and presence of a vaginal foreign body.

2. Behavioral signs and symptoms: often the first signs noted by those close to the child, but not unique to sexual abuse, being present in other forms of severe stress; include temper tantrums or running away from home, developmentally regressive behaviors (thumbsucking or bedwetting), obsessive cleanliness or neglect, self-mutilating or self-stimulating behaviors, poor school attendance and performance, delinquency, substance abuse, and premature participation in sexual relationships.
3. Psychiatric signs and symptoms: depression, evidenced by social withdrawal and the inability to form or maintain meaningful peer relations; profound grief in response to losses of innocence, childhood, and trust in oneself, trust in adults; sleeping disorders with fear of the dark and nightmares; changed eating habits (anorexia, overeating, avoiding certain foods); and suicide.

Support Systems

- Specialty divisions, special police units, social workers, and multidisciplinary child abuse evaluation teams or child advocacy centers where representatives of all the involved fields are gathered may be employed in evaluating childhood sexual abuse cases.
- Protocols have been developed to improve the

accuracy and thoroughness of evaluation, the recommended management of the child, and the provision of legal services, including the appointment of a guardian ad litem as needed.

• Key roles are played by the pediatrician and family practitioner in the assessment of a child sexual abuse case. The practitioner is often the person the family feels most comfortable with and to whom they turn; the person to whom they may disclose the abuse.

• Physicians are mandated reporters and must be familiar with state law regarding reportable offenses and the process to be followed in reporting suspicions.

• The primary care physician provides emotional as well as medical support for the child and family and must be aware of potential resources to which referrals can be made as well as consultants who are available.

• Primary care physicians are also responsible for parental education through anticipatory guidance, teaching young children about good touches and bad touches; alerting families to behaviors or physical signs that are cause for concern; and reassuring in cases of normal childhood play and curiosity.

Outcomes

Finkelhor and Browne describe 4 traumagenic dynamics as a framework for understanding the link between the experience of sexual abuse and its sequelae (the traumagenic model).

• Traumatic sexualization: the inappropriate and dysfunctional development of a victim's sexuality as a result of the abuse; marked by confusion and misconceptions concerning sexuality, with distorted

perceptions of sexual activities, victims develop sexual preoccupations (compulsive masturbation, sexualized play, sexual aggression, seductive behaviors), gender identity conflict and cross-gender behavior, prostitution, and sexual dysfunction as adults. Invasive abuse is more sexualizing than using the child to masturbate, and older children who can understand the implications of the abuse are more likely to suffer traumatic sexualization than other victims.

• Sense of betrayal: often 3-fold, with first, betrayal by the perpetrator in the form of manipulations and misconceptions about sex and love; second, betrayal by the child's own body, since their body responded to the sexual stimulation then they must have somehow wanted the abuse; and third, betrayal of the child by the family who disbelieves the child's allegations or attempts to suppress them, further violating the child's trust. Responses to betrayal include anger expressed in risk-taking behavior or delinquency, dissociation in which the child separates himself from his body and from the world, or excessively clingy behavior in an effort to restore trust and security in redeeming relationships (may continue into adulthood). If the sexual abuse is within the family, the sense of betrayal is heightened and remains for a much longer time; if the offender is not held accountable for the crime, the victim suffers a strong sense of betrayal by the legal system and the norms of society.

• Powerlessness leading to somatization: the loss of power that develops when the child's body is repeatedly misused or invaded without consent and failed attempts to end the abuse lead to fear and anxiety, which are then expressed in nightmares, phobias, eating disorders, and somatic complaints. Somatization is the preoccupation with bodily dysfunction that many sexual abuse victims experience; among the manifestations are headaches, nausea and vomiting, heart palpitations, dizziness, fatigue, and muscle aches. The victim may respond to the sense of powerlessness by running away, self-mutilation, or suicide attempts; aggressive and dominating behaviors; or posttraumatic stress disorder (PTSD).

• Stigmatization: refers to the negative connotations that become part of the child's self-image after the abuse. These may result from demeaning comments made directly to the child by the offender; the message of badness and shame that accompanies pressure from the perpetrator to keep silent; or the child's internal stigma of guilt. Stigmatization may be magnified if the family reacts with disgust or blames the child for the abuse. Victims identify with other stigmatized groups in society and may involve themselves in substance abuse, delinquency, and prostitution, viewing themselves as damaged goods and alienating themselves from family and friends.

Coping Mechanisms

Avoidant Coping

• Involves distraction, wishful thinking, and cognitive restructuring

• Used more often by children who received greater social support after disclosure

• Produces short-term benefits but long-term problems, with victims using this strategy developing more negative attitudes and anxieties about sexuality

• Associated with fewer behavioral problems than other coping mechanisms

Internalized Coping

- Includes social withdrawal, self-blame, and resignation
- Used more commonly by children who received negative reactions from others after disclosure; may be linked to hyperreactive behaviors that lead to the development of posttraumatic stress reactions
- Found more frequently in female victims, who display internalized behaviors (dissociation and depression), phobias, regressive behaviors, and multiple somatic complaints
- Rated the least helpful of the strategies by victims

Angry Coping

- Involves the cathartic release of emotions and the tendency to blame others; also termed externalization
- Instigated often when the perpetrator had a more distant relationship to the child
- High frequency of abuse interactions and forceful abuse also noted as antecedents to this coping strategy
- Seen more in older victims and in male victims
- Associated with the greatest number of behavioral problems, including physical as well as sexual aggression in males and sexually reactive behaviors in females (which puts them at increased risk for revictimization)

Active/Social Coping

- Uses child's problem-solving abilities as well as social support resources
- Most commonly implemented by children who experienced less severe sexual experiences
- Only strategy not linked to negative abuse-related behaviors
- Does not produce measured benefits

INTERVENTIONS

- Ensuring child's safety from further abuse.
- Family therapy to facilitate a supportive and protective environment for the child.
- Developmentally appropriate personal therapy for the child.
- Comparison of abuse-specific cognitive behavior therapy and nondirective supportive therapy shows both to be appropriate for posttraumatic stress symptoms, although significantly greater improvement occurred with cognitive behavior therapy.
- Influence on long-term effects of child sexual abuse is unknown.

ADOLESCENT AND ADULT SEXUAL ABUSE

Rape is generally defined as meeting 3 criteria:

1. Any vaginal, anal, or oral penetration by a penis, object, or other body part
2. Lack of consent, communicated with verbal or physical signs of resistance, or if the victim is unable to consent by means of incapacitation because of age, disability, or drug or alcohol intoxication
3. Threat of or actual use of force

Modern definitions of rape also include taking advantage of incapacitated individuals, such as children, the disabled, or the elderly. Drug-facilitated rape has also recently been addressed, with increased penalties where this takes place. Sexual assault has a broader characterization, including any unwanted sexual contact, thus encompassing rape, incest, molestation, fondling or grabbing, or forced viewing

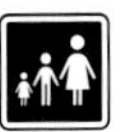

of or involvement in pornography as well as other less definable behaviors.

Scope

- An estimated 1 million rapes or attempted rapes occur annually in the United States: 876 000 in women and 111 000 in men, meaning that 1 in 6 women has been the victim of an attempted or completed rape in her lifetime.
- Most rapes are never reported to either the police or healthcare providers, with adolescents and males the least likely to report.
- The majority of males who rape males are not homosexual and the majority of males who are raped are not homosexual.
- Youths and adolescents are sexually assaulted in disproportionate numbers compared to the population.
- A reported 22% of women are raped by strangers ("blitz" rapes), 29% by acquaintances, 9% by ex-husbands, 11% by stepfathers, 10% by boyfriends, and 16% by other relatives.
- Victims who know their assailant are less likely to report the crime or receive medical care.

Why Victims Don't Report (and Remain "Silent Victims")

- Fear of family, friends, and others finding out
- Fear of the assault being made public by the media
- Fear of being blamed
- Fear of retaliation
- Perceived shame or actual stigma associated with being the victim of a sexual assault
- Victim does not fit into the classic definition of a rape victim as a woman raped by a stranger

Victim-Assailant Relationships

While rape is an act of violence, it is also an act of opportunity. The one common link that identifies rape victims is that the rapist has access to the victim.

- A known assailant perpetrates 80% of rapes.
- Most victims and perpetrators are of the same race.
- Many rapists prey on vulnerable victims who may be seen as less likeable or credible (eg, homeless or substance abusers).
- More attractive, provocatively dressed individuals are not more likely to be victims of rape.
- Classic rape victim is a victim of blitz rape, but this is actually fairly uncommon.
- "Confidence rape" in which the victim has had a previous nonviolent relationship with the assailant occurs more commonly than blitz rape. This may involve the following 3 situations:

1. Friend or acquaintance who uses deceit, such as offering a ride home
2. Assailant who controls the victim by age or rank
3. Assailant who exploits someone unable to give consent

- In the "stress-sex" situation, the victim initially consents to contact, but the assailant becomes abusive and violent, forcing further sexual activity without consent; this often occurs in date rape or situation (prostitute as victim) rape.

Public Health Implications

Most cost calculations only consider short-term tangible costs, which focus on property and productivity lost or medical bills. Intangible costs

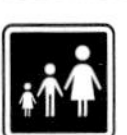

include pain, suffering, risk of death, disability, and long-term emotional trauma.

- Considering tangible costs, from 1987 to 1990, the tangible cost to society was $5100 per sexual assault, making rape the most costly crime in the United States.
- Adding intangible costs over the same period, the cost escalates to $87 000 annually per assault, or more than $425 for each man, woman, and child in the United States.

With regard to healthcare, sexual assault victims:

- Are more likely to develop mental health problems, with an estimated 3.8 million adult American women having rape-related PTSD.
- Have higher rates of alcohol and drug use.
- Use the healthcare system at a higher rate even for problems not related to sexual assault, with outpatient costs 2.5 times greater than for nonvictims.
- May become pregnant, with an estimated 32 000 unwanted pregnancies resulting annually contributing to the cost of treating survivors.

Populations at Risk

- Greatest risk factor for sexual assault is female gender; 70% to 90% of victims are female and 10% to 30% are male.
- Second greatest factor is young age, with studies suggesting that 50% to 60% of victims are under age 17 years, over 80% under age 25 years, and only 6% over age 29 years.
- Adolescents and young women are most at risk for acquaintance and date rape.

- Women attending college have a risk of rape 3 times greater than the general population; they are often raped by someone they know.
- Past victimization is a strong risk factor for revictimization, with sexual assault in childhood a powerful risk factor for sexual assault as an adult.
- Women in physically and emotionally abusive relationships are more likely to experience rape and sexual assault, especially repeated rape and serious physical injuries. They are also less likely to report to healthcare providers and law enforcement agencies.
- Mental incapacitation is a risk factor, possibly targeted by predators because mentally incapacitated individuals are unable to perceive dangerous situations, they are vulnerable, and they are less likely to be taken seriously if they report the incident.
- The sexual assault rates of women in the military and institutionalized women are significantly higher than in the general population.

Immediate Reactions to Sexual Trauma

- Most rape victims do not seek immediate medical assistance.
- There is no normal or abnormal response to sexual victimization, but immediate reactions may include shock and disbelief, shame, and self-blame; anger toward the assailant, healthcare workers, advocates, or law enforcement personnel is also seen.
- Outward behaviors range from crying and sobbing to a quiet, calm demeanor; inwardly the victim may feel anxiety, helplessness, and guilt.
- Fear of death is the most intense fear during and immediately after a rape.

- Other initial concerns:

1. Fear of contracting an STD
2. Fear of pregnancy
3. Fear of serious genital injury that would affect sexual functioning
4. Fear of transmission of human immunodeficiency virus (HIV)

- The rape trauma syndrome consists of a group of "behavioral, somatic, and psychological reactions, which are an acute stress reaction to a life-threatening situation." Its 2 phases are as follows:

1. Acute "disorganization phase": lasts several weeks; survivor experiences somatic reactions, such as pain from physical trauma, headaches, sleep disturbances, gastrointestinal symptoms, and genitourinary symptoms; may also continue to display initial emotional reactions of fear, humiliation, self-blame, anger, and revenge; recall of the event is often clouded by intense feelings of guilt, helplessness, and fear.
2. "Reorganization phase": lasts several weeks to years; survivor often continues to have somatic symptoms, with nonspecific anxiety that can be associated with phobias; may fear being indoors if he or she was raped inside or may fear crowds; survivor often changes addresses and phone numbers frequently.

Delayed Effects on the Survivor

- Survivors often experience PTSD, depression, suicidal ideation, substance abuse, and physical complaints (pelvic pain, abdominal pain, headaches).

- Posttraumatic stress disorder (PTSD):

1. Among the most debilitating after-effects of sexual assault
2. Hallmarks: persistent reliving of event and behavioral changes to avoid stimuli associated with the trauma
3. Occurs in up to one third of sexual assault survivors

- Major depression:

1. Extremely common, with almost 30% of survivors experiencing at least 1 episode
2. Occurs in 3 times more rape survivors than nonvictims

- Substance abuse:

1. May involve alcohol or other drugs
2. Attempt to self-medicate the painful emotions linked to sexual victimization
3. Often places survivor at increased risk for further victimization
4. PTSD often associated with increased rates of drug- and alcohol-related problems

Components of an Effective Response

Ideal care of a sexual assault victim includes compassionate treatment by knowledgeable professionals, which encompasses the rape crisis hotline personnel, police and law enforcement personnel, and prehospital providers as well as specially trained detectives, skilled medical staff, trained sexual assault examiners, and rape crisis counselors.

Rape Crisis Centers

- First established in San Francisco and Washington, DC as an outgrowth of the feminist movement in the 1970s

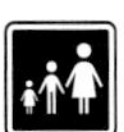

- Staff are usually lay people who are often sexual assault survivors
- Function in prevention, acute treatment, and ongoing follow-up
- Provide public education to prevent rape, confidential emergency assistance for victims and family members or friends, and short-term follow-up crisis counseling

Prehospital Personnel

- Must be aware that rape or sexual assault is not specific to one gender, race, or socioeconomic status
- Require training in evidence preservation and the importance of saving the sheet the patient is transported on as well as avoiding cutting the patient's clothes and destroying evidence whenever possible
- Need to listen to patient with empathy and remind the patient that the assault is never the victim's fault
- Establish a safe environment to transfer the patient, including removing the patient from the scene as soon as possible

Emergency Department Personnel

- Victim should be given top priority, brought back from triage immediately, and provided a safe, nonthreatening environment
- Should have immediate screening to see if serious injuries are present
- Avoid undressing the patient so that clothing can be collected during the forensic examination
- Instruct the patient not to eat, drink, or urinate if possible

• Offer appropriate postexposure prophylaxis for pregnancy and STDs, including HIV and hepatitis

• Recognize that there is no appropriate survivor response and be able to respond appropriately and effectively to the range of survivor reactions, providing a supportive, nonthreatening patient interaction that allows the patient to retain control, thus preventing further anxiety

• Be able to address concerns that rape victims may not always express, such as whether the injuries will cause permanent damage and the likelihood of becoming pregnant or acquiring an STD, especially HIV

• Focus on examining the victim, collecting evidence if the patient consents, offering support, and giving medical treatment

Specially Trained Personnel

• Sexual assault detectives: conduct interview in nonjudgmental, sensitive, and compassionate manner while obtaining vital information

• Sexual assault nurse examiners (SANEs) and rape crisis counselors: most helpful in evaluating and treating the victim, with SANEs able to counsel the patient, collect a history, examine and obtain forensic evidence compassionately, and evaluate the patient's physical and psychological injuries

• Arrange for follow-up services: mental health care counselors, rape crisis center referral, medical follow-up including testing for pregnancy, HIV, hepatitis, and STDs

Prevention

Primary Prevention Programs

• Interventions aimed at decreasing the number of sexual assaults

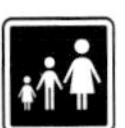

- The most effective means of decreasing the sequelae of sexual victimization
- Must be aimed at younger population (under age 18 years), with special programs targeted toward college-age populations
- Include rape-myth–based programs, victim empathy programs, lecture format courses, discussion groups, interactive improvisational theater presentations, and self-defense strategies
- Programs for women should focus on increasing women's awareness, addressing rape myths and risk perception, and decreasing risky behaviors
- Programs for men should focus on increasing awareness, increasing respect for women, dispelling rape myths, and enhancing empathy for victims

Secondary Prevention Programs

- Focus on early screening and identification of sexual assault survivors and decreasing future assaults and the sequelae of sexual assault once an assault has already occurred
- Include efforts to improve care of rape survivors immediately after the crime and follow-up services

Tertiary Prevention Programs

- Focus on interventions to treat and alleviate advanced disease or the late effects, such as the physical and mental health sequelae of sexual assault
- Include educating medical providers about the importance of asking questions about previous trauma and recognizing the signs and symptoms of previous sexual victimization and rape trauma syndrome

• Train providers to recognize signs of sexual and physical abuse, respond effectively, and refer to resources available in the area

References

Acierno R, Resnick HS, Kilpatrick DG, Saunders B, Best CL. Risk factors for rape, physical assault and posttraumatic stress disorder in women: examination of differential multivariate relationships. *J Anxiety Disord.* 1999;13:541-563.

American Academy of Pediatrics, Committee on Child Abuse and Neglect. Guidelines for the evaluation of sexual abuse in children. *Pediatrics.* 1999;103:186-191.

Bachman R, Saltzman LE. *Violence Against Women: Estimates from the Redesigned Survey.* Washington, DC: US Dept of Justice; 1995. Report NCJ-154348.

Bass E, Thornton L, eds. *I Never Told Anyone: Writings by Women Survivors of Sexual Abuse.* New York, NY: Harper & Row; 1983.

Botash A. What office-based pediatricians need to know about child sexual abuse. *Contemp Pediatr.* 1994;11:83-100.

Briere J, Runtz M. Symptomatology associated with childhood sexual victimization in a nonclinical adult sample. *Child Abuse Negl.* 1988;12:51-59.

Burgess AW, Holmstrom LL. Rape trauma syndrome. *Am J Psychiatry.* 1974;131:981-986.

Chaffin M, Wherry JN, Dykman R. School age children's coping with sexual abuse: abuse stresses and symptoms associated with four coping strategies. *Child Abuse Negl.* 1997;21:227-240.

Child Abuse Prevention and Treatment Act (CAPTA). 1974;PL 93-247.

Cosentino CE, Collins M. Sexual abuse of children: prevalence, effects, and treatment. *Ann NY Acad Sci.* 1996;789:45-65.

Deblinger E, Lippman J, Steer R. Sexually abused children suffering posttraumatic stress symptoms: initial treatment outcome findings. *Child Maltreat.* 1996;1:310-321.

Feldhaus KM, Houry D, Kaminsky R. Lifetime sexual assault prevalence rates and reporting practices in an emergency department population. *Ann Emerg Med.* 2000;36:23-27.

Finkelhor D. Sexual abuse: a sociological perspective. *Child Abuse Negl.* 1982;6:95-102.

Finkelhor D, ed. *Child Sexual Abuse: New Theory and Research.* New York, NY: Free Press; 1984.

Finkelhor D. Epidemiological factors in the clinical identification of child sexual abuse. *Child Abuse Negl.* 1993;17:67-70.

Finkelhor D, Baron L. High-risk children. In: Finkelhor D, ed. *Sourcebook on Child Sexual Abuse.* Beverly Hills, Calif: Sage Publications; 1986: 60-88.

Finkelhor D, Browne A. The traumatic impact of child sexual abuse: a conceptualization. *Am J Orthopsychiatry.* 1985;55:530-541.

Finkelhor D, Hotaling G, Lewis IA, Smith C. Sexual abuse in a national survey of adult men and women: prevalence, characteristics, and risk factors. *Child Abuse Negl.* 1990;14:19-28.

Friedrich WN, Urquiza AJ, Beilke R. Behavioral problems in sexually abused young children. *J Pediatr Psychol.* 1986;11:57-67.

Guidry HM. Childhood sexual abuse: role of the family physician. *Am Fam Physician.* 1995;51:414.

Herendeen PM. Evaluating for child sexual abuse. *Adv Nurse Pract.* 1999;7:54-58.

Hilton MR, Mezey GC. Victims and perpetrators of child sexual abuse. *Br J Psychiatry.* 1996;169:408-415.

Holmes MM, Resnick HS, Kilpatrick DG, Best CL. Rape-related pregnancy rate: estimates and descriptive characteristics from a national sample of women. *Am J Obstet Gynecol.* 1996;175:320-325.

Holmes WC, Slap GB. Sexual abuse of boys. *JAMA.* 1998;280:1855-1860.

Justice B, Justice R, eds. *The Broken Taboo: Sex in the Family.* New York, NY: Human Sciences; 1979: 109-202.

Kempe CH. Sexual abuse, another hidden pediatric problem: the 1977 C. Anderson Aldrich lecture. *Pediatrics.* 1978;62:382-389.

Kendall-Tackett KA, Simon AF. A comparison of the abuse experiences of male and female adults molested as children. *J Fam Violence.* 1992;77:57-62.

Kerns DL, Terman DL, Larson CS. The role of physicians in reporting and evaluating child sexual abuse cases. *Future Child.* 1994;4:119-134.

Kilpatrick DG, Saunders BE. *Prevalence and Consequences of Child Victimization: Results From the National Survey of Adolescents, Final Report.* Washington DC: US Dept of Justice, Office of Justice Programs, National Institute of Justice; 1997.

Kilpatrick DG, Saunders BE, Seymour AK. *Rape in America: A Report to the Nation.* Charleston, SC: Crime Victim Research and Treatment Center; 1992.

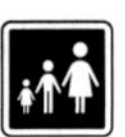

Koss MP, Dinero TE, Seibel CA. Stranger and acquaintance rape: are there differences in the victim's experience? *Psychol Women Q.* 1988;12:1-24.

Koss MP, Gidycz CA, Wisniewski N. The scope of rape: incidence and prevalence of sexual aggression and victimization in a national sample of higher education students. *J Consult Clin Psychol.* 1987;55:162-167.

Leventhal JM. Epidemiology of sexual abuse of children: old problems, new directions. *Child Abuse Negl.* 1998;22:481-491.

Nadelson CC, Notman MT, Zackson H, Gornick J. A follow-up study of rape victims. *Am J Psychiatry.* 1982;139:1266-1270.

National Institute of Justice. *The Extent and Costs of Crime Victimization: A New Look* (research preview). Washington, DC: US Dept of Justice; 1996.

Nieves-Khouw FC. Recognizing victims of physical and sexual abuse. *Crit Care Nurs Clin North Am.* 1997;9:141-148.

Pierce R, Pierce LH. The sexually abused child: a comparison of male and female victims. *Child Abuse Negl.* 1985;9:191-199.

Sanford J, Cryer L, Christensen BL, Mattox KL. Patterns of reported rape in a tri-ethnic population: Houston, Texas, 1974-1975. *Am J Public Health.* 1979;69:480-484.

Sansonnet-Hayden H, Haley G, Marriage K, Fine S. Sexual abuse and psychopathology in hospitalized adolescents. *J Am Acad Child Adolesc Psychiatry.* 1987;26:753-757.

Sedlak AJ, Broadhurst DD. *Third National Incidence Study of Child Abuse and Neglect.*

Washington, DC: US Dept of Health and Human Services (contract #105-94-1840); 1996. HIS-3 Final Report.

Tjaden P, Thoennes N. *Prevalence, Incidence and Consequences of Violence Against Women: Findings From the National Violence Against Women Survey.* Washington, DC: National Institute of Justice; 1998. Report NCJ-172837.

Tjaden P, Thoennes N. *Full Report of the Prevalence, Incidence and Consequences of Violence Against Women.* Washington, DC: National Institute of Justice and Centers for Disease Control; 2000. Report NCJ-183781.

US Department of Health and Human Services, Administration on Children, Youth and Families. *Child Maltreatment 1998: Reports From the States to the National Child Abuse and Neglect Data System.* Washington, DC: US Government Printing Office; 2000.

Violence Against Women: Estimates from the Redesigned Survey. Washington, DC: Bureau of Justice Statistics, US Dept of Justice; 1995. Special Report NCJ-154348.

Walker EA, Gelfand AN, Gelfand MD, Koss MP, Katon WJ. Medical and psychiatric symptoms in female gastroenterology clinic patients with histories of sexual victimization. *Gen Hosp Psychiatry.* 1995;17:85-92.

Walker EA, Katon WJ, Roy-Byrne PP, Jemelka RP, Russo J. Histories of sexual victimization in patients with irritable bowel syndrome or inflammatory bowel disease. *Am J Psychiatry.* 1993;150:1502-1506.

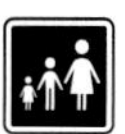

Whetsell-Mitchell J. Indicators of child sexual abuse: children at risk. *Issues Compr Pediatr Nurs.* 1995a;18:319-340.

Whetsell-Mitchell J. The many faces of child sexual abuse. *Issues Compr Pediatr Nurs.* 1995b;18:299-318.

Chapter 2

Anogenital Anatomy

William J. Reed, MD, FAAP

Medical Embryology of the External Genitalia

- Genetic sex is determined at the time the ovum is fertilized, but during the first 12 weeks of embryonic life, both male and female primordial tracts are present and develop in unison.
- In the female: cortex develops into the ovary at 10 to 11 weeks, with medullary regression.
- In the male: medulla differentiates into the testis, with regression of the cortex.
- Gonadal primordia are influenced by the sex-determining region (SRY) on the Y chromosome.
- If a functioning testis is present, the phenotype is male, whereas in the absence of the sex-determining region, with or without the presence of an ovary, the phenotype is female.

Development of External Genitalia in Boys

- External genital development occurs between 10 and 16 weeks of gestation and requires the conversion of 6% to 8% of the total testosterone to 5-dihydrotestosterone. The genital tubercle grows into a penis and the urogenital folds fuse to enclose the penile urethra.
- At 28 weeks, the "inguinal scrotal" stage of descent begins, with the testis descending into the scrotal sac between 28 and 32 weeks of gestation.
- Testosterone is responsible for the evolution of the mesonephric duct system into the vas deferens,

epididymis, ejaculatory ducts, and seminal vesicle. Dihydrotestosterone results in the development of the male external genitalia, including the prostate gland, and the bulbourethral glands of Cowper.

• At puberty, testosterone leads to spermatogenesis and the development of the secondary sexual characteristics as well as a 5- to 7-fold enlargement of the prostate gland, epididymis, and testes.

Anatomic Variations in Boys

Many variations of normal and some previously unrecognized problems may be noted in the examination of the male from infancy through puberty stage Tanner G5. The more common variations in genital findings are as follows: Leydig cell aplasia or hypoplasia; partial androgen insensitivity; phimosis; paraphimosis; hypospadias; circumcision adhesions; erythema or hyperpigmentation; smegma; uric acid crystals; pink pearly papules of the penis; urethral meatal stenosis; epispadias; exstrophy of the bladder; shawl defect; micropenis; diphallia; (rarely) urethral duplication, atresia, fistula, parameatal cysts, and megalourethra; and penile torsion.

Development of External Genitalia in Girls

• Female external genitalia develop from the genital groove and urogenital sinus between 6 and 11 to 12 weeks of gestation.

• Among the principal structures are the mons pubis, labia minora and majora, symphysis pubis, clitoral prepuce, vulva, vagina, and hymen.

Anatomic Variations in Girls

An appreciable number of congenital abnormalities pass undetected in the newborn, becoming clinically

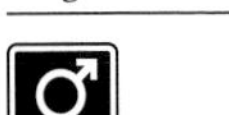

apparent only later or remaining partially expressed and found only incidentally during surgery or other procedures. The more prevalent variant entities are as follows: partial or complete virilization; labial agglutination or fusion and premenarchal lichen sclerosis; labial hypertrophy; hydrocolpos; midline perineal fusion defect; vaginal prolapse or procidentia; vaginal agenesis or caudal müllerian agenesis (Mayer-Rokitansky-Kuster-Hauser syndrome); vaginal atresia; vaginal duplication; linea vestibularis; Skene's duct cysts; prolapse of the circular eversion of the urethral mucosa through the urethral meatus; paraurethral cysts; urethral caruncle; unilateral or bilateral absence of the ovaries; supernumerary ovaries; ovarian cysts; ovarian tumors; streak ovaries; duplication of the uterine body; incomplete or didelphys vagina and uterus; bicornuate uterus with a single vagina and cervix; epispadias; and hypospadias.

The Hymen

The hymen is a recessed structure at the entrance to the vaginal opening. It may occur in at least 6 well-described and anatomically differing configurations, and its appearance may be influenced by estrogenization, aging, and development, as well as the patient's position during the examination, the examiner's experience and/or bias, the patient's degree of relaxation, and the use of labial traction or labial separation. Three basic hymenal types are recognized:

1. Fimbriated: denticulate, sleeve-like, or scalloped **(Figures 2-1 and 2-2)**
2. Annular: concentric or symmetrical **(Figure 2-3)**
3. Posterior rim: crescentic or semilunar **(Figure 2-4)**

These may be seen in 7 configurations:

1. Fimbriated

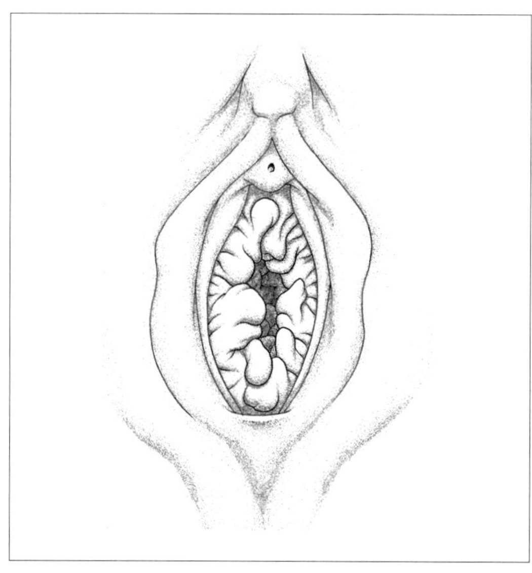

Figure 2-1. *A fimbriated or denticulate hymen.*

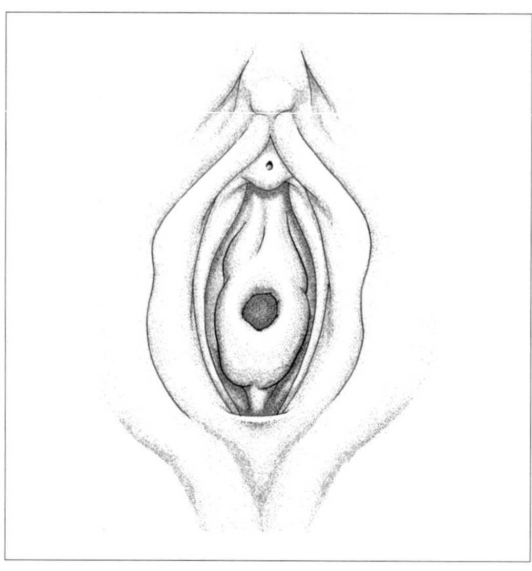

Figure 2-2. *The redundant or sleeve-like hymen.*

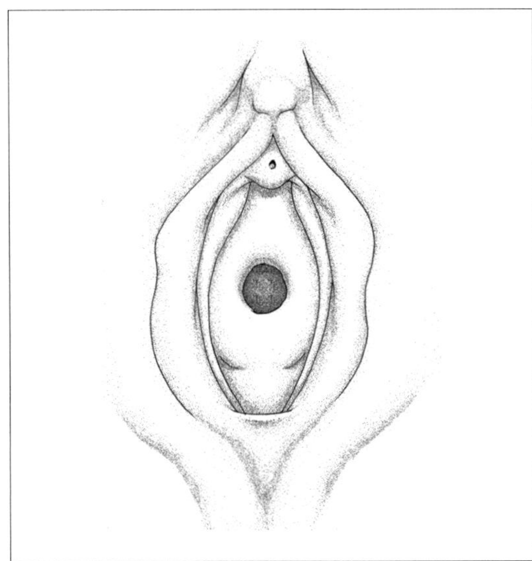

Figure 2-3. The annular hymen.

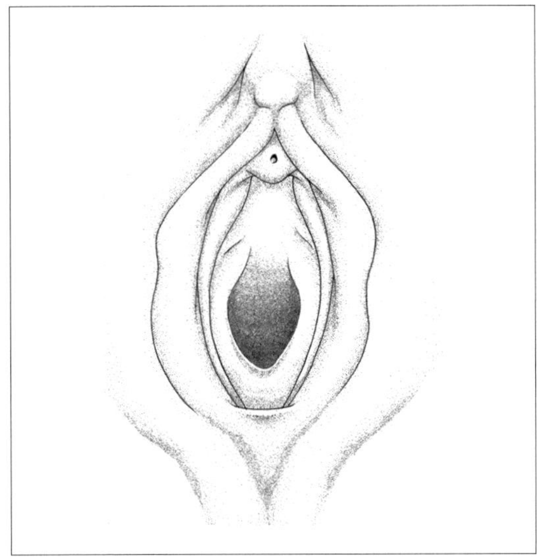

Figure 2-4. The crescentic hymen.

2. Annular
3. Redundant
4. Crescentic
5. Septate
6. Cribriform
7. Imperforate

• Annular or fimbriated configuration is most common at birth. Fimbriated hymen is more often noted in African American infants and decreases with age. The incidence of crescentic hymen increases with age and is the most prevalent by age 3 years. Septal remnants are common, and imperforate hymen occurs in over 1 in 1000 live female births.

• Nonspecific clinical features of the normal and recognized variants of hymenal anatomy include variations in morphology; presence of an external vaginal ridge; presence of a hymenal tag; presence of a longitudinal intravaginal ridge; hymenal notches or clefts **(Figure 2-5)**; vaginal rugae; periurethral and perihymenal vestibular bands; labial agglutination/adhesions; erythema of the vestibular sulcus; linea vestibularis; hymenal bumps or mounds; and lymphoid follicles.

• Hymenal measurements are made of the posterior or inferior portion of the hymenal rim and the transhymenal diameter **(Table 2-1)**.

• The effects of estrogen on the hymen are first noted in the newborn female and result from maternal estrogen that has crossed the placenta. The labia minora, clitoris, and paraurethral tissue are prominent; hymenal tissue is thickened, pale, and has few surface capillaries.

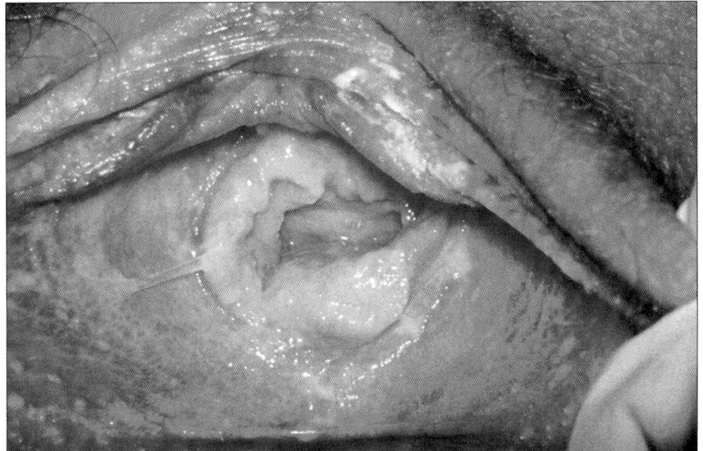

Figure 2-5. *Hymenal cleft at 8 o'clock. (Contributed by Nancy D. Kellogg, MD; San Antonio, Tex.)*

- At birth and during puberty, changes occur in the morphology, size, mucosa, secretions, environmental pH, and bacterial flora of the hymen.
- In the first 4 to 6 weeks of life, about 10% of newborn girls have pigmentation of the external genitalia, a thick white creamy discharge, and withdrawal vaginal bleeding.
- Genitalia begin to appear prepubertal by age 1 to 2 months.
- By age 8 to 10 years, early changes in the hymen show estrogen effects again. The labia minora mature, periurethral tissue increases, and the hymen thickens.

Female Puberty

- Breast budding (thelarche) is the first sign of puberty traditionally, although hymenal changes (just described) may occur earlier.

Table 2-1. Transhymenal Diameters

AGE	DIAMETER
Preschool children (2 to 4 yrs 5 mos)	3.9–5.2 mm (range 1–8.5 mm)
Early school (5 to 7 yrs 11 mos)	4.2–5.6 mm (range 1–9 mm)
Preadolescent (8 yrs to Tanner 2)	5.7–7.3 mm (range 3–11 mm)

Adapted from McCann J, Wells R, Simon M, Voris J. Genital findings in prepubertal children selected for nonabuse, a descriptive study. Pediatrics. *1990b;86:428.*

- Lack of breast development by age 14 years or lack of any development by age 13 years is considered abnormal and deserves further evaluation.
- Pubic hair appears (pubarche) at the same time as breast development or within 5 to 6 months thereafter.
- In the prepubertal female the uterus/cervix ratio is 1:2 or 1:3, but this reverses to 2:1 after puberty. Other internal genital changes are as follows:

1. Myometrium thickens markedly.
2. Uterine lining becomes multilayered columnar and mucocolumnar.
3. Uterine length becomes 3.5 cm on average.
4. Ovaries increase in size.
5. The cervix undergoes anteflexion, placing it into the posterior vaginal vault.
6. Ectopy of the columnar epithelium into the vaginal vault occurs.

• Changes in the external genitalia include the following:

1. The hymen and tissue in the periurethral area thicken.
2. Vagina lengthens and epithelium lining thickens.
3. Mucus-secreting cells and Skene's and Bartholin's glands produce watery mucus.
4. Vaginal epithelium becomes lighter pink in color and tissue rugation and protrusion increase.
5. Elasticity increases and sensitivity to pain decreases.
6. The vaginal pH becomes 3.5 to 5, which may be protective against vulvovaginitis.
7. Labia majora and labia minora enlarge.

Pubertal Variations in Girls

Among the normal variations are the following: adolescent vestibular growths; elongation of the vestibule in obese girls; intravaginal and paraurethral cysts; and myrtiform caruncles (usually in sexually active girls).

Male Puberty and Variations in Male Sexual Development

• The first sign of puberty in the male is enlargement of the testes at a mean age of 9.5 years, accompanied by tenderness with referred pain to the ipsilateral lower quadrant. Testicular size is the most accurate method of assessing male puberty.

• The average length of puberty is 2.5 to 3 years, with progression from spermarche to ejaculation to fertility.

• At a mean age of 11.6 years, the penis grows in length and pubic hair appears at its base. Next, axillary hair grows, then bony growth occurs, and finally muscle mass increases.

• Variations found at physical examination include the following: gynecomastia, spermatocele; varicocele; and pink pearly papules of the penis.

Sexual Maturity Rating

• The Tanner stages of maturity are strictly guidelines used in assessing the progression of pubertal development in adolescents **(Table 2-2)**. They are not criteria for use in video review of probable chronological age.

• The alternative use of the Garn-Falkner system for breast changes includes the following 4 stages:

1. Prepubertal
2. Palpable areola and increased pigmentation
3. Growth and separation of the areola with an increase in papillae
4. Regression of the areola as nipple papillae enlarge

Development of the Anorectum

The main event in normal development is a shift of the dorsal part of the cloaca and hindgut to the body surface of the tail groove. The hindgut develops at 4 weeks of gestation and ultimately forms the spleen, bladder, descending colon, sigmoid, and rectum as far inferiorly as Hilton's white line. At 5 to 6 weeks of gestation, the anorectal bar of mesenchyme coronally bisects the cloaca into the dorsal anorectal compartment and ventral urogenital sinus, then forming the perineal body. At 6 weeks, the dorsal anal fossa terminates the gastrointestinal tract and gives rise to the distal anal canal and anus.

Table 2-2. Tanner Stages of Maturity

BREAST SEXUAL MATURITY RATING	
Stage 1 (prepubertal)	Elevation of the papilla
Stage 2	Breast budding with areolar enlargement and later tenderness
Stage 3	Enlargement with no separation of breast/nipple contour
Stage 4	Projection of the areola and papilla to form a clear mound (nipple)
Stage 5	The mature stage with areolar recession
PUBIC MATURITY RATING	
Stage 1 (preadolescent)	Only vellus over the pubes, no pubic hair
Stage 2 (pubarche)	Sparse growth downy hair, straight, little curl, hairs easily counted
Stage 3	Hair darker, coarser, curlier, mainly over the pubes, still countable
Stage 4	Adult type hair over the mons and labia, counting now requires compulsive behavior
Stage 5	Mature stage spreads to medial thighs and forms the female escutcheon (inverted triangle)

(continued)

Table 2-2. *(continued)*

Boys Sexual Maturity Rating	
Stage G1 (preadolescent)	Infantile, no enlargement of penis, testicular volume 1.5 mL
Stage G2	Testes enlarge (volume 1.6–6 mL), early sparse pubic hair
Stage G3	Hair increases, both testes (volume 6–12 mL) and penis grow
Stage G4	Hair now thickened, scrotum more rugated, volume of testes 12–20mL
Stage G5	Adult male hair on the thighs; penis and testes (volume >20 mL) full size; male escutcheon is triangular shaped

Testicular size may be measured by comparing the graduated sized testes on the orchidometer, developed by Austrian ephebiatrician and endocrinologist Dr. Andrea Prader.

The anorectal septum divides the cloacal sphincter into the anterior part (ischiocavernous and bulbocavernosus muscles) and a posterior part (external anal sphincter). At 8 weeks, the membrane ruptures, forming the anal canal. In adults the superior two thirds of the hindgut measures 2.5 cm and the inferior third about 13 mm. The junction of these two is called the pectinate line. About 2 cm superior to the pectinate line is the anocutaneous line, where columnar epithelium meets stratified squamous epithelium.

Normal Perineum and Anorectum

- Anus is normally located in the middle of any pigmentation and has circumferential rugal folds formed by the corrugator cutis ani muscle.
- Perianal tissue overlying the external anal sphincter at the most distal part of the anal canal is the anal verge, which extends from the edge of the primitive proctoderm to the margin of the anal canal.
- The pectinate or dentate line is where the anoderm meets the rectal ampulla.
- Circumferentially and deep to this tissue in the perianal space are the inferior or external hemorrhoidal veins; because they have no valves, they are easily distended and obstructed.
- Color changes that may be noted in children but are within norms are as follows:

1. Red = erythema
2. Brown = hyperpigmentation
3. Blue = venous congestion
4. White = lichen sclerosus or autoimmune disorders

Anatomic Variations

Among the variations that are noted are the following: diastasis ani; anal tags; symmetrical or asymmetrical anal opening; superficial fissures; imperforate anus; fistulous formation; and cloacal exstrophy.

Healing After Anogenital Injury

- Evidence of tissue injury in childhood anogenital trauma heals rapidly. Therefore, sexual misuse may result any of the following 3 findings:

1. No injury to the victim
2. Acute injury with rapid healing and no evident residual
3. Evidence of chronic and recurrent abuse

• Serious tissue injury or deformation is more often seen in sexual assault cases than child sexual abuse.

• Scarring can distort the predicted clinical prognosis and lead to a faulty conclusion.

• Pain and bleeding correlate with an increased probability of finding evidence of significant injury in child sexual abuse.

• The more protection from estrogenization, glycogen production, and secretion content, the less clinically observable the injury over time.

• Using the colposcope and a green filter, even subtle interruptions in vascular supply are easily recognized, and any neovascularization that occurs in the healing process is readily observed.

• Wound resolution is the reverse action of original structure and function and involves 2 overlapping phases, taking place only if tissue damage is minor, complications do not ensue, and damaged or destroyed tissue has the ability to proliferate the remaining cells. Resolution may require up to 2 years, depending on the tissue injured.

• Healing occurs in 2 ways:

1. Regeneration

   a. Generation of cellular debris as thrombosis, platelet degradation, and inflammation occur rapidly (noticeable within 24 hours).

   b. Regeneration of denuded epithelial cells (48 to 72 hours).

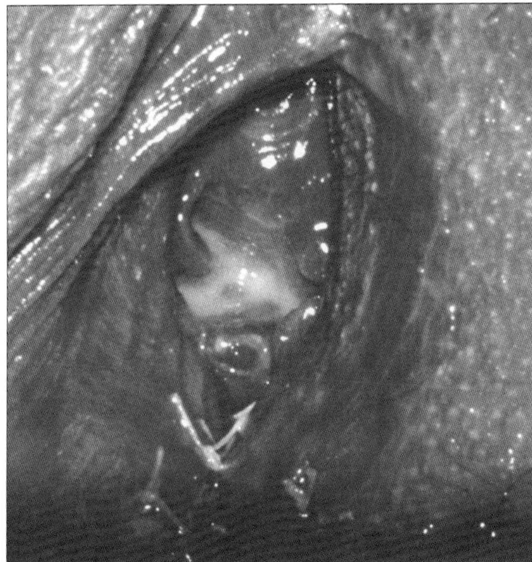

Figure 2-6. *Subacute trauma, 9 days postinjury.*

c. Production of new immature cells (5 to 7 days).

d. Differentiation and maturation of new cells (several weeks).

e. Most superficial anogenital injuries cannot be seen with the unaided eye by 4 to 5 days **(Figure 2-6)**.

2. Repair

a. Angiogenesis of new capillaries.

b. Migration and proliferation of fibroblasts.

c. Synthesis of extracellular matrix by fibroblasts.

d. Maturation and remodeling of fibrous tissue scar.

e. The wound appears reddened from neo-vascularization, then contracts and pales as the scar matures at about 60 days. Very little repair healing occurs in the anogenital area, possibly because of mucosal surface qualities, but narrowing of the hymenal rim at the point of injury is not uncommon. A V-shaped cleft or notch occurs when the elastic tissue in the separating edges of the hymen retracts during injury.

References

Adams JA, Knudson S. Genital findings in adolescent girls referred for suspected sexual abuse. *Arch Pediatr Adolesc Med.* 1996;150:850-857.

Biro FM, Falkner F, Khoury P. Areolar and breast staging in adolescent girls. *Adolesc Pediatr Gynecol.* 1992;5:271.

Bukowski TP, Zeman PA. Hypospadias: of concern but correctable. *Pediatrics.* 2001;18:89-109.

Cantwell HB. Vaginal inspection as it relates to child sexual abuse in girls under thirteen. *Child Abuse Negl.* 1987;11:545-546.

Cowell CA. The gynecological examination of infants, children, and young adolescents. *Pediatr Clin North Am.* 1981;28:247-266.

Cupoli JM, Sewell PM. One thousand fifty-nine children with a complaint of sexual abuse. *Child Abuse Negl.* 1988;2:151-162.

Emans SJ, Woods ER, Flagg NT, Freeman A. Genital findings in sexually abused, symptomatic and asymptomatic girls. *Pediatrics.* 1987;79:778-785.

Finkel MA. Anogenital trauma in sexually abused children. *Pediatrics.* 1989;84:317-322.

Fleischer AC, Shawker TH. The role of sonography in pediatric gynecology. *Clin Obstet Gynecol.* 1987;30:735-746.

Gorsch RV. *Proctological Anatomy.* Baltimore, Md: Williams & Wilkins; 1955:56-57.

Heger A, Emans SJ. Introital diameter as the criterion for sexual abuse [commentaries]. *Pediatrics.* 1990;85:222-223.

McCann J, Voris J, Simon M, Wells R. Comparison of genital examination techniques in prepubertal girls. *Pediatrics.* 1990a;85:182-187.

McCann J, Voris J, Simon M, Wells R. Perianal findings in prepubertal children selected for nonabuse; a descriptive study. *Child Abuse Negl.* 1989;13:179-193.

McCann J, Wells R, Simon M, Voris J. Genital findings in prepubertal girls selected for nonabuse; a descriptive study. *Pediatrics.* 1990b;86:428-439.

Mittwoch U, Burgess AMC, Baker PJ. Male development in a sea of oestrogen. *Lancet.* 1993;342(8863):123-124.

Moore KL. The urogenital system. In: *The Developing Human: Clinically Oriented Embryology.* 3rd ed. Philadelphia, Pa: WB Saunders; 1982:255-256.

Pokorny SF. Configuration of the prepubertal hymen. *Am J Obstet Gynecol.* 1987;157:950-956.

Pokorny SF, Kozinetz CA. Configuration and other anatomic detail of the prepubertal hymen. *Adolesc Pediatr Gynecol.* 1988;1:97.

Pokorny SF, Murphy JG, Preminger MK. Circumferential hymen elasticity: a marker of physiologic maturity. *J Reprod Med.* 1998;43(11):943-948.

Rapaport R. Disorders of the gonads. In: Behrman RE, Kliegman RM, Jenson HB, eds. *Nelson Textbook of Pediatrics.* 16th ed. Philadelphia, Pa: WB Saunders; 2000:1760-1766.

Rapaport R. Gynecomastia. In: Behrman RE, Kliegman RM, Jenson HB, eds. *Nelson Textbook of Pediatrics.* 16th ed. Philadelphia, Pa: WB Saunders; 2000:1752.

Simpson JL. Disorders of sexual differentiation. In: Sanfilippo JS, Muram D, Dewhurst J, Lee PA, eds. *Pediatric and Adolescent Gynecology.* 2nd ed. Philadelphia, Pa: WB Saunders; 2000:87-115.

Styne DM. Normal growth and pubertal developmental. In: Sanfilippo JS, Muram D, Dewhurst J, Lee PA, eds. *Pediatric and Adolescent Gynecology.* 2nd ed. Philadelphia, Pa: WB Saunders; 2000:31.

Teixeria WR. Hymenal colposcopic examination in sexual abuse. *Am Med Pathol.* 1981;3:209-214.

Usta IM, Awwad JT, Usta JA, Makarem MM, Karam KS. Imperforation of the hymen: report of an unusual familial occurrence. *Obstet Gynecol.* 1993;82:655-656.

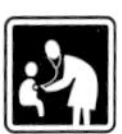

Chapter 3

PHYSICAL EVALUATION OF CHILDREN

Jacqueline M. Sugarman, MD

The child who comes to medical attention in the acute medical setting because he or she made a specific disclosure of developmentally inappropriate sexual contact or who has either physical or behavioral symptoms that cause concern for such contact should undergo a history, physical examination, diagnostic and forensic testing as needed, and referrals as appropriate.

HISTORY

- Most children who are sexually abused have normal examinations, so the diagnosis of sexual abuse usually rests solely on the history given by the child.
- Obtaining and documenting an accurate account of what happened are crucial in diagnosing sexual abuse.
- Make every attempt to interview the child separate from the parents, guardians, or accompanying caregivers so his or her full disclosure of the events is not hindered.
- Do not assume that the child's caregiver believes the child and will protect the child from further abuse.
- It may be easier to first interview the accompanying caregiver separate from the child, so you can obtain a history and better understand the child's world. Obtain from the caregiver:

1. The child's names for body parts

2. How long ago the abuse took place and the possible extent of the abuse
3. Any unusual living situations
4. The child's past medical history
5. Changes in the child's behavior
6. Medications that the child is taking

• If the child has been brought to medical attention because of behavior or physical symptoms that seem suspicious for sexual abuse, ask specifically what is being questioned. Be aware that most signs and symptoms in abused children are nonspecific (**Table 3-1**).

1. Sexual behaviors that appear most frequently in nonabused children include self-stimulating behaviors, exhibitionism, and behaviors related to personal boundaries.
2. Infrequent behaviors in nonabused children are more intrusive, such as putting the mouth on sex parts or putting objects into the vagina or rectum.
3. Behavior that suggests a child's explicit or inappropriate knowledge of adult sexual behavior and compulsive masturbation warrant further investigation.

• Form an impression as to whether the caregiver is protective of the child and if the child is at risk for being abused in the future. Ask if the perpetrator resides in the home and if there are other children at risk.

• Conduct the interview of the child in an unhurried manner and in an unthreatening environment (**Table 3-2**). Be sensitive to the child's desire for an

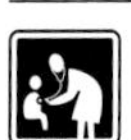

Table 3-1. Common Presenting Complaints of Sexually Abused Children and Adolescents in the Medical Setting

PHYSICAL SIGNS AND SYMPTOMS	
Genital discharge, bleeding	Recurrent urinary tract infections
Genital pruritis (itching)	Drug overdose
Pregnancy, including pregnancy with genetic disorders	Abdominal pain
Other genital infections	Numbing of body parts
Muscle weakness	Seizures
Migraine headache	Short stature
Genital skin lesions	Appetite disturbance
Genital or urethral trauma	Sleep disturbance
STDs: typical, atypical, or disseminated	Fatigue or exhaustion
	Enuresis and/or encopresis
PSYCHOSOMATIC DISORDERS	
Diffuse somatic complaints	Abdominal pain
Hysterical or conversion reactions	Anorexia
SEXUAL PROBLEMS	
Sexualized play	Sexual dysfunction
Sexual self-abuse	Sexual revictimization
Excessive masturbation	Fear of intimacy
Sexual perpetration to others	Promiscuity or prostitution

(continued)

Table 3-1. *(continued)*

SOCIAL AND BEHAVIORAL PROBLEMS	
School adjustment problems	Social withdrawal
Taking on parental roles	Aggressive behavior
Phobias, avoidance behavior	Family conflicts
Temper tantrums	Impulsive behavior
Substance abuse	Self-mutilating behavior
Suicidal ideation, gestures, or attempts	Truancy or runaway behavior
Neurotic or conduct disorders	
OTHER PSYCHOLOGIC PROBLEMS	
Excessive guilt	Mistrust
Irritability	Hyperalertness
Feelings of helplessness	Terrified of rejection
Low self-esteem	Anxiety
Amnesia	Multiple personalities
Fear of criticism or praise	Identity diffusion
Rage	Dissociation
Altered states of consciousness	Obsessive ideas
Depression	Flashbacks
Self-hate, self-blame	
OTHER	
Asymptomatic sibling of a victim	
Association with a known offender (Schmitt, 1982a)	

Data from Hunter et al. (1983), Krugman (1986), and Massie & Johnson (1989). Reprinted with permission from Jenny C. Medical issues in sexual abuse. In: Briere J, Berliner L, Buckley JA, Jenny C, Reid T, eds. The APSAC Handbook on Child Maltreatment. *Thousand Oaks, Calif: Sage Publications; 1996:197-199.*

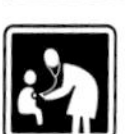

impartial third party to be present. Allow the parent to remain while you establish rapport with the child before asking questions related to the alleged abuse.

- Tailor your attempts to establish rapport to the child's developmental status.
- Avoid long, complex questions and the use of pronouns instead of names. Be direct.
- In building rapport, gauge the child's developmental level.
- Ask about daily living and intimate relationships.
- Ask the child to identify body parts by either pointing to them on a diagram or drawing a crude stick figure, usually starting with the head and working downward.
- Once rapport has been established, ask about abuse using open-ended or nondirective questions **(Table 3-3)**.
- Note spontaneous responses regarding sexual details, such as ejaculation, because most children have no knowledge of them unless they have experienced them.
- Be aware that not every child will be cooperative. Some have been threatened by the perpetrator, some may feel guilty because they believe the abuse was their fault, some may not want to betray the perpetrator, some may fear no one will believe them, some may be too embarrassed or shy, and some simply do not want to talk at that particular time.

1. It may be necessary to defer further interviewing and proceed with the examination or reschedule both.

Table 3-2. Interview Protocol	
Initial procedure	Obtain information from caretaker or social worker. Determine child's terminology for genitalia.
Interview child alone in nonthreatening environment Establish rapport with child	What's your name? How old are you? Who lives at your house? Do you have any pets? What school do you attend?
Ask about daily living and intimate relationships Ask child to identify body parts/ ascertain names for genitalia	Where do you sleep? Who gives you a bath? Identify hair, eyes, nose, belly button, private parts.
Try to determine what happened Begin with open-ended questions (may need to ask more specific questions for younger children)	Why did you come to see the doctor? Did something happen to you? Did something happen to your bottom?
More specific questions	Where were you when it happened? Where was Mommy? Daddy? Who did it? What did he/she do? Where were your clothes? Did you tell anyone? Who did you tell? What did he or she say when you told?

(continued)

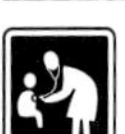

Table 3-2. *(continued)*

Conclude the interview	Tell the child she did a good job. Reassure her that it was not her fault and nobody blames her.
Explain the examination	"Now I'm going to check you out, listen to your heart and lungs, feel your tummy, and look at your private parts."
Document	Document questions asked and answers given. Record exact words and phrases.
Modifications for adolescents	Obtain more specific information: date and time of assault, history of assault (oral, rectal or vaginal penetration, oral contact by the offender, ejaculation [if known by the victim], digital penetration or penetration with foreign object). Obtain history of any self-cleaning activities (bathing, teeth brushing, urination, douching, changing clothes). Obtain menstrual history and whether patient uses contraceptives. Were any lubricants or a condom used?

Adapted with permission from Midwest Children's Resource Center Interview Protocol, Carolyn Levitt, MD, Director, Midwest Children's Resource Center.

2. If the abuse occurred in the past 72 hours, physical findings or forensic evidence may be found, so it may be necessary to proceed despite the child's reluctance.

• At the conclusion of the interview, tell the child that he or she did well and did the right thing by telling. Reassure the child that the abuse was not his or her fault. Finally, tell the child what will happen next—the physical examination.

The Physical Examination

Purposes

1. Document the condition of the patient.
2. Diagnose and treat injuries and sexually transmitted diseases (STDs).
3. Collect and preserve evidence.
4. Reassure the patient and address concerns about his or her physical and psychologic well-being.

Procedure (Table 3-4)

• Integrate any forensic evidence collection with the medical testing and examination.

• Ensure that the patient feels comfortable with you and can anticipate what the examination will entail.

• Respect the patient's modesty and allow her to feel she has some control over the examination.

• Begin with overall inspection of the patient, usually those areas that provoke the least anxiety, and progress to the most sensitive areas.

• Note nongenital as well as genital injuries.

• Determine when the alleged abuse occurred.

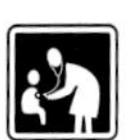

Table 3-3. A Continuum of Types of Questions Used in Interviewing Children Alleged to Have Been Sexually Abused and Confidence in Responses (Faller, 1990)

OPEN-ENDED

This type of question allows the child to respond with the most confidence.

Q: How are you?

A: Sad, 'cause my dad poked me in the pee-pee.

FOCUSED

Children respond with a little less confidence than the open-ended questions.

Q: How do you get along with your dad?

A: OK, except when he pokes me in the pee-pee.

Q: Did anything happen to your pee-pee?

A: My daddy poked me there.

Q: What did he poke you with?

A: He poked me with his ding-dong.

MULTIPLE CHOICE

Children respond to this type of question with more confidence than the yes/no and leading questions but with less confidence than a focused or open-ended question.

Q: Did he poke with his finger, his ding-dong, or something else?

A: He used his ding-dong.

Q: Did this happen in the daytime or nighttime?

A: In the day and night.

(continued)

Table 3-3. *(continued)*

YES/NO

Q: Did he tell you not to tell?
A: No, he didn't say anything like that.
Q: Did you have your clothes off?
A: No, just my panties.

LEADING

Q: He took your clothes, didn't he?
A: Yes.
Q: Didn't he make you suck his penis?
A: Yes.

Reprinted with permission from The Advisor. *1990;3(2).* The Advisor *is a quarterly publication of the American Professional Society on the Abuse of Children, Chicago, Ill.*

Table 3-4. Equipment for Sexual Assault Examination

EQUIPMENT	COMMENTS
Drapes, gowns	Preserve patient's modesty
Books, videos, pictures	Distract young patient while examination is being performed
Small dacron swabs, sterile saline	May be needed to "float" hymen
Warmed *N. gonorrhoeae* culture plates (up to 3 for vaginal/urethral, anal, and pharyngeal specimens)	Culture is the gold standard for detecting *N. gonorrhoeae* in children

(continued)

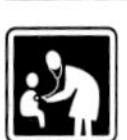

Table 3-4. *(continued)*

EQUIPMENT	COMMENTS
C. trachomatis culture tubes (for vaginal/urethral, anal, and pharyngeal specimens)	Culture is the gold standard for detecting *C. trachomatis* in children
Saline solution for wet prep, microscope slides	When vaginal discharge needs to be tested for *T. vaginalis*
Viral culture media	If lesion is suspicious for herpes
Forensic evidence collection kit	If abuse occurred within last 72 hours and medical discretion determines need. Available from police.
Additional sterile dacron swabs	May be necessary to collect additional forensic evidence
Colposcope with camera	Optional; magnification is helpful, not required. Photographs may help examiner describe findings; not essential.
Blood drawing supplies	If blood for serology or rape kit is to be obtained
Measuring tape	Should any lesions need to be measured

- Examine genital areas with or without a colposcope and taking photographs. Use the Tanner stage to communicate sexual maturity.
- Prepubertal female genitalia are examined without a speculum; if there is unexplained vaginal bleeding, the examination should usually be accomplished under anesthesia by a pediatric gynecologist or surgeon.
- Generally, thorough visual inspection of the external genitalia, vaginal vestibule, and hymenal structures is sufficient.

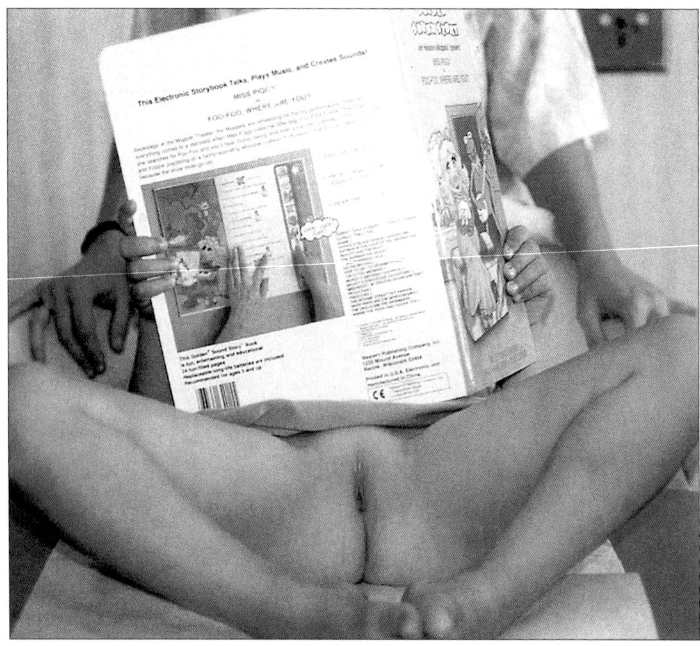

Figure 3-1. *Child in a frog-leg supine position with a book on her abdomen to distract her attention away from the exam.*

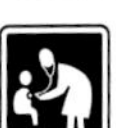

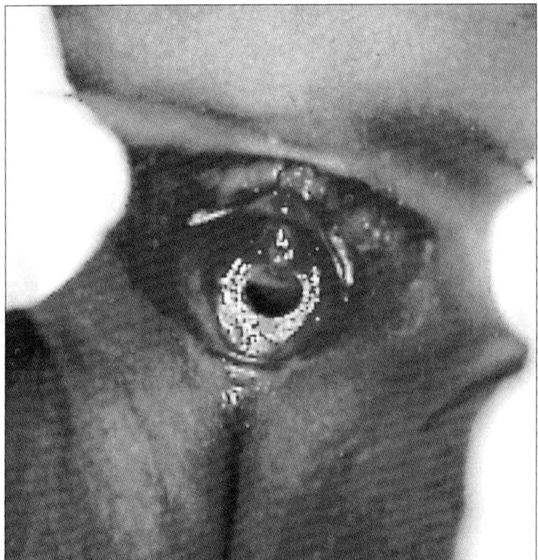

Figure 3-2. *Labial traction for a child in the supine frog-leg position. Examiner is gently pulling outward and downward on labia majora with gloved hands. In view is a normal crescentic hymen of a Tanner stage 1 girl. Hymen has attachments at the 11 and 1 o'clock positions without tissue being present between the two attachments.*

1. Visual inspection in the prepubertal female is done with her lying in a frog-leg supine position **(Figure 3-1)**.
2. In the supine frog-leg position, the hymen is best visualized using gentle traction on the labia majora **(Figure 3-2)**. Pull the labia majora outward and downward.
3. In the knee-chest position, the labia majora is lifted upward and outward to visualize the hymen; this allows you to see the posterior hymen, vagina, anus, and often the cervix as well **(Figure 3-3)**.

4. For redundant or folded hymenal tissue, use a swab moistened with saline solution to tease the tissue apart **(Figure 3-4)** or apply a few milliliters of warm saline solution to make the hymenal edges float **(Figure 3-5 a and b)**.
5. Describe findings related to the hymen with relationship to the face of a clock **(Figure 3-6)**, always noting whether the patient is prone or supine.
6. Male genitalia are examined while the patient is sitting or standing. Retract the foreskin if possible and examine the glans. Also examine the scrotum and testes.
7. For either sex, the anus can be examined while the child is supine with the knees drawn up to the chest, in a lateral decubitus position, or in the prone knee-chest position. The anus is seen by spreading the gluteal folds. Note rectal sphincter tone. Digital rectal examination is not needed, but endoscopic examination is indicated if deeper rectal injury is suspected because of severe or unexplained bleeding.

Findings of Concern in Sexual Abuse Evaluations

• Findings noted on physical examination are classified in **Table 3-5**.

• If an STD is suspected, follow the screening recommendations given in **Table 3-6**.

Forensic Evidence

A sexual assault examination kit provides an organized means of collecting forensic evidence. Though they vary from state to state, they gener-

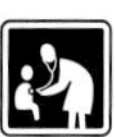

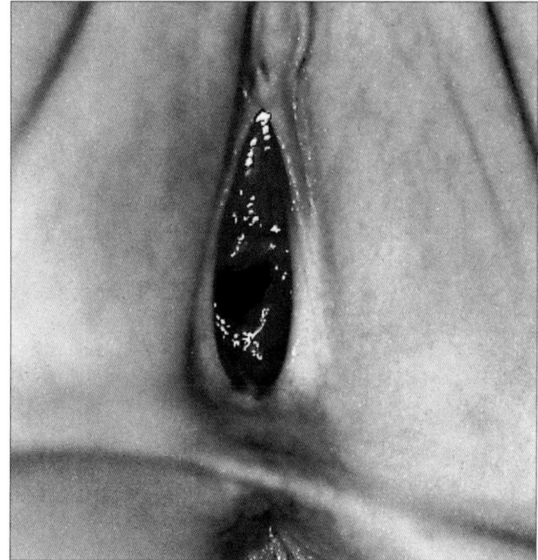

Figure 3-3. *Labial traction for a child in the prone knee-chest position. Examiner is gently pushing the labia majora upward and outward.*

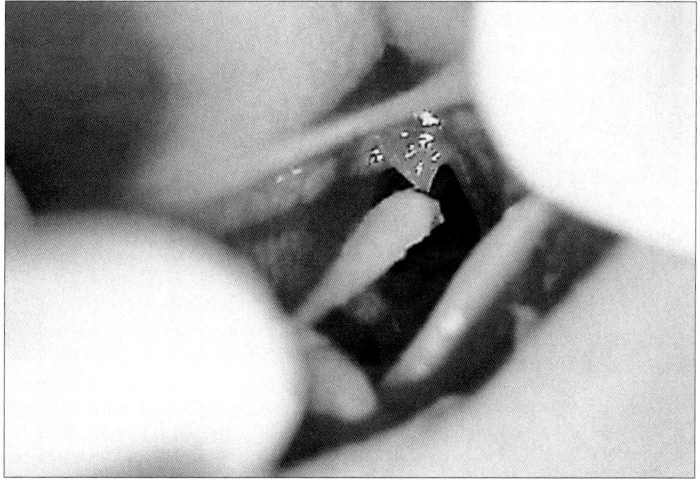

Figure 3-4. *The examiner is using a cotton swab moistened with saline solution to assess a bump (probably a septal remnant) on the hymen at 6 o'clock in the supine position.*

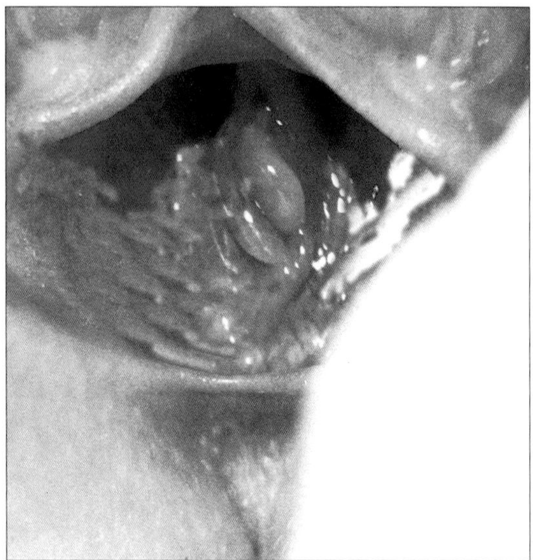

Figure 3-5-a. *Supine view.*

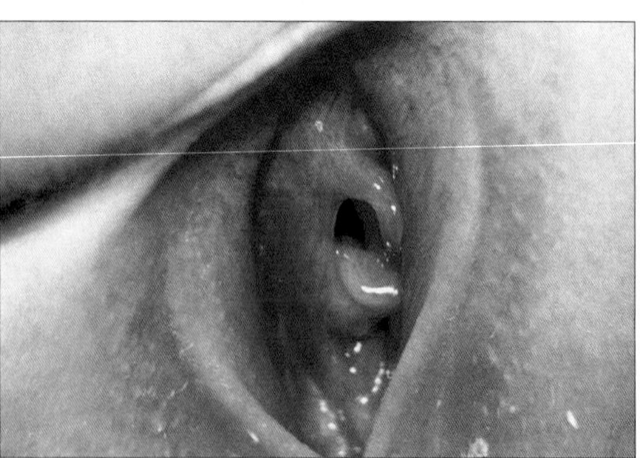

Figure 3-5-b. *Knee-chest view.*

Figure 3-5. *Supine and knee-chest views of a Tanner stage 1 hymen. It is difficult to access the hymen supine. In the prone knee-chest position, however, the hymen is seen to be slightly redundant and annular, with a tag present at 6 o'clock. This is a normal examination. While the knee-chest position does not add much if the hymen is normal and well visualized in the supine position, it is helpful if results in the supine position are abnormal or equivocal. The knee-chest position is also helpful to assess whether the hymen is folded onto itself and therefore merely looks abnormal.*

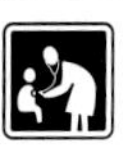

Figure 3-6. *Face of a clock.*

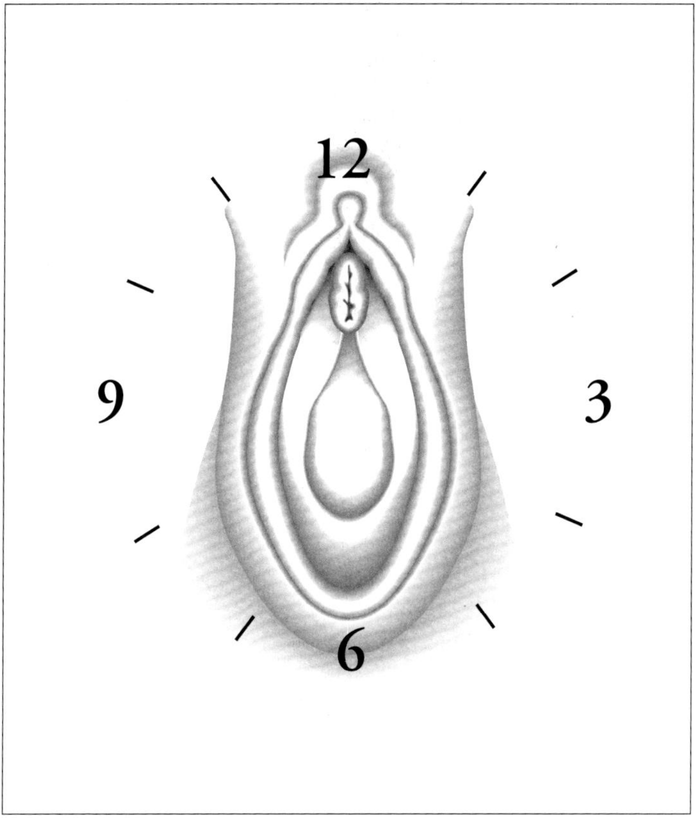

ally provide the means to collect clothing worn by the victim, debris from the assaulted genital area, pubic hair (if the patient is prepubertal), swabs for collecting dried secretions left on the victim's genital area, head hair, saliva, and blood from the victim. **Table 3-7** outlines the procedure to be followed.

Table 3-5. Revised Classification of Anogenital Findings in Suspect Sexual Abuse

CLASSIFICATION OF FINDINGS

Class 1: Normal

Found in newborns

— Periurethral or vestibular bands
— Longitudinal intravaginal ridges or columns
— Hymenal tags
— Hymenal bumps or mounds
— Hymenal clefts in the anterior (superior) half of hymenal rim, above the 3 to 9 o'clock line, with patient supine
— Estrogen changes, when hymenal tissue appears thickened, redundant, and pale
— Linea vestibularis (a flat, white, midline streak in posterior vestibule)

Class 2: Nonspecific

Findings that may result from sexual abuse, depending on timing of examination with respect to abuse, but that may also be normal variants or result from other causes

— Perianal skin tags
— Increased perianal skin pigmentation
— Diastasis ani, or a smooth area at 6 or 12 o'clock in perianal area, where there are no anal folds or wrinkles
— Erythema (redness) of vestibular or perianal tissues
— Increased vascularity, or dilation of existing blood vessels, in the vestibule
— Labial adhesions, or agglutination or fusion of labia minora in midline
— Hymenal rim that appears narrow, but is 1 mm wide or less, with measurements taken from magnified photographs by means of calibrated measuring device

(continued)

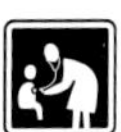

Table 3-5. *(continued)*

Class 2: (cont.)

— Vaginal discharge (this is a nonspecific finding unless appropriately obtained cultures confirm the presence of a sexually transmitted infection)
— Lesions of condyloma acuminata in child less than 2 years of age
— Anal fissures
— Flattened or thickened anal folds
— Anal dilatation, or the opening of internal and external anal sphincters, which demonstrates stool in the rectal vault
— Venous congestion or venous pooling in perianal tissues causing a purple coloration, which may be localized or diffuse

Class 3: Suspicious

Findings that have rarely been described in nonabused children, but have been noted in children with documented abuse, and would prompt examiner to investigate carefully the possibility of abuse

— Enlarged hymenal opening, with measurements more than 2 standard deviations above mean for age and examination method
— Hymenal notch/cleft/partial transection, which appears as sudden narrowing in hymenal rim to less than 1 mm in width, located on or below 3 to 9 o'clock line (patient supine)
— Acute abrasions, lacerations, or bruising of labia or perihymenal tissue, with no history of accidental injury
— Apparent condyloma acuminata in child less than 2 years old
— Distorted anal folds, which are irregular in appearance and may have signs of edema of the tissues
— Immediate (within 30 seconds) anal dilatation of 20 mm or more, with no stool visible or palpable in the rectal vault

(continued)

Table 3-5. *(continued)*

Class 4: Suggestive of Abuse or Penetration

Findings, or combination of findings, that can be reasonably explained only by postulating abuse or penetrating injury of some type

— Combination of 2 or more suspicious genital findings or 2 or more suspicious anal findings
— Scar or fresh laceration of posterior fourchette, not involving the hymen
— Perianal scar

Class 5: Clear Evidence of Blunt Force or Penetrating Trauma

Findings that can have no explanation other than trauma to hymen or perianal tissues

— Complete hymenal transection (healed): hymen has been torn through to the base, so that no measurable hymenal tissue remains between vaginal wall and fossa or vestibular wall
— Areas, more extensive than transections, where there is complete absence of hymenal tissue below the 3 to 9 o'clock line (patient supine)
— Acute laceration of hymen: recent tear through full thickness of hymenal tissue, which may also extend into the vagina and/or posterior fourchette
— Ecchymosis or bruising on the hymen
— Perianal lacerations extending deep to the external anal sphincter

OVERALL ASSESSMENT OF LIKELIHOOD OF ABUSE

Class 1: No Evidence of Abuse

— Normal results of examination, no history, no behavioral changes, no witnessed abuse
— Nonspecific findings with another known or likely explanation, and no history of abuse or behavior changes
— Child considered at risk for sexual abuse, but gives no history and has only nonspecific behavior changes
— Physical findings of injury consistent with history of accidental injury, which is clear and believable

(continued)

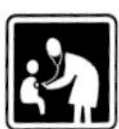

Table 3-5. *(continued)*

Class 2: Possible Abuse

- Class 1 or 2 findings in combination with marked behavior changes, especially sexualized behaviors, but child unable to give history of abuse
- Presence of condyloma acuminata in a child less than 2 years old or herpes type 1 genital lesions with history of abuse, and with otherwise normal results of examination
- Child has made a statement, but it is not sufficiently detailed or is not consistent
- Class 3 findings with no disclosure of abuse

Class 3: Probable Cause

- Child gives a clear, consistent, and detailed description of being molested, with or without physical findings
- Class 4 findings in a child with or without a history of abuse, and with no history of accidental penetrating injury
- Positive culture (not rapid antigen test) for *C. trachomatis* from genital area in child less than 2 years old
- Positive culture for herpes simplex type 2 from genital lesions
- Confirmed condyloma acuminata, when lesions first appeared in a child 2 years old or younger
- Trichomonas infection, diagnosed by wet mount or culture

Reprinted with permission from Adams J. Evolution of a classification scale: [appendix]. Child Maltreat. *Thousand Oaks, Calif: SAGE Publications, Inc. 2001;6(1):34-35.*

Table 3-6. STD Screening Recommendations

INITIAL EXAMINATION

Prepubertal Children

Decision to evaluate for STDs must be made on an individual basis. Situations involving a high risk for STDs include symptomatic child, child with abnormal genital findings on examination, high STD prevalence in community, and suspected offender at high risk for having STD.

CULTURES FOR *N. GONORRHOEAE* AND FOR *C. TRACHOMATIS*

Adolescents

Cultures should be obtained from any sites of penetration or attempted penetration.

Prepubertal Children

Cultures should be obtained from any sites of penetration or attempted penetration, including (when indicated): pharyngeal, anal, vaginal or urethral cultures. In evaluating for chlamydia, a urethral specimen should be obtained only if urethral discharge is present. In evaluating for *N. gonorrhoeae*, a specimen of urethral meatal discharge can be substituted for intraurethral swab. Pharyngeal specimens not recommended for *C. trachomatis*.

WET MOUNT AND CULTURE FOR *T. VAGINALIS*

Adolescents and Prepubertal Children

Wet mount and culture of vaginal swab specimen for *T. vaginalis*. Examine wet mount for evidence of bacterial vaginosis and yeast infection if vaginal discharge or malodor is evident.

(continued)

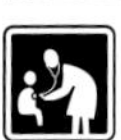

Table 3-6. *(continued)*

SERUM FOR HIV, SYPHILIS, AND HEPATITIS B

Adolescents and Prepubertal Children
Preservation of a serum sample for subsequent analysis if follow-up serologic tests are positive.

FOLLOW-UP 2 WEEKS AFTER ASSAULT

Adolescents
Repeat physical examination. Cultures should be repeated unless prophylaxis was given.

Prepubertal Children
Repeat physical examination. Cultures (if indicated) should be repeated unless prophylaxis was given. If abuse was chronic, testing for STDs once may suffice.

FOLLOW-UP 12 WEEKS AFTER ASSAULT

Adolescents and Prepubertal Children
Serologic tests for HIV and syphilis.

Adapted from Centers for Disease Control and Prevention. 1998 guidelines for treatment of sexually transmitted diseases. MMWR Morb Mortal Wkly Rep. *1998;47:1-116.*

Table 3-7. Sexual Assault Examination Protocol and Evidence Collection for Adults and Adolescents

— Examine for nongenital trauma
— Inspect buccal cavity
— Search hair for foreign material and blood
— Inspect for bite marks
— Inspect for bruises

— Collect relevant clothing and underwear in a paper bag

Comments:

— Avoid plastic bags because mold can form
— Damaged or torn clothing may be significant
— Clothing provides surface on which traces of foreign material may be found
— Each garment should be placed in a separate bag to prevent cross-contamination

Modifications for Prepubertal Children:

— Collect underwear or diaper in a paper bag

— Examine genital area

Modifications for Prepubertal Children:

— A speculum examination is not performed
— If the examiner suspects a vaginal laceration or tear because the patient has unexplained vaginal bleeding, then a speculum examination will need to be done, most likely under anesthesia

---

— Comb hair from pubic area

Comments:

— May contain specimens from assailant and may, in some cases, help to identify race, sex, blood type, and hair color of suspect

(continued)

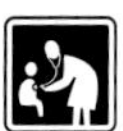

Table 3-7. *(continued)*

Modifications for Prepubertal Children:
- — No pubic hair to comb
- — Debris can be collected from pubic area

— Pluck head and pubic hair from victim

Comments:
- — Must be plucked, not cut
- — Differentiates hair debris of assailant found on victim from victim's own
- — May choose to obtain these specimens after all other evidence is collected because many victims find this unpleasant
- — Patient may choose to pluck own hair

Modifications for Prepubertal Children:
- — Omit pubic hair, collect head hair

— Vaginal fluid: wet mount of material from posterior fossa for motile sperm

— Fixed smear from the vagina or vulva or both for sperm

Comments:
- — Wet mount may not be required in all states
- — If penetration to the anus or mouth occurred, anal and/or oral swabs should be collected
- — For male victim or penile trauma, the external shaft and glans of the penis should be swabbed with cotton swabs that are slightly moistened with distilled water or saline solution

---

— Endocervical culture for *N. gonorrhoeae* and *C. trachomatis*

— Swab from vaginal pool

— Swab from any area that fluoresces with UV lamp (Wood's lamp) or appears to have dried secretions on it, (vulva, rectum, inner thighs)

(continued)

Table 3-7. *(continued)*

Comments:
- — State crime laboratory can analyze for acid phosphatase, ABO(H) antigen, and sperm preciptins

Modifications for Prepubertal Children:
- — Culture obtained by swabbing vagina for *N. gonorrhoeae* and *C. trachomatis*

— Collect debris from beneath fingernails if victim scratched assailant

---

— Note dried secretions on skin by examination or fluorescing on Wood's lamp examination

Comments:
- — State crime laboratory can analyze for acid phosphatase, ABO(H) antigen, and sperm precipitins

---

Serum

— Serology for hepatitis B, syphilis, and HIV

— Beta HCG

— Blood typing

Comments:
- — Repeat in 4 to 6 weeks

— Collect saliva sample

Comments:
- — Sample will determine if the victim secretes blood group antigens in body fluids other than blood

---

Adapted from American College of Obstetricians and Gynecologists. Technical Bulletin, Sexual Assault. *1987;101:1-5.*

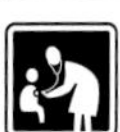

Table 3-8. Prophylaxis Regimens

CHLAMYDIAL, GONOCOCCAL, AND TRICHOMONAL INFECTIONS AND FOR BACTERIAL VAGINOSIS

Adolescents Prepubertal
Recommended regimen:
Ceftriaxone 125 mg intramuscularly
or
Cefixime 400 mg once orally
or
Spectinomycin 2 g intramuscularly
PLUS
Metronidazole 2 g once orally
PLUS
Doxycycline 100 mg orally twice daily for 7 days or
Azithromycin 1 g once orally

Children*
Recommended regimen:
Ceftriaxone 125 mg intramuscularly
or
Spectinomycin 40 mg/kg intramuscularly
PLUS
Erythromycin base 50 mg/kg/d (max 2 g/day) orally 4 times/day for 10 to 14 days
or
(for children over 8 years of age) Azithromycin 1 g once orally or Doxycycline 100 mg orally twice daily for 7 days

PREGNANCY

Adolescents Prepubertal
Please see chapter 11 for pregnancy prophylaxis information.

(continued)

Table 3-8. *(continued)*

HEPATITIS B

Adolescents Prepubertal
Postexposure hepatitis B vaccination (without hepatitis B immune globulin) should adequately protect against hepatitis B. Hepatitis B vaccine should be administered to victims of sexual assault at the time of the initial examiniation. Follow-up doses of vaccine should be administered 1-2 months and 4-6 months after the first dose if not previously vaccinated.

Children*
Consider vaccination if nonimmune.

*Prophylaxis is generally offered to adolescents. Presumptive treatment for sexually abused children is not routinely done. (Often, they are not seen acutely or the nature of the abuse may make it unlikely that an STD has been transmitted; prepubertal girls appear to be at lower risk for ascending infections than are adolescent or adult women, and regular follow-up can usually be assured.) Treatment should be considered for prepubertal girls (after cultures for STDs are obtained) who are likely to have acquired an STD, have signs of a penetrating injury, are symptomatic (abdominal pain, vaginal discharge, or dysuria), or whose parents or guardians are very concerned about the possibility of contracting an STD (Muram, 1989).

Adapted from Centers for Disease Control and Prevention (CDC). 1998 guidelines for treatment of sexually transmitted diseases. MMWR Morb Mortal Wkly Rep. *1998;47:110.*

Drug dosage recommendations listed herein are those of the authors and are not endorsed by the US Public Health Service or the US Department of Health and Human Services.

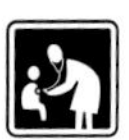

Table 3-9. Sexual Assault Examination Checklist
—History documented
—Physical examination documented (may use drawings)
—Documentation that photographs were taken (if indicated)
—Sexual assault evidence collection kit obtained, correctly labeled, sealed, locked up until retrieved by law enforcement
—Cultures and serologic tests for STDs obtained
—Prophylaxis for STDs and pregnancy discussed with patient and provided
—Mental health follow-up arranged
—Follow-up medical examination arranged
—Appropriate authorities (law enforcement, child protective services) notified
—Documentation of person to whom child was released

Definitive Care

• Offer antibiotic prophylaxis for STDs to selected pubertal children; **Table 3-8** provides antibiotic treatment regimens.

• For acute assaults, human immunodeficiency virus (HIV) prophylaxis may be required. (See Chapter 6.)

• Medical follow-up is generally recommended for all patients at 2 weeks and 12 weeks after an assault.

• Emotional and mental well-being should also be addressed. Stress that healing will come over time and ensure that adequate follow-up with the resources available in the community is in place before the patient leaves the examination site.

• **Table 3-9** offers an assault examination check-list to follow in approaching a child sexual assault examination.

References

Adams JA, Harper K, Knudson S, Revilla J. Examination findings in legally confirmed child sexual abuse: it's normal to be normal. *Pediatrics.* 1994;94:310-317.

American Academy of Pediatrics: Committee on Child Abuse and Neglect. Guidelines for the evaluation of sexual abuse of children. *Pediatrics.* 1999;103:186-191.

American Academy of Pediatrics: Committee on child abuse and neglect. Oral and dental aspects of child abuse and neglect. *Pediatrics.* 1999;104(2):348-350.

American College of Obstetricians and Gynecologists. *Technical Bulletin, Sexual Assault.* 1987;101:1-5.

American Professional Society on the Abuse of Children (APSAC). *Practice Guidelines, Descriptive Terminology in Child Sexual Abuse Evaluations.* San Diego, Calif: APSAC; 1995.

Bays J, Chadwick D. Medical diagnosis of the sexually abused child. *Child Abuse Negl.* 1993;17:91-110.

Centers for Disease Control and Prevention (CDC). 1998 guidelines for treatment of sexually transmitted diseases. *MMWR Morb Mortal Wkly Rep.* 1998;47(No. RR-1):1-116.

Frasier LD. The pediatrician's role in child abuse interviewing. *Pediatr Ann.* 1997;26:306-311.

Giardino AP, Finkel MA, Giardino ER, Seidl T, Ludwig S. *A Practical Guide to the Evaluation of Sexual Abuse in the Prepubertal Child.* Thousand Oaks, Calif: Sage Publications; 1992.

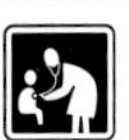

Hymel KP, Jenny C. Child sexual abuse. *Pediatr Rev.* 1996;17:236-250.

Jenny C. Medical issues in sexual abuse. In: Briere J, Berliner L, Buckley JA, Jenny C, Reid T, eds. *The APSAC Handbook on Child Maltreatment.* Thousand Oaks, Calif: Sage Publications; 1996:197-199.

Meyers JEB. Role of physician in preserving verbal evidence of child abuse. *J Pediatr.* 1986;109:409-411.

Siegel RM, Schubert CJ, Meyers PA, Shapiro RA. The prevalence of sexually transmitted diseases in children and adolescents evaluated for sexual abuse in Cincinnati: rationale for limited STD testing in prepubertal girls. *Pediatrics.* 1995;96:1090-1094.

Chapter 4

Forensic Evaluation of Children

Sarah Anderson, RN, MSN
Pamela Ross, MD

The forensic evaluation of a prepubescent child is designed to collect, document, and preserve evidence in a law enforcement investigation of a crime or possible crime. In the event of a crime, the systematic manner of collecting, documenting, and preserving evidence is referred to as *processing the scene.*

Principles of Evidence Collection

- Determination of team composition: establish a team to provide contamination control; document accurately; prioritize the collection of evidence; and collect, preserve, package, transport, and submit the evidence by established protocols. Team members may come from law enforcement, child protective services (CPS), social work, medical personnel, psychologists, forensic interviewers, and district attorneys' office; all need specialized training in pediatric sexual abuse.

- Contamination control: ensure that the integrity of the evidence is maintained. Use sterile, non-reusable items to collect specimens and observe universal precautions.

- Documentation: assess what needs to be documented and establish the types of equipment needed, considering photography, video, diagrams, measurements, and notes.

1. Take photographs with and without scale and evidence identifiers.
2. Videotape to give a broader perspective and demonstrate correct technique during evidence collection.
3. Draft preliminary sketches with measurements to document location of injuries and evidence collected in relation to the body.
4. Note location of the examination, times of arrival and completion of the examination, general information before evidence collection begins, transient evidence (smells, sights, conditions), and deviations from usual standards of practice or care.

• Prioritization of evidence collection: prevent the loss, destruction, or contamination of evidence.

1. Conduct a careful, methodical evaluation, considering all physical evidence possibilities.
2. Focus on easily accessible areas in open view first, then proceed to out-of-view locations.
3. Follow a systematic search pattern based on size, type, and location of the evidence.
4. Move from least intrusive to most intrusive processing and collection methods.
5. Assess continually environmental and other factors that may affect evidence.

• Collection and preservation of evidence: maintain evidence security throughout the process.

1. Note location of evidence collection, date and time collected, who collected it, and who had access to it.
2. Establish a chain of custody—document the

handling and account for all specimens through each step of the evidence processing. Begin with initial collection and follow all the way to the courtroom. This ensures validity and admissibility of forensic evidence in court.

3. Obtain reference and control samples and consider obtaining elimination samples.
4. Secure any electronically recorded evidence immediately.
5. Establish policies and procedures and maintain them.

Limitations of the Forensic Evaluations

It is important not to overinterpret genital or anal anomalies because the percentage of changes attributable to sexual abuse is low. Remember that the forensic evaluation and report of findings have social and legal consequences for the child and family.

When to Collect Evidence

Only after an investigation by a law enforcement or CPS agency is initiated is forensic evidence collected. The American Academy of Pediatrics recommends forensic evidence collection when sexual abuse is believed to have occurred within the previous 72 hours or when there is bleeding or acute injury.

Process of Collection

- A head-to-toe physical examination with a detailed genital examination should be done with the patient in the frog-leg position, either supine or on the caregiver's lap, and in the prone knee-chest position. Written documentation of evidence, diagrams, and photographs are recommended.

• Physical evidence recovery kits specifically for sexual assaults are usually supplied by law enforcement agencies or can be obtained through a state forensic laboratory **(Figure 4-1)**. Most are destined for adults but are routinely modified for pediatric use. Follow the kit's instructions on how the evidence should be collected and how to handle used and unused supplies **(Table 4-1)**.

• Collect evidence using normal saline solution, distilled water, or sterile water based on the recommendations of the local forensic laboratory. Open a sealed bottle of the fluid chosen during the actual evidence collection and take a control sample to ensure that nothing was added to the evidence collected.

• Collect and separately package each piece of clothing worn during and immediately after the assault.

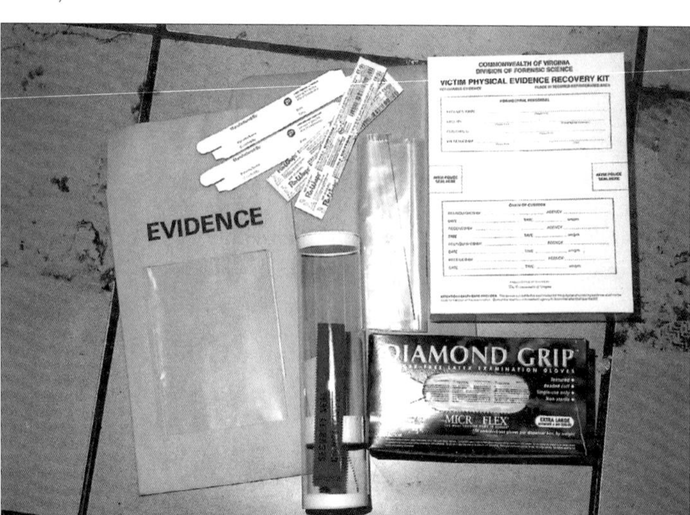

Figure 4-1. *The contents of a physical evidence recovery kit.*

Table 4-1. Forensic Evidence Collection and Preservation

SPECIMEN: CLOTHING

— Garments
— Bedding (includes sheets and paper drapes used to lay clothing on)
— Diaper

Evidence Collection Items
— Paper envelopes—various sizes
— Evidence tape
— Permanent marker
— Examination table paper

Method of Preservation
— Remove clothing one piece at a time.
— Avoid cutting through any holes, tears, or stained areas.
— If clothing is damp or wet, place a piece of paper between the layers.
Rationale: Blood and body fluids, if not allowed to dry, will cause the fabric to break down.
— Place each item in its own paper envelope or package.
Rationale: If clothing is packaged together, the trace evidence may be transferred to other items.
— Seal with a piece of evidence tape labeled with the date, time, and initials.
— If items are saturated and are soaking through the package, the package can be placed in a plastic bag, but it must be left open.
Rationale: If the items are placed in a sealed plastic bag, bacteria and fungus growth will be increased.

(continued)

Table 4-1. *(continued)*

SPECIMEN: DEBRIS

— Hair
— Paint chips
— Grass, leaves, vegetation
— Fibers

Evidence Collection Items
— Paper envelopes—various sizes
— Evidence tape
— Permanent marker

Method of Preservation
— Collect and place in separate envelopes.
Rationale: These items may connect the suspect with the child or the child and/or suspect with the crime scene.
— Write a description of the item and where it was collected on the outside of the envelope before placing the item inside.
— Seal the envelope with evidence tape labeled with the date, time, and initials.

SPECIMEN: BODY FLUIDS

— Seminal fluid
— Blood
— Urine
— Gastric contents

(continued)

Table 4-1. *(continued)*

Evidence Collection Items
— Specimen containers and tubes
— Sterile cotton swabs
— Sterile water
— Paper envelopes—various sizes
— Evidence tape
— Permanent marker

Method of Preservation
— If large quantities, collect in specimen containers or tubes. The containers should be sealed with evidence tape that has been initialed with date, time, location collected. The container should be placed in a plastic bag. The fluid specimens must be refrigerated.
Rationale: These items may connect the suspect with child or the child and/or the suspect with the crime scene.
— Areas of suspected body fluids or stains should be collected using the double swab technique. Swabs need to be either dried before packaging or placed in air-dry boxes. The swabs are placed in a paper envelope sealed with evidence tape, labeled with date, time and initials.
— If clothing is damp or wet, place a piece of paper between the layers.

1. If the child is still wearing the original clothes, undress the child over a paper sheet placed on a clean hospital bed sheet.
2. If the clothing is damp or wet, place examination table paper between the layers and notify the police so the articles of clothing are stored properly.
3. Label each package to identify the child, date, time, and your signature, then seal it securely.
4. Initial the seal through the seal.

5. Collect linens and bedding (whether they are brought to the emergency room or are at the scene), packaging them individually in paper bags, sealing them, and turning them over to the police.
6. Instruct the child's caregivers to minimize bathing, brushing the teeth, voiding, defecating, vomiting, eating, drinking, and changing clothes after an assault if at all possible.

Process of Forensic Evaluations

More Than 72 Hours After Incident or in Chronic Abuse

• Do not use a forensic evidence collection kit.

• Perform a head-to-toe physical examination and detailed genital examination as for acute abuse.

• Document findings and provide diagrams and photographic evidence.

Chronic Abuse With the Most Recent Occurrence Within 72 Hours

• Perform forensic evidence collection and a full evaluation.

• Look for evidence of acute injuries as well as old injuries.

Interview Process

See Chapter 3 for specifics of the interview.

Physical Examination

• See Chapter 3 for a general overview of the physical examination.

• The physical examination and evidence collection are performed at the same time.

• Look for signs of injury from abuse that are acute, healing, or chronic.

• Perform the genital examination with the child as directed in Chapter 3. In the female child, the genital examination should include initially direct visualization, then gentle labial separation, and finally labial traction.

• During visualization, identify and inspect the following: medial thighs, mon pubis, labial minora, labia majora, clitoris, urethra, navicularis, and posterior commissure/fourchette.

• View the anus with and without traction.

• Note the presence or absence of stool in the rectal vault.

• In the male child, carefully inspect the medial thighs, scrotum, testicles, penis, and urethra along with the anal examination.

• Unless they facilitate the removal of a foreign body, speculum and digital examinations of prepubertal children are not needed.

Special Evidence Collection Techniques in the Evaluation of Sexual Abuse

• Forensic photography

1. A 35-mm camera with a macro lens gives the best resolution but pictures cannot be viewed immediately for accuracy and technique; Polaroid or digital cameras allow immediate review and reduce the risk of obtaining inadequate photographs or none at all.
2. Take an overview or full body picture, an orientation or medium range shot, and then a close-up of the area to be emphasized; all close-ups should be taken with and without a scale,

which should be held parallel to and in the same plane as the injury and camera.

3. Repeat photographs may be required in a few days when bruises are more pronounced and patterns easier to identify; these can also help discern whether anomalies seen in the initial examination have changed or remained the same.
4. Colposcopy magnifies the genitalia and can increase the ability to see genital and perineal abnormalities. Photographs of colposcopy findings facilitate consultation between examiners in peer review, discussion with child abuse experts, and presentation in court. Take them with and without a scale.
5. A Wood's lamp may be used to identify suspicious areas for more definitive testing. Semen, urine, and other oily substances fluoresce a blue-green to orange color. Examine the child's body under a Wood's lamp in a darkened room and swab, package, and send to the laboratory any areas of fluorescence.
6. Alternate light sources also help identify old, healed bruises and bite marks, but this is a highly technical procedure that requires specialized equipment and lighting.

- Double swab technique

1. The double swab technique should be used for any areas that fluoresce under the alternate light source or where you suspect that a body fluid is present.
2. The first swab is obtained with a dampened cotton-tipped applicator, and the second with a dry cotton-tipped applicator.
3. The swabs are then placed on a slide and allowed to air dry.

- Saline float/irrigation of hymenal tissue

1. If hymenal tissue is folded over and the edges not easily identified even with positioning of the child, gently dribble saline solution over the edges of the hymen and reexamine the child.
2. Be sure to inform the child that this will be done beforehand because of the extreme sensitivity of the prepubescent hymen.

- Foley catheter technique

1. Only used in pubertal and postpubertal girls, the Foley catheter technique allows the identification of forensically significant abnormalities in the hymenal tissue by allowing the examiner to see the floppy, redundant edges.
2. A Foley catheter is inserted just past the vaginal opening, the balloon is inflated with 10 mL of sterile water, and traction is gently applied to help spread hymenal tissue edges.

- Toluidine blue

1. Toluidine blue dye is applied to the external genitalia to identify acute lacerations and abrasions.
2. Use the dye sparingly, applying it with a cotton swab or piece of gauze.
3. Remove the dye after a few seconds using lubricating jelly and examine the area for lacerations. Only damaged skin cells take up the dye.
4. Perform all DNA swabs of the external genitalia before applying toluidine blue dye.

- Bite mark impressions

1. Bite marks can be mistaken as a bruise or normal childhood mishap.

2. Breaks in the skin are more likely with animal bites than human bites.
3. Shape can vary depending on amount of force, surface area, and amount of contact made with the area involved.
4. If the bite mark is suspected to be acute, test the area using the double swab technique and dry or package the specimen in a self-drying box.
5. If indentations are noted in the skin, a bite mark impression can be made using a casting compound. Photograph all suspected bite marks with and without a scale.

- Documentation

1. Use a form that allows for the following information: basic demographic information, history from the child, data from the physical examination, and evidence collected in written form plus schematic diagrams of the whole child and genitalia.
2. Label photographs on the back with the following information: child's name, date, time, and examiner's initials as well as position of the child and a number to correspond with their locations on the diagrams.

- Peer review of cases

1. All cases should be reviewed by the team members to ensure consistency in the interpretation of findings and as a continued learning experience.
2. Feedback is also given regarding the written and photographic documentation of examinations.

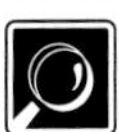

• Testing for sexually transmitted diseases (STDs). (See also Chapter 6.)

1. Reserve STD testing for cases in which vaginal or penile discharge is evident.
2. Decide to obtain cultures and perform serologic testing based on the likelihood of oral, genital, or anal penetration and the presence of symptoms. Also consider the local prevalence of STDs and the risk factors of the child and the alleged perpetrator.
3. In cases of acute sexual assault, tests for gonorrhea, *Chlamydia*, *Trichomonas*, and bacterial vaginosis are done 2 weeks after the assault if the patient received no prophylactic treatment during the initial examination.
4. Serologic testing for syphilis, human immunodeficiency virus (HIV) infection, and hepatitis B is done 6, 12, and 24 weeks after the assault.
5. When testing for *Chlamydia* and gonorrhea, true cultures must be obtained. If only nonculture methods are available, refer the patient to a location where true cultures can be obtained.
6. Do not initiate antimicrobial treatment until cultures are obtained.
7. Generally, the results of nonculture methods are not admissible in court.
8. A positive culture for gonorrhea or *Chlamydia* and a positive serologic test for syphilis or HIV provide the basis for medical certainty for sexual abuse, even without a disclosure, if neonatal transmission has been ruled out.

References

American Academy of Pediatrics. Guidelines for the evaluation of sexual abuse of children. *Pediatrics.* 1991;87:254-260.

American Academy of Pediatrics: Committee on Child Abuse and Neglect. Guidelines for the evaluation of sexual abuse of children: subject review. *Pediatrics.* 1999;103:186-191.

Centers for Disease Control and Prevention (CDC). Sexually transmitted diseases treatment guidelines 2002. *MMWR Recomm Rep.* 10 May 2002;51(RR-6);1-78.

Christian CW, Lavell JM, De Jong AR, Loiselle J, Brenner L, Joffee J. Forensic evidence findings in prepubertal victims of sexual assault. *Pediatrics.* 2000;106:100-104.

Ferrell J. Foley catheter balloon technique for visualizing the hymen in female adolescent sexual abuse victims. *J Emerg Nurs.* 1995;21:585-586.

Gabby T, Winkleby MA, Boyce WT, Fisher DL, Lancaster A, Sensabaugh GF. Sexual abuse of children: the detection of semen on skin. *Am J Dis Child.* 1992;146:700-703.

Jessee SA. Recognition of bite marks in child abuse cases. *Pediatr Dent.* 1994;16:336-339.

Lauber AA, Souma JL. Use of toluidine blue for documentation of traumatic intercourse. *Obstet Gynecol.* 1982;60:644-648.

McCauley J, Gysinski G, Welch R, Gorman R, Osmers F. Toluidine blue in the corroboration of rape in the adult victim. *Am J Emerg Med.* 1987;5:105-108.

Starling SP, Jenny C. Forensic examination of adolescent female genitalia: the Foley catheter technique. *Arch Pediatr Adolesc Med.* 1997;151:102-103.

Sweet D, Lorente JA, Valenzuela A, Lorente M, Villanueva E. PCR-based DNA typing of saliva stains recovered from human skin. *J Forensic Sci.* 1997;42:320-322.

US Department of Justice. *Crime Scene Investigation: A Guide for Law Enforcement.* Washington, DC: US Dept of Justice; 2000.

Chapter 5

DIFFERENTIAL DIAGNOSIS

Philip Scribano, DO, MSCE
Barbara W. Girardin, RN, PhD
Diana K. Faugno, RN, BSN, CPN, FAAFS, SANE-A
Carolyn J. Levitt, MD
Malinda Waddell, RN, MN, FNP
Mary J. Spencer, MD

Examination findings may result from any of the following:

- A variation in normal anatomy of a prepubertal child
- Nonabusive traumatic injury resembling an abusive injury
- Medical conditions

VARIATIONS OF NORMAL ANATOMY

GENITALIA

- Vestibular bands **(Figure 5-1)**

1. Includes skin tags, septa, and notches and clefts of the hymen
2. Congenital absence of the hymen
3. Superficial notches on the inferior half of the hymen; however, notches extending through more than 50% of the membrane have been seen only in abused children
4. Vaginal columns

- Linea vestibularis
- Median raphae
- Failure of midline fusion

ANUS

- Skin tags, particularly midline tags; lateral skin tags may be viewed with concern

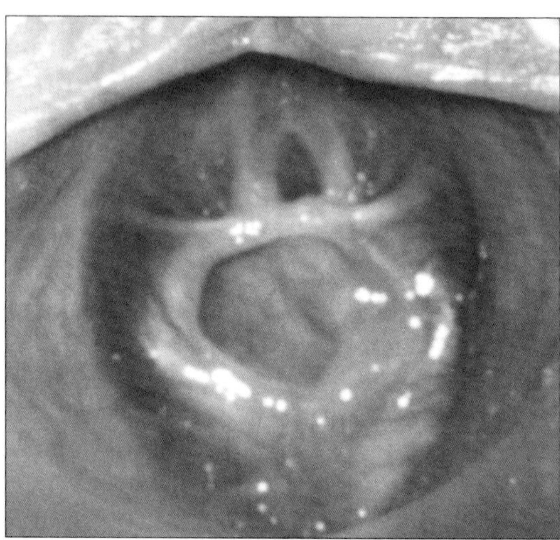

Figure 5-1. *Vestibular bands. (Contributed by Lori D. Frasier, MD; Salt Lake City, Utah.)*

- Smooth midline external sphincter with a fan-shaped area in the posterior midline
- Perianal erythema
- Degree of anal dilation; significant dilation can result from retained stool or chronic constipation or neurogenic patulous anus; postmortem dilation may also confuse the issue

Nonabusive Trauma

- Straddle injury **(Figures 5-2 and 5-3 a to d)**; however, these are extremely unlikely mechanisms of injury in children under age 9 months
- Penetrating injuries caused by falls onto pointed objects
- Excessive bleeding with a minor injury; occurs because of the rich blood supply to the external genitalia
- Vulvar hematomas, which result from straddle

injury and are very painful, cause swelling and prevent the child from urinating

- Vaginal injuries resulting from impalement from a sharp object or high-pressure water that insufflates the vagina; most of these injuries are probably abusive however
- Urogenital injuries in females are generally nonabusive
- Scrotal trauma in males
- Penile ecchymoses and/or lacerations
- Anal trauma that is isolated; when localized to the 10 to 2 o'clock and/or the 5 to 7 o'clock positions, these should cause concern for abuse
- Zipper entrapment
- Motor vehicle crashes that produce pelvic fracture,

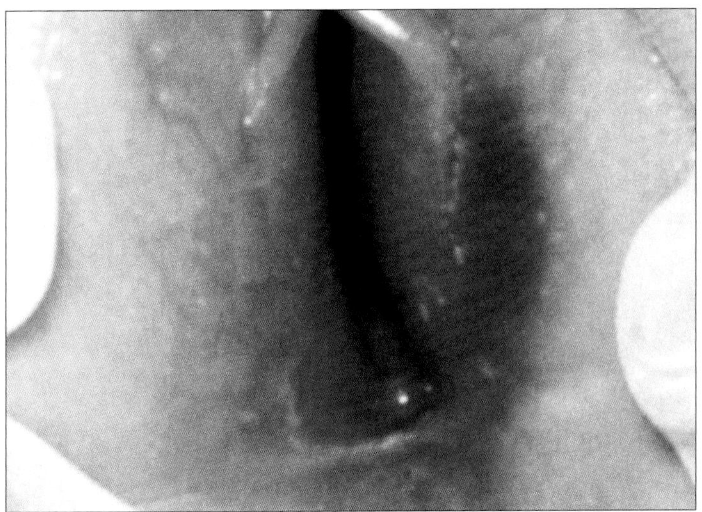

Figure 5-2. *Straddle injury. (Contributed by Lori D. Frasier, MD; Salt Lake City, Utah.)*

Case Study

This 2-year-old Caucasian was jumping on the bed when she fell, straddling the side rail. Her mother's boyfriend was watching her while the mother was out running errands. The child was dressed and wearing a diaper while jumping on the bed. She was brought in within 12 hours of the accident.

Figure 5-3-a. *The diaper she wore on arrival for the exam (35mm).*

Figure 5-3-b. *A laceration of the posterior fourchette (35mm).*

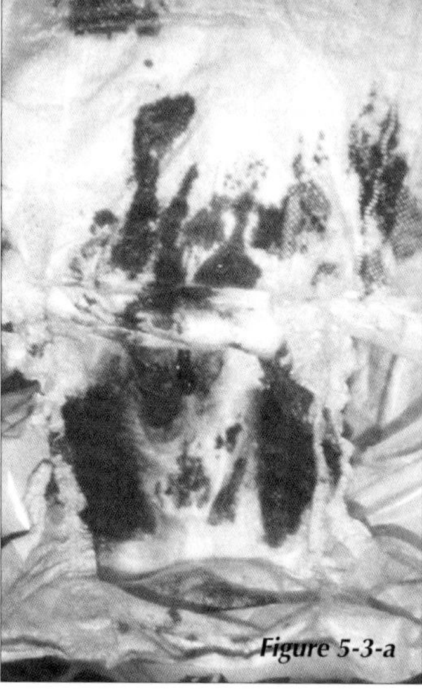

Figure 5-3-a

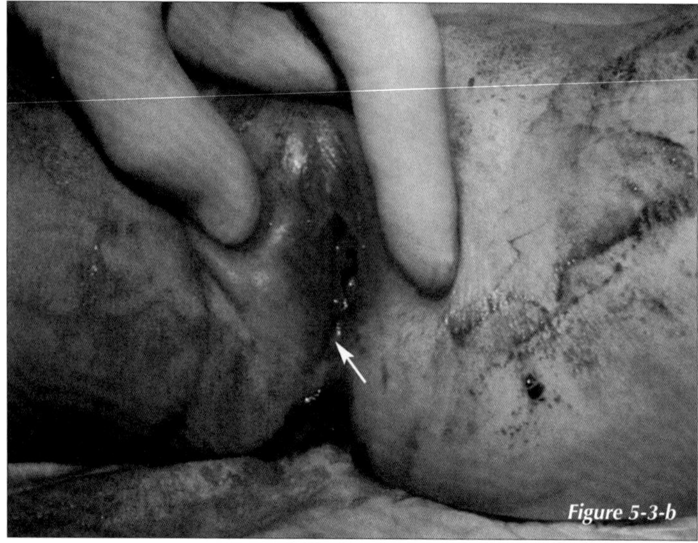

Figure 5-3-b

Figure 5-3-c. *The child is draped for a surgical repair (35mm).*

Figure 5-3-d. *A deep posterior fourchette laceration. There is focal erythema of the hymen at 3 to 5 and 7 to 10 o'clock. The labia majora and minora are free of injury that might be expected from a straddle fall.*

This case was canceled because it lacked elements of a crime.

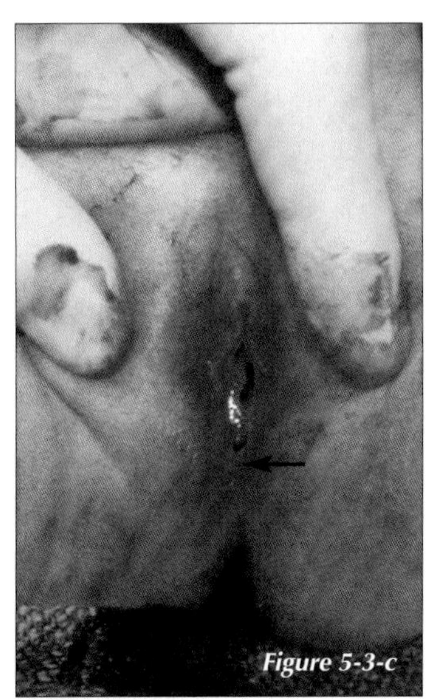

Figure 5-3-c

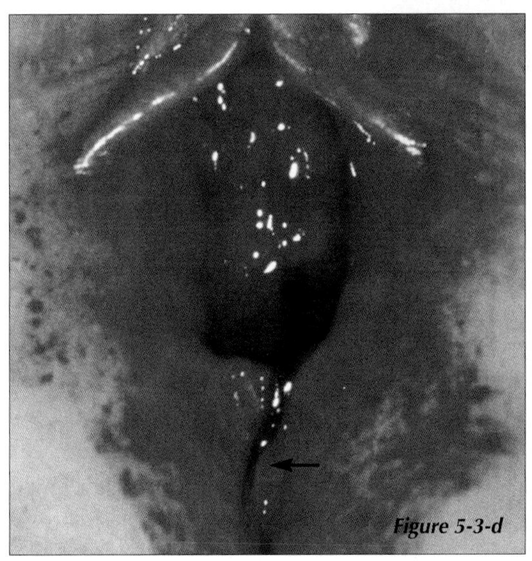

Figure 5-3-d

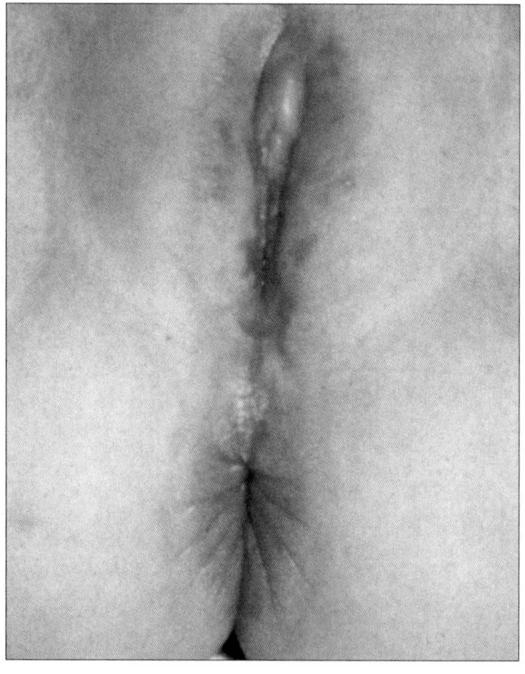

Figure 5-4. Lichen sclerosus et atrohicus. (Contributed by Lori D. Frasier, MD; Salt Lake City, Utah.)

wherein a sharp bony fragment may penetrate the vagina and lower urinary tract

• Fissures of the posterior fourchette or anus produced during an examination that included traction of the labia or buttocks

• A sharp foreign body that traverses the gastrointestinal tract and causes trauma on passage from the anus (rare)

• Childhood masturbation does not generally cause genital injury

• Injury to the perineum with perianal bruising, rectal prolapse, or evisceration of the bowel from sitting on suction drain vents in swimming pools

Dermatologic Disorders

- Lichen sclerosus et atrophicus **(Figure 5-4)**

1. Hemorrhagic, bullous lesions, fissures, or ulcers lead to confusion with traumatic injuries caused by a sexual assault.
2. Typical symptoms are anogenital itching, pain, and bleeding.

- Seborrheic dermatitis (diaper rash); severe cases may involve postinflammatory hypopigmentation and possible fissures.
- Allergic reactions that cause contact dermatitis on any region of the body.
- Bedwetting; the use of a bedwetting alarm has produced a genital rash that was vesicular over the labia and inner thigh.
- Psoriasis of the diaper area; examine the nails and other skin areas to assist in diagnosis.

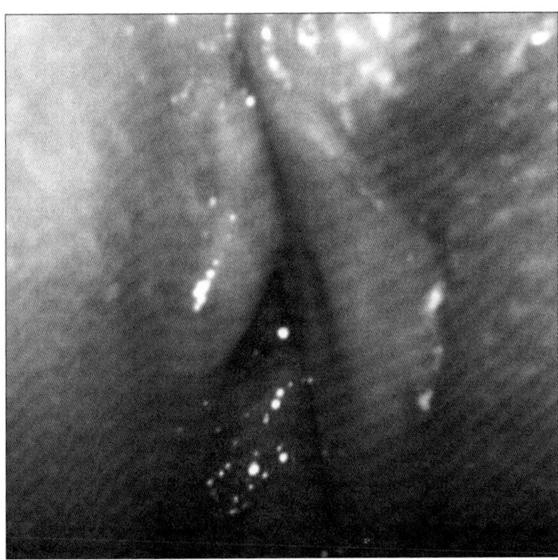

Figure 5-5. *Strawberry hemangioma. (Contributed by Lori D. Frasier, MD; Salt Lake City, Utah.)*

- Cavernous or strawberry hemangiomas **(Figure 5-5)**

1. The most common benign vascular tumors of infancy.
2. Present at birth, these tumors grow in proportion to the growing infant and appear as small, red masses with an irregular border.

- Pemphigus disorders

1. Bullous pemphigoid is rare in children but can appear as large, tense bullae on normal-appearing or erythematous skin.
2. Associated bullae may be seen in the mouth, lower abdomen, and thighs.
3. Symptoms include mild pruritus, pain, and occasional bleeding.
4. Pemphigus vulgaris: autoimmune disorder with flaccid vesiculobullous lesions measuring 1 to 3 cm with persistent erosions on the face, scalp, neck, and anogenital regions.

Infectious Disorders

- Vulvovaginitis

1. Most often caused by *Staphylococcus aureus* (which may also cause impetigo in the anogenital region), group *A Streptococcus*, *Enterococcus*, and *Shigella*.
2. Even if there are no identified risk factors and no disclosure of sexual abuse, consider *Neisseria gonorrhoeae* in the differential diagnostic evaluation of bacterial vaginitis.

- Group A streptococcal infection can also manifest as intense perianal erythema or, in males, balanitis, generally in early childhood.

- Vulvar or anal human papillomavirus (HPV) warts

1. Typically soft, less than 0.5 mm and have a papular or more verrucous shape **(Figure 5-6)**.
2. In males the scrotal region is the predominant site of infection.
3. Children are usually asymptomatic but may complain of itching or bleeding.
4. Disease has extremely high frequency in adults (10% to 80% of asymptomatic, sexually active young women), so increasing prevalence of HPV infection in children is predictable, but concern for sexual transmission should exist.
5. Anogenital condyloma accuminata may result from infection with HPV types 6 and 11.

- Varicella infection

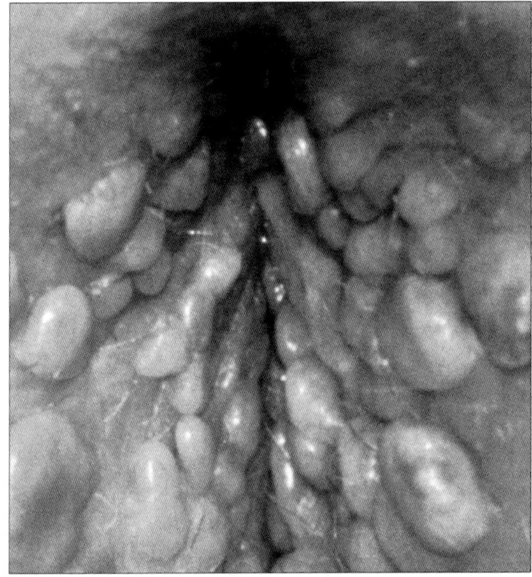

Figure 5-6. *Human papillomavirus: anal. (Contibuted by Lori D. Frasier, MD; Salt Lake City, Utah.)*

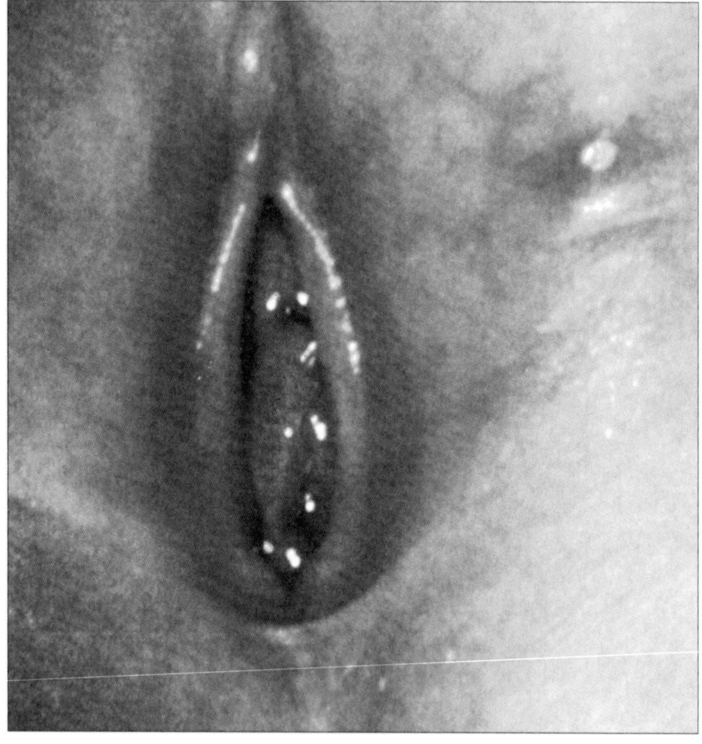

Figure 5-7. Molluscum contagiosum. (Contributed by Lori D. Frasier, MD; Salt Lake City, Utah.)

• Epstein-Barr infection has been associated with genital ulcers.

• Herpes simplex virus (HSV) infection may be the result of autoinoculation from oral lesions with gingivostomatitis or infection of the digit (herpetic whitlow); a child presenting with genital herpes requires a child protection investigation in most cases.

• Molluscum contagiosum **(Figure 5-7)**

1. Produces characteristic pale, umbilicated papules and is self-limiting.

2. Rarely seen on palms, soles, and mucous membranes, but can be localized to the inner thighs and perineum, causing concern for sexual abuse.

- Schistosomiasis
- Pinworm infestation *(Enterobius vermicularis)*

1. May cause vulvar bleeding or vulvar and/or anal itching.
2. Diagnosed by characteristic small, white adult worms easily visualized on examinations.

- Scabies

1. May be localized to anogenital region in addition to more common areas of web spaces of fingers, wrists, elbows, axillae, abdomen, and waist.
2. Characterized by pruritic, erythematous, papular rash, usually worst at night when adult female mites are most active.

- Retained foreign body, while uncommon, may cause recurrent urinary tract infection.
- Candidal diaper dermatitis

Inflammatory Disorders

- Perianal lesions of Crohn's disease

1. Skin tags, fissures, thickened perianal skin, fistulas and abscesses, and scarring can result from complications of Crohn's disease.
2. Intestinal manifestations of Crohn's disease may be absent, with vulvar lesions (erythema, edema, and ulceration) the first presentation of the disease in children.

- Kawasaki disease (mucocutaneous lymph node syndrome)

Case Study

This 9-month-old male was cared for by an uncle while the mother went away for 3 days. When the mother returned, she found blood in the child's diaper. It was determined that this child had perianal fissures from a combination of diaper dermatitis and constipation. The mother brought in the large (4 cm diameter) "rock-hard" ball of stool that the child passed, while he was screaming in pain.

Figure 5-8-a. *Perianal erythema, an abrasion at 12 o'clock, and macular lesions along the edge of the erythema.*

Figure 5-8-b. *This is the same area as in Figure 5-8-a, but the edges of the fissures are separated. There are 3 fissures at the superior end of the anus and at least 3 fissures around the 6 o'clock area.*

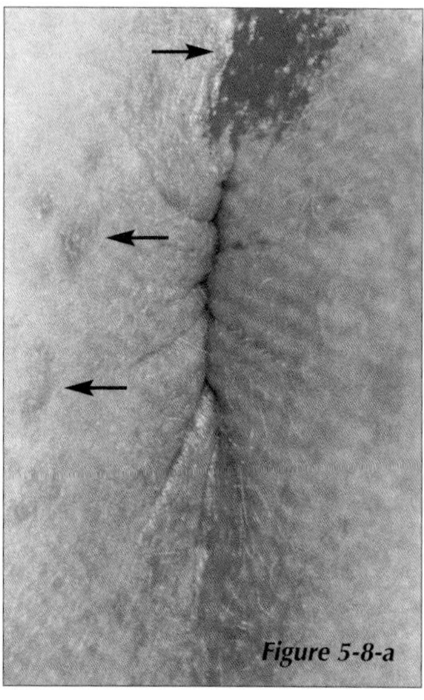
Figure 5-8-a

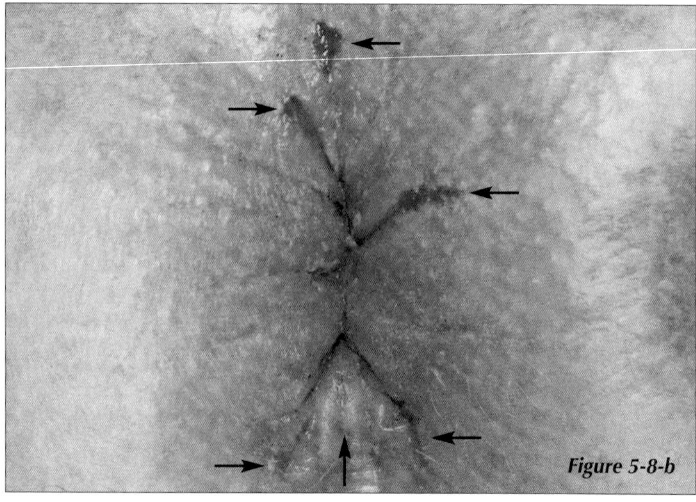
Figure 5-8-b

Figure 5-8-c. *This is the uptake of toluidine blue dye by some of the fissures.*

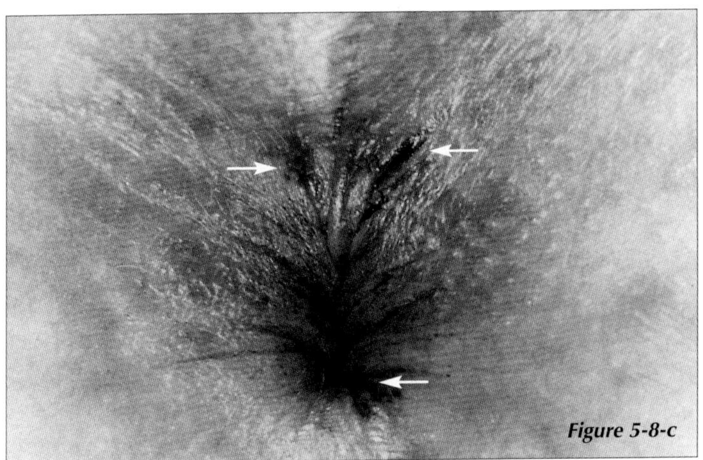

Figure 5-8-c

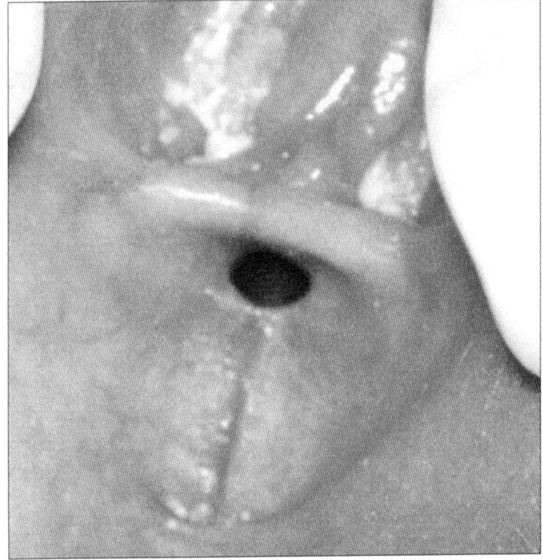

Figure 5-9. *Labial agglutination. (Contributed by Lori D. Frasier, MD; Salt Lake City, Utah.)*

1. Vasculitis characterized by fever for 5 or more days and cervical adenopathy, bilateral conjunctival infection, changes to the mucus membrane (dry, cracked lips and strawberry anal skin), changes to the extremities (edema, erythema, and desquamation).
2. Erythematous rash of the perineum that progresses to desquamation of the region can precede the onset of the more diagnostic findings.

- Behçet's syndrome

1. Triad of oral aphthous stomatitis, ulcers of the external genitalia, and inflammatory disease of the eye structures (uveitis, iritis, iridocyclitis) is characteristic.
2. Genital ulcers occur in 10% of patients and are often painless and may heal with scarring by 7 to 14 days; recurrence is common.

Miscellaneous Disorders

- Idiopathic calcinosis cutis
- Erythema multiforme
- Idiopathic thrombocytopenic purpura and other bleeding diatheses
- Henoch-Schönlein purpura
- Mongolian spots
- Disorders causing urethral bleeding or abnormalities of the urethra (hemangioma, polyps, ureterocele, prolapse of the urethra)
- Rectal prolapse: predisposing medical conditions include cystic fibrosis, myelomeningocele, prune belly syndrome, or other conditions that require straining (chronic constipation or excessive cough; **Figures 5-8 a to c**)

- Hair tourniquet syndrome
- Labial agglutination or fusion of the labia minora **(Figure 5-9)**

1. Occurs commonly in infants and results from any inflammatory condition of the vulvar region.
2. Denuded labial epithelium becomes agglutinated as the labia closely appose in the diapered child.

References

Agnarsson U, Warde C, McCarthy G, Evans N. Perianal appearances associated with constipation. *Arch Dis Child.* 1990;65:1231-1234.

Bays J. Conditions mistaken for child sexual abuse. In: Reece RM, Ludwig S, eds. *Child Abuse: Medical Diagnosis and Management.* 2nd ed. Philadelphia, Pa: Lippincott Williams & Wilkins; 2001:287-306.

Cain WS, Howell CG, Ziegler MM, Finley AJ, Asch MJ, Grant JP. Rectosigmoid perforation and intestinal evisceration from transanal suction. *J Pediatr Surg.* 1983;18:10-13.

Centers for Disease Control. Suction-drain injury in a public wading pool—North Carolina, 1991. *MMWR Morb Mortal Wkly Rep* 1992;41:333-335.

Dodds ML. Vulvar disorders of the infant and young child. *Clin Obstet Gynecol.* 1997;40:141-152.

Dowd MD, Fitzmaurice L, Knapp JF, Mooney D. The interpretation of urogenital findings in children with straddle injuries. *J Pediatr Surg.* 1994;29:7-10.

Gibbon KL, Bewley AP, Salisbury JA. Labial fusion in children: a presenting feature of genital lichen sclerosus? *Pediatr Dermatol.* 1999;16:388-391.

Hurwitz S, ed. *Clinical Pediatric Dermatology: A Textbook of Skin Disorders of Childhood and Adolescence.* 2nd ed. Philadelphia, Pa: WB Saunders Co; 1993.

Kadish HW, Schunk JE, Britton H. Pediatric male rectal and genital trauma: accidental and nonaccidental injuries. *Pediatr Emerg Care.* 1998;14:95-98.

McCann J, Voris J, Simon M, Wells R. Perianal findings in prepubertal children selected for nonabuse: a descriptive study. *Child Abuse Negl.* 1989;13:179-193.

McCann J, Wells R, Simon M, Voris J. Genital findings in prepubertal girls selected for nonabuse: a descriptive study. *Pediatrics.* 1990;86:428-439.

Merritt DF. Evaluation of vaginal bleeding in the preadolescent girl. *Pediatr Surg.* 1998;7:35-42.

Powell J, Wojnarowska F. Childhood vulval lichen sclerosus and sexual abuse are not mutually exclusive diagnoses. *BMJ.* 2000;320:311.

Siegfried EC, Frasier LD. Anogenital skin diseases of childhood. *Pediatr Ann.* 1997;26:322-331.

Stratakis CA, Graham W, DiPalma J, Leibowitz I. Misdiagnosis of perianal manifestations of Crohn's disease. *Clin Pediatr.* 1994;33:631-633.

Wood PL, Bevan T. Lesson of the week: child sexual abuse enquiries and unrecognised vulval lichen sclerosus et atrophicus. *BMJ.* 1999;319:889-890.

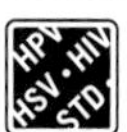

Chapter 6

Evaluations in Special Situations

Charles J. Schubert, MD
Kathi Makaroff, MD
William C. Holmes, MD, MSCE
Sharon W. Cooper, MD, FAAP

Sexually Transmitted Diseases

As implied by the term, a sexually transmitted disease (STD) is generally transmitted by sexual contact although other routes of transmission are possible **(Table 6-1)**. The overall incidence of STDs in victims of child abuse is relatively low. Even if a perpetrator of a sexual assault has an STD, the victim may not be infected because of the following:

- Perpetrators have a high incidence of sexual dysfunction so there may not be the intimate contact required to transmit an STD.
- The organism carried by the perpetrator may not be easily transmitted.
- The environment of the prepubertal vagina is not as conducive to the survival of STD organisms.
- Disclosure of an episode of sexual abuse often occurs months to years after the abuse, which means that some STDs will resolve spontaneously or be asymptomatic.

The following factors should be considered in determining what degree of workup is needed:

- Regional prevalence
- Likelihood of preexisting disease in the perpetrator
- How recently the episode occurred

Table 6-1. Modes of Transmission of STDs in Children

Organism Body	Sexual Assault	Autoinoculation/ Heteroinoculation	Fomites	Infected Fluids†
Bacterial vaginosis	X			
Chlamydia trachomatis	X			
Gonorrhea	X		?*	
Hepatitis B	X			X
HIV	X			X
HPV	X	X		
HSV	X	X		
Syphilis	X			
Trichomonas vaginalis	X		?*	

** No study has directly documented this in children.*
† Excluding genital secretions.
Abbreviations: HIV, human immunodeficiency virus; HPV, human papillomavirus; HSV, herpes simplex virus.

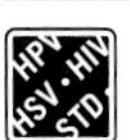

- Type of abuse
- Child's age or Tanner stage
- The specific organism

If an STD is found, an evaluation for sexual abuse must be undertaken **(Table 6-2)**.

For treatment, see **Table 6-3**.

Chlamydia Trachomatis

- Bacterial agent; obligate intracellular parasite
- Currently the most common STD in the United States; highest rates are in sexually active adolescents
- Infants acquire via vertical transmission, with 50% to 75% of children of infected women becoming infected
- Sites: conjunctiva, nasopharynx, rectum, vagina
- If not perinatally acquired, considered a marker for sexual abuse because no evidence supports a postnatal nonsexual acquisition
- Signs/symptoms: rectal and vaginal cases often asymptomatic in children; epididymitis, urethritis, and vaginitis noted in postpubertal individuals; women may have pelvic inflammatory disease (PID), ectopic pregnancy, or infertility
- Diagnosed by history, physical examination, and laboratory findings (tissue culture)

Neisseria Gonorrhoeae

- Gram-negative diplococcus
- Acquired vertically by newborn infant; when found in prepubertal children beyond the newborn period, strongly consider sexual abuse
- Usually affects the eye but can involve disseminated

Table 6-2. Laboratory Investigation for STDs in the Evaluation of Sexually Abused Children

SEXUALLY TRANSMITTED DISEASE	DIAGNOSTIC TEST
Gonorrhea	— Only acceptable method is a bacterial culture — A positive culture must be confirmed by 2 other identifying tests of different biologic principles — NAA tests (LCR, PCR)*
Chlamydia infection	— Only acceptable method is a bacterial culture — NAA tests (LCR, PCR)*
Syphilis	Serologic blood tests: Positive nontreponemal test — RPR — VDRL — ART — In addition to: Positive treponemal tests Fluorescent treponemal antibody absorption Microhemagglutination test for *T. pallidum*

(continued)

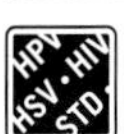

Table 6-2. *(continued)*

Sexually Transmitted Disease	Diagnostic Test
HPV	— Usually made by appearance on physical examination — Virus type can be determined, but identification of virus type does not differentiate sexual from nonsexual transmission
***Trichomonas* infection**	— Microscopic identification — Bacterial culture of vaginal secretions — Must differentiate from other types of *Trichomonas* organisms if identified in urine or stool
HSV	— Usually made by appearance on physical examination — Virus can be cultured if diagnosis is in question — Virus type can be determined, but identification of virus type does not differentiate sexual from nonsexual transmission
HIV	Serologic blood tests — EIA — If EIA is positive: Western blot or immunofluorescence antibody test is used for confirmation

(continued)

Table 6-2. *(continued)*

SEXUALLY TRANSMITTED DISEASE	DIAGNOSTIC TEST
Bacterial vaginosis	Diagnosis made clinically by presence of 3 of following symptoms or signs: — Homogeneous gray or white discharge on examination — Vaginal fluid pH > 4.5 — Positive amine test: mixing vaginal fluid with 10% potassium hydroxide results in a fishy odor — Presence of "clue cells": vaginal epithelial cells massively coated with coccobacilli
Hepatitis B	Serologic blood tests — Hepatitis B surface antigen (HBsAg) detects acutely or chronically infected individuals — Anti-HBs identifies individuals who have had infections with HBV; determines immunity after vaccination — Anti-HBc identifies individuals with acute past HBV infection; is not present after immunization

** NAA tests are not approved for use in prepubertal children or for medicolegal purposes. Abbreviations: ART, automated reagin test; EIA, enzyme immunoassay; HBV, hepatitis B virus; HIV, human immunodeficiency virus; HPV, human papillomavirus; HSV, herpes simplex virus; LCR, ligase chain reaction; NAA, nucleic acid amplification; PCR, polymerase chain reaction; RPR, rapid plasma reagin test; VDRL, Venereal Disease Research Laboratory.*

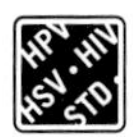

Table 6-3. Treatment Options for STDs in Children

ORGANISM	TREATMENT OPTIONS
Gonorrhea[a] Uncomplicated vulvovaginitis, cervicitis, urethritis, proctitis, or pharyngitis	— Prepubertal children who weigh <100 lb: ceftriaxone 125 mg IM in a single dose or spectinomycin 40 mg/kg IM in a single dose (maximum 2 g)[b] — Prepubertal children who weigh >100 lb and are 8 years old or older: ceftriaxone 125 mg IM in a single dose or cefixime 400 mg orally in a single dose or ciprofloxacin 500 mg orally in a single dose
Chlamydia Uncomplicated genital tract infection	— Prepubertal children: erythromycin 50 mg/kg orally in divided doses for 14 days (maximum daily dose 2 g) or azithromycin 20 mg/kg orally as a single dose (maximum 1 g) — Adolescents: doxycycline 100 mg orally twice daily for 7 days or azithromycin 1 g orally as a single dose

(continued)

Table 6-3. *(continued)*	
ORGANISM	TREATMENT OPTIONS
Syphilis	— Primary, secondary, and early latent disease in children: benzathine penicillin G 50,000 U/kg IM in a single dose (not to exceed the adult dose of 2.4 million U) — Late latent syphilis in children: benzathine penicillin G 50,000 U/kg IM weekly for 3 weeks (not to exceed the adult dose of 7.2 million U)
***Trichomonas* infection**	— Prepubertal children: metronidazole 15 mg/kg orally in 3 divided doses for 7 days (maximum daily dose 2 g) — Adolescents: metronidazole 2 g orally as a single dose
HPV	— Consultation with a dermatology specialist is recommended
HSV	— Consultation with an infectious disease specialist is recommended[c]

(continued)

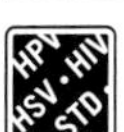

Table 6-3. *(continued)*

Organism	Treatment Options
HIV	— Consultation with an infectious disease specialist is recommended
Bacterial vaginosis	— Metronidazole 1 g orally in 2 divided doses for 7 days
Hepatitis B	— No specific therapy for acute HBV infection is available

a) Patients should also receive concurrent treatment for presumptive chlamydial infection.
b) Spectinomycin is not effective for the treatment of pharyngeal gonorrhea.
c) Acyclovir is the only approved antiviral drug for children.
Adapted from American Academy of Pediatrics (AAP). In: Pickering LK, ed. 2000 Red Book: Report of the Committee on Infectious Diseases. *25th ed. Elk Grove Village, Ill: American Academy of Pediatrics; 2000. Centers for Disease Control and Prevention (CDC). 2002 guidelines for treatment of sexually transmitted diseases.* MMWR Morb Mortal Wkly Rep. *2002;47:110.*

Drug dosage recommendations listed herein are those of the authors and are not endorsed by the US Public Health Service or the US Department of Health and Human Services.

disease and result in bacteremia, meningitis, endocarditis, or arthritis

• Transmission occurs from intimate contact with the organism found in secretions of infected mucosal surfaces; survives up to 24 hours on toilet seats and towels but is very susceptible to drying and cool temperatures, making transmission from fomites unlikely.

• Signs/symptoms: children are usually symptomatic, having vaginal discharge; adolescents can have more ascending disease, such as Fitz-Hugh-Curtis syndrome, or be asymptomatic.

• Diagnosis is based on cell culture confirmed by other tests; all positive cultures must be confirmed by at least 2 bacteriologic tests.

Human Immunodeficiency Virus

• A retrovirus that causes acquired immunodeficiency syndrome (AIDS) and is found in 2 types; type 1 is the most common in the United States.

• Transmission by 4 means: vertical, breastfeeding, percutaneous or mucous membrane exposure to infected blood or body fluids, or sexual contact.

• Signs/symptoms: in children include failure to thrive, generalized lymphadenopathy, hepatomegaly, splenomegaly, diarrhea, oral candidiasis, central nervous system (CNS) disease, cardiomyopathy, hepatitis, and recurrent invasive infections; opportunistic infections are common.

• Consider testing for HIV in the following circumstances:

1. The perpetrator has known HIV infection or known risk factors for HIV infection.
2. The victim has had multiple assailants, another STD, a history of vaginal or rectal penetration, or known risk factors for HIV infection.
3. The child/adolescent or parent requests testing.

• Tests must be repeated at 6 weeks and 3 and 6 months after the initial visit.

• Arrange for pretest and posttest counseling.

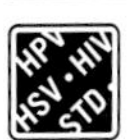

SYPHILIS

• Caused by a thin, mobile spirochete, *Treponema pallidum*

• Incidence has increased greatly, with neonates and children affected to a degree similar to that found in adults.

• Transmitted to children in utero (congenital syphilis) or through intimate contact (acquired syphilis); *T. pallidum* is fragile and survives only briefly outside the host.

• Signs/symptoms: at birth, infected infants may or may not show signs of disease, but these may occur after as long as 2 years and include hepatosplenomegaly, snuffles, lymphadenopathy, rash, and hemolytic anemia; after age 2 years, late manifestations may develop (40% of untreated cases), involving the CNS, bones, teeth, skin, and eyes; symptoms occur in 3 stages:

1. Primary syphilis: one or multiple indurated painless ulcers or chancres at the site of inoculation and lasting 1 to 5 weeks
2. Secondary syphilis: generalized maculopapular rash of the palms and soles, with condyloma lata (flat, gray-white coalescent papular lesions of the vulva or anus) possible
3. Latent period and then tertiary syphilis, which involves dermal and cardiovascular manifestations

• Diagnosed by serologic testing, with definitive diagnosis by microscopic darkfield examination

• Testing may be done for the following situations:

1. Child has evidence of other STDs
2. Adolescent victim

3. Child lives with a family member or the perpetrator who has syphilis
4. Child lives in an area with a high incidence of syphilis

Herpes Simplex Viruses

• Double-stranded DNA viruses that occur in 2 types, with HSV-1 usually involving the face and skin above the waist and HSV-2 involving the genitalia and skin below the waist; however, either type may be found in either location

• Transmitted to infants during birth through an infected maternal genital tract or by ascending infection; may also be transmitted postnatally from a caregiver via nongenital contact; transmitted to children via contact with infected lesions either sexually or nonsexually

• Signs/symptoms: for newborns, localized CNS disease, disseminated disease, or localized skin disease; for children and infants beyond the neonatal period, genital herpes involves tender vesicular or ulcerative lesions of the genitalia, perineum, or both plus systemic symptoms (fever, malaise) and tender inguinal adenopathy

• Diagnosed by visual inspection of the lesions and confirmed by cell culture

Trichomonas Infection

• Caused by *Trichomonas vaginalis*, a flagellated protozoa; common STD in adolescents and adults, but uncommon in prepubertal girls beyond the first few weeks of life due to the hostile vaginal environment of this age group

• Acquired during birth or through sexual contact

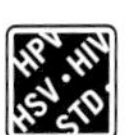

in adults; therefore, the presence in a prepubertal girl is strongly suspicious for sexual abuse

• Signs/symptoms: may be asymptomatic; infants, a vaginal discharge; prepubertal girls, vaginitis; adolescent and adult females, a pale yellow or green vaginal discharge and vulvovaginal itching, dysuria, abdominal pain; infected males, urethritis, epididymitis, or prostatitis

• Diagnosis based on examination of a wet mount preparation of the discharge; these are only 40% to 80% accurate, so a culture should also be considered

Human Papillomavirus Infection

• A nonenveloped, icosahedral, double-stranded DNA virus comprising nearly 70 virus types

• Signs/symptoms: anogenital warts in adults and children (condylomata acuminata), which can cause itching, burning with urination, pain, or bleeding

1. These may range from clinically inapparent infection to obvious symptoms.
2. Males have lesions on the shaft of the penis, urethral meatus, scrotum, or perianal area.
3. Females have lesions on the labia and perianal area and less commonly in the vagina and cervix.

• Among adults, almost exclusively transmitted sexually, but children may acquire vertically or perinatally, through digital autoinoculation or heteroinoculation, via fomites or casual contact, or through sexual abuse.

• Diagnosis must be based on history as well as clinical findings:

1. Check for history of cutaneous warts in caregivers or maternal history of genital warts or abnormal Papanicolaou (Pap) smears.

2. Do complete forensic interview and physical examination of the child to help determine if the HPV infection was acquired via sexual or nonsexual contact.
3. Confirmation is made with tissue biopsy, but biopsy is only required when the diagnosis is in doubt.

• Because evidence supports a link between anogenital HPV infection and anogenital neoplasm, regular follow-up on a long-term basis is recommended.

Bacterial Vaginosis

• An abnormal condition of the vagina characterized by a shift in the vaginal flora from the normally predominant *Lactobacillus* to an overgrowth of *Gardnerella vaginalis*, *Mycoplasma hominis*, and anaerobic bacteria

• Signs/symptoms: vaginal discharge that is nonviscous, homogeneous, white, and malodorous (fishy) without abdominal pain, dysuria, or significant pruritus; may also be asymptomatic

• Transmission is controversial but its presence should prompt testing for other sexually transmitted pathogens.

• Diagnosed on clinical grounds based on the presence of 3 of the following 4 signs or symptoms (Amsel's criteria):

1. Homogeneous gray or white discharge
2. Vaginal fluid pH over 4.5
3. Positive amine test
4. Presence of vaginal epithelial cells that appear moth-eaten or massively coated with coccobacilli on gram stain ("clue cells")

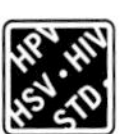

Hepatitis B Infection

- Caused by a DNA-containing hepadnavirus
- Transmitted through blood or bodily fluids, including semen, cervical secretions, and saliva; may be through infusion of blood or blood products, percutaneous or mucous membrane exposure to blood or body fluids, or sexual activity; mother-to-infant transmission occurs to infants born to hepatitis B-infected mothers; when prevalence of HBV is high, horizontal transmission during early childhood is possible.
- Signs/symptoms: range from asymptomatic to nonspecific (anorexia or malaise) to clinical hepatitis with jaundice; about 10% of individuals develop chronic infection, which increases the risk of chronic liver disease or primary hepatocellular carcinoma.
- Diagnosis based on serologic antigen tests for the hepatitis B surface antigen; incubation period is 45 to 120 days, so testing should be repeated 3 and 6 months after exposure.
- When found in a child beyond the perinatal period, should prompt suspicion for sexual abuse.

Sexual Abuse in Boys and Male Adolescents

Understanding the cultural norms of masculine gender socialization is the first task to pursue when evaluating issues specific to sexually abused boys and male adolescents.

- One of the core moves in male development is the movement away from the feminine.
- If the abuse occurs at the hands of a male perpetrator, the boy faces having to disclose participating

in a homosexual act while avoiding homosexuality as an overriding concern of the "Boy Code." Thus he often hides the truth.

- Incidence rates of sexual abuse among males range from 4% to 16% or higher.

Understanding the types of acts that happen to a boy and being able to discuss this information frankly in front of the boy or adolescent who has experienced the activity is important in beginning care. Types of abuse include the following:

- Noncontact interactions: exhibitionism, masturbation in front of the boy, asking the boy to expose himself, verbally or visually stimulating the boy sexually via pornography
- Contact interactions: in addition to the obvious (deep kissing, sexualized touch, manual-genital contact, orogenital contact, oroanal contact, anal penetration, or vaginal penetration), contact interactions do not necessarily involve actual touching of the skin, but include any noncontact interaction that culminates in the perpetrator touching the boy's genitals or other eroticized body parts through clothing

Because boys are unlikely to disclose abuse, a screening strategy is important to identify abuse histories and manage them clinically. Steps to consider are as follows:

- Create an environment that demonstrates willingness to consider male sexual abuse as a common reality; a suggestion is to provide reading material in the waiting room.
- Employ direct, verbal screening within the safety of a private clinical interaction; do not use a paper screening form.

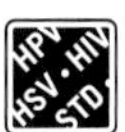

• Provide an explanatory and normalizing introduction to all abuse- and/or violence-related screening questions.

• Recognize that both you and the boys you treat may prefer silence to the discomfort of disclosure.

• Ask screening questions at each visit.

If the boy and/or male adolescent discloses an abusive history in response to screening:

• The provider's first response should be a nonjudgmental, validating, empowering, and advocating comment or series of comments. Examples are as follows:

"I think you are a brave person to have told me what you did. It's like what a superhero would do, and I'm particularly glad you did because I can help you."

"I'm sorry this happened to you."

"It was not your fault."

"I'm here to help you."

"It's my job, along with your family member [family member's name], to make sure that you are safe from now on."

These initial comments affirm the boy's decision to tell and the provider's willingness to help and provide a supportive environment.

• The boy may experience extreme ambivalence with fear, regret, anticipation, exhilaration, worry, loss, relief, happiness that someone finally knows, and anxiety about the future. These feelings may manifest as bodily symptoms: tachycardia, sweating, dizziness, or blushing.

• If the boy is uncomfortable, proceed with simple questions concerning other topics, staying attuned to reported changes in all areas of the boy's life that may raise red flags for abuse or its aftermath.

• When you return to the topic of abuse, acknowledge the boy's feelings and reassure him to initiate a sense of trust.

• Establish common ground with regard to the use of names for different body parts. It is also possible to show the boy anatomical dolls or draw pictures and use these guides for him to explain what happened.

• Remember that the process of disclosure often occurs in stages and be patient.

• Keep the focus on acknowledging the boy's experience and exhibit empathy without visible emotion.

• Be aware that females may also be perpetrators and be sensitive to this possibility.

• Make it clear that you are required by law to report known sexual abuse of a minor. Any plan for reporting must ensure the safety of the boy and allow no further abuse to occur.

• An examination is an important component of the evaluation of sexual abuse. Guidelines include the following:

1. Have both male and female providers available from which the victim may choose.
2. If you are not prepared to complete this part of the assessment, refer the patient to a site where the needed expertise is available.
3. Broadly describe what he will experience at the specialty site.
4. Keep a sexual assault examination kit available.
5. Refer the boy to a therapist with expertise in treating sexually abused boys as well as girls.

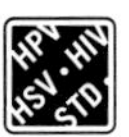

• If you must refer the boy elsewhere, assure him that he can and should continue to see you after he receives care at the other site. It is also helpful to mention the individuals who will complete the examination there.

• Parents/family members of the sexually abused boy play an important role **(Table 6-4)**.

Disability and Sexual Violence

The child or adult with a disability is a special patient when sexual assault is the concern. Often disclosure of the event is delayed or expressed behaviorally or with physical evidence rather than verbally. As in the case of victims without disabilities, the most likely offender is known to the victim.

Why Abuse of the Disabled Occurs

• Disability-related abuse occurs when the perpetrators withhold needed equipment and assistance to coerce sexual conduct.

• The effects of sexual assault are the same for victims with disabilities as with other patients, although reporting is less likely to be believed or investigated.

• The incidence of abuse and assault among persons with disabilities is significantly higher than in the general population.

• Children may be at higher risk because of the increased burden of care associated with their condition. The presence of a physical or mental disability is a recognized risk for victimization from a hate crime.

• Myths that propagate the development of psychological justification of a hate crime include the following:

Table 6-4. Recommendations for Parents/Family Members of Sexually Abused Boys

Do Not

1. Pry into physically intimate details of experiences, but be fully accepting of these details should victim choose to divulge them.
2. Ask questions that begin with "Why?" These can easily be misconstrued as blaming questions.
3. Minimize the gravity of what has happened, such as making jokes about abuse events.
4. Encourage threats of revenge against perpetrator. Victim may worry about the the safety of those exacting revenge, and threats may affect legal remedies.
5. Seek the "remedy" of distraction, or "taking his mind off it." The victim should be the one to request distraction. However, distraction should not be the primary mode of resolving abuse history.
6. Assume that because the victim is quiet, stoic, and seemingly unharmed by the abuse that he is not upset, angry, hurt, confused, and in other ways harmed by the abuse.
7. Take personally increased concerns by the male victim surrounding communication about either the event, the confusion after the event, or even generalizing this to all things in the relationship. He may be establishing boundaries.
8. Become demeaning if school performance declines. Inform school personnel on a "need to know" basis and then only with discussion about this with victim.

(continued)

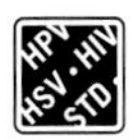

Table 6-4. *(continued)*

Do

1. Allow victim to talk about details he would like to talk about.
2. Reassure him that he isn't responsible for what happened, you don't blame him, and you don't think that he is weak. At the same time, encourage discussion of self-blaming beliefs and other self-doubts.
3. Be careful about attempts to reduce tension (humor that reflects one's own discomfort is inappropriate).
4. Respect victim's wishes with regard to disclosure. He should determine, when possible, who is and is not told, how, when, why, and so forth.
5. Remind family and friends to be careful in comments they make that could be understood, misunderstood, or purposely meant to imply blame.
6. Remind family/friends that the victim has privacy needs. At the same time, don't isolate the victim because this can confirm beliefs he is damaged.
7. Be careful about how the victim is "protected." Disclosure can be regretted if it leads to restrictive rules having more to do with fears than real threats. Encourage him to resume his normal life.
8. Be aware of behavioral change, such as loss of appetite, withdrawal, sleep disturbance, fears of being alone or being touched, excessive crying, bedwetting, sexual preoccupations, or alcohol and drug use, that may indicate difficulties victim is unable to articulate.

Adapted from McEvoy AW, Rollo D, Brookings JB. If He Is Raped: A Guidebook for Parents, Partners, Spouses, and Friends. *Holmes Beach, Fla: Learning Publications, Inc; 1999.*

1. The "dehumanization" myth: perpetrators may feel their abusive behavior is not really injuring another person because the person with a disability is less than a full member of society.
2. The "damaged merchandise" myth: the individual with a disability is worthless and has nothing to lose.
3. The "feeling no pain" myth: people with disabilities have no feelings or are immune to pain and suffering.
4. The "disabled menace" myth: individuals with disabilities are different, unpredictable, and dangerous, promoting fear in others.
5. The "helpless" myth: individuals with disabilities are helpless and therefore unable to take care of themselves, making them vulnerable to abuse and manipulation.

Evaluation of the Child or Adult With a Disability

If a victim with a disability comes for health care with evidence of severe physical bodily harm and genital trauma, the practitioner must provide a concise but extremely detailed account of both the history as related by the victim and that offered by any other reliable observer. Interviews of multiple caregivers may be required.

• Make a call to law enforcement immediately to secure the crime scene before intentional or unintentional tampering of evidence occurs.

• Obtain verbal evidence from the victim whenever possible, using such aids as photographs of various rooms in the facility, interpreters, or family members or other persons familiar with the disabled victim.

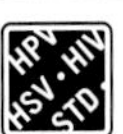

• Document the method and content of any disclosure that is forthcoming.

• Note any extremely sexually explicit information that is well outside the normal range of the victim's psychosexual development and knowledge.

• Carefully document sensory information such as tastes, smells, sounds made by the perpetrator, or tactile descriptions.

• Be aware that individuals with disabilities are at risk to behave in a more compliant manner than nondisabled individuals in attempts to ensure that they will be liked and included by others. Carefully explore and document all aspects of your interaction.

• Fit your evaluation to the individual's disability, as follows:

1. Hearing-impaired victim: obtain a cursory history even if a certified sign language interpreter is not readily available. Even with an interpreter, make eye contact with the victim and follow the standard method of interviewing (build rapport, allow free association conversation, then embark on the sexual assault history). Review the behaviors of the victim with a supportive family member or care provider as well as with the victim.
2. Visually impaired victim: be aware that most of the data will be nonvisual sensory information. Details such as time of day or place of assault will require greater explanation, proceeding in a step-by-step fashion. Children and adolescents with visual impairment may also have language delay. Screen the child for language concepts and ensure that the child is responding reliably,

consistently, and with expressive understanding. Tactile defensiveness is a common response in multiply impaired individuals after a sexual assault; it should not be assumed that no sexual assault could have occurred based on this behavior.

3. Cognitively or behaviorally impaired victim: be aware the nonverbal documentation may constitute the essence of the history, requiring the assistance of a care provider who is familiar with the habits and behaviors of the victim. The change in behavior is the most important timeline event. Among the behavioral changes being observed are the following:

   Irrational fearfulness of a person, place, or object

   Emotional lability

   Problems with arousal such as hypersomnolence or insomnia

   Changes in activity level (hyperactive or withdrawn)

   Distractibility

   Angry outbursts

   Separation anxiety behaviors

   Increased masturbation

   Sexualized behaviors

4. Motor-impaired victim: depending on the etiology of the motor delay, cognition may be spared, with the exception of the traumatic brain injury victim, who may have significant gaps in motor, cognitive, and behavioral function. A family member or individual accustomed to the victim's communication style is invaluable to assist in understanding what is being communicated.

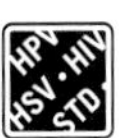

Interview Techniques

• Frame questions with a certain topic once rapport has been established, enabling the victim to focus on specific facts.

• Once the individual has described various locations in or around the scene of the crime, specify that you want to discuss "the place where you got hurt, at school."

• Be aware that redundancy in questioning for children and adults with disabilities increases the chance that examiner and victim will be talking consistently about the same thing at the same time.

• Talk slowly and choose your words carefully. Clarify what terms the victim uses for anatomic parts of the body.

• Use simple picture board symbols or allow the victim to draw what happened.

• Allow the victim to describe the perpetrator within the context, for example, "the man who always takes us to the lunchroom."

• Consider a gradual approach to seeking information.

• Perform a brief test of mental status and short-term memory as part of the evaluation.

• Ask questions about daily routines to encourage free association conversation in building rapport.

Physical Examination

• Examinations in institutionalized settings may be very difficult and require sedation to complete evidence collection. Examination under anesthesia is also an option.

• If it is necessary to move the victim to another facility for the physical examination, be aware that several barriers may limit access for the victim with a disability and make adjustments or accommodations as required.

• Note that disabled women are less likely to have regular pelvic examinations than other women and provide for dignified and independent access to the examination.

1. Make accommodations to avoid injury to the staff or victim during transfer onto the examination table.
2. Ask the woman what would make the examination more comfortable and respond accordingly.

• A more comfortable examination experience can be achieved by considering the following:

1. Positioning of the patient's legs
2. Warming the temperature of the room and table
3. Positioning the table in a 45-degree angle to avoid pulmonary compromise
4. Administering oxygen
5. Examining the patient on a bed rather than a firm examination table if that is desired
6. Employing extra personnel to assist with the examination

• Use a rape kit to collect evidence and consider the possibility of the victim having acquired an STD.

• Violence associated with sexual assault requires close surveillance for head and neck injury, facial trauma, and other bodily injuries. Be thorough, as if examining a young child, to be assured of discovering every affected site.

DNA Testing

A DNA result falls into 1 of the 3 categories:

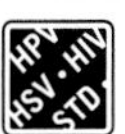

1. Inclusion: the DNA profile of a known individual matches the DNA profile from the crime scene.
2. Exclusion: there is no DNA match between the suspect and the crime scene.
3. Inconclusive: DNA testing did not produce information that would allow the individual to be included or excluded as the source of the biological evidence.

Sexual Assault and Homicide

Generally, the cause of death in a homicide of a disabled child or youth is strangulation, often associated with blunt trauma to the head and/or stabbing. Other findings are as follows:

- Severe tearing through the vagina or rectum or both in children
- Less severe genital trauma in youths, with abrasions, superficial lacerations, or contusions at the introitus of the vagina, usually the 6 o'clock position; bruising of the inner thighs; and bite marks on the breasts
- Anal injuries are generally minor and on the anal verge.
- Seminal deposits may be noted on the perineum, perianal area, and the thighs; these are nonspecific but require further analysis.
- Preexisting medical problems often contribute to the victim's death.

Multidisciplinary Considerations

- A team decision-making process is indicated particularly when the victim has a disability.
- The sexual assault response team (SART) is composed of specially trained sexual assault investigators, a sexual assault nurse examiner

(SANE), and possibly a prosecutor with advanced training in sexual assault cases.

• With a nonverbal or verbal child victim, review of custody or other extenuating concerns that might support a coerced or spontaneous false allegation should be considered. If such an allegation is discounted, it lends support to the credibility of the final decision.

• All should be documented in the medical record according to jurisdictional considerations.

• In an institutional setting, the caregiver histories may be contaminated; law enforcement questioning is important to determine what is rumor and what acts actually occurred.

• The most important factors to be documented for legal considerations in a case involving a sexual assault survivor are as follows:

1. The child's method and content of disclosure
2. A history of changes in the child's behavior
3. Physical examination findings, including the child's behavior during the examination

• Establish that you are a healthcare professional and the encounter is a "check-up." Document that the patient expresses the understanding that he or she is present to "see the doctor and make sure that their body is all right."

• Establish that the victim is competent to give a medical history; this is possible if the person's cognitive developmental level is at least age 4 years or is an adult capable of self-care and has mastered activities of daily living.

• Gather information from a familiar care provider regarding the child's or youth's short-term and long-

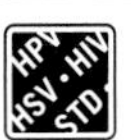

term memory, reliability to recount normal facts, and expressive and receptive language abilities.

• Recognize the importance of the social worker's role in the emergency room setting; he or she can offer information regarding the victim's functional levels and language comprehension, allowing the practitioner to craft appropriate questions.

• Note if sexually explicit language is used in describing events, which indicates environmental exposure of a chronic nature or sexual experiences that have been explained in this way.

• Note the individual's behavior (as listed earlier).

• Address the issue of consent:

1. This includes not just volition but also the victim's ability to understand the nature of the sexual act and its consequences.
2. Without confirmation of an understanding of these areas, the individual cannot satisfy the legal criteria for distinguishing between a consensual sex act and sexual abuse.

• Be aware that competency to testify in court has legal ramifications and includes the following 4 factors:

1. A present understanding of the difference between a truth and a lie as well as an indication that the person feels compelled to speak the truth
2. The mental capacity at the time of the event to observe or receive accurate impressions of the event
3. Memory sufficient to retain an independent recollection of the observations
4. The capacity to communicate that memory into words and to understand questions about the event

References

American Academy of Pediatrics (AAP). Bacterial vaginosis. In: Pickering LK, ed. *2000 Red Book: Report of the Committee on Infectious Diseases.* 25th ed. Elk Grove Village, Ill: American Academy of Pediatrics; 2000a:149-150.

American Academy of Pediatrics (AAP). Hepatitis B. In: Pickering LK, ed. *2000 Red Book: Report of the Committee on Infectious Diseases.* 25th ed. Elk Grove Village, Ill: American Academy of Pediatrics; 2000b:289-302.

American Academy of Pediatrics (AAP). Human immunodeficiency virus infection. In: Pickering LK, ed. *2000 Red Book: Report of the Committee on Infectious Diseases.* 25th ed. Elk Grove Village, Ill: American Academy of Pediatrics; 2000c:325-350.

Bagley C, Bolitho F, Bertrand L. Mental health profiles, suicidal behavior, and community sexual assault in 2112 Canadian adolescents. *Crisis.* 1995;16:126-131.

Bays J, Chadwick D. Medical diagnosis of the sexually abused child. *Child Abuse Negl.* 1993;17:91-110.

Boney-McCoy S, Finkelhor D. Prior victimization: a risk factor for child sexual abuse and for PTSD-related symptomatology among sexually abused youth. *Child Abuse Negl.* 1995;19:1401-1421.

Crowe C, Forster GE, Dinsmore WW, Maw RD. A case of acute hepatitis B occurring four months after multiple rape. *Int J STD AIDS.* 1996;7:133-134.

DiMaio VJM, Dana S. *Handbook of Forensic Pathology.* Austin, Tex: Landes Bioscience; 1998.

Faller KC. Characteristics of a clinical sample of sexually abused children: how boy and girl victims differ. *Child Abuse Negl.* 1989;13:281-291.

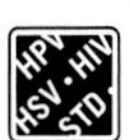

Federal Bureau of Investigation (FBI). *Summary of Hate Crime Statistics.* Washington, DC: Federal Bureau of Investigation; 2000.

Finkelhor D, Hotaling G, Lewis IA, Smith C. Sexual abuse in a national survey of adult men and women: prevalence, characteristics, and risk factors. *Child Abuse Negl.* 1990;14:19-28.

Frasier LD. Human papillomavirus infection in children. *Pediatr Ann.* 1994;23:354-360.

Gardner M, Jones JG. Genital herpes acquired by sexual abuse of children. *J Pediatr.* 1984;104:243-244.

Gil E, Johnson C. *Sexualized Children: Assessment and Treatment of Sexualized Children and Children Who Molest.* Rockville, Md: Launch Press; 1993.

Groth AN, Burgess AW. Sexual dysfunction during rape. *New Engl J Med.* 1977;297:764-766.

Hammerschlag MR. Chlamydia trachomatis in children. *Pediatr Ann.* 1994;23:349-353.

Jenny C. Sexually transmitted diseases and child abuse. *Pediatr Ann.* 1992;21:497-503.

Harrison PA, Fulkerson JA, Beebe TJ. Multiple substance use among adolescent physical and sexual abuse victims. *Child Abuse Negl.* 1997;21:529-539.

Hernandez JT, Lodico M, DiClemente RJ. The effects of child abuse and race on risk-taking in male adolescents. *J Natl Med Assoc.* 1993;85:593-597.

Hibbard RA, Ingersoll GM, Orr DP. Behavioral risk, emotional risk, and child abuse among adolescents in a nonclinical setting. *Pediatrics.* 1990;86:896-901.

Jones JG, Yamauchi T, Lambert B. Trichomonas vaginalis infestation in sexually abused girls. *Am J Dis Child.* 1985;139:846-847.

Kohan MJ, Pothier P, Norbeck JS. Hospitalized children with history of sexual abuse: incidence and care issues. *Am J Orthopsychiatry*. 1987;57:258-264.

Levitt CJ. Sexual abuse of boys: a medical perspective. In: Hunter M, ed. *The Sexually Abused Male*. Vol 1. Lexington, Mass: Lexington Books; 1990:227-240.

Lodico MA, Gruber E, DiClemente RJ. Childhood sexual abuse and coercive sex among school-based adolescents in a midwestern state. *J Adolesc Health*. 1996;18:211-217.

MacMillan HL, Fleming JE, Trocme N, et al. Prevalence of child physical and sexual abuse in the community: results from the Ontario Health Supplement. *JAMA*. 1997;278:131-135.

McEvoy AW, Rollo D, Brookings JB. *If He Is Raped: A Guidebook for Parents, Partners, Spouses, and Friends*. Holmes Beach, Fla: Learning Publications, Inc; 1999:112.

Nagy S, Adcock AG, Nagy MC. A comparison of risky health behaviors of sexually active, sexually abused, and abstaining adolescents. *Pediatrics*. 1994;93:570-575.

Nelson DE, Higginson GK, Grant-Worley JA. Using the youth risk behavior survey to estimate prevalence of sexual abuse among Oregon high school students. *J Sch Health*. 1994;64:413-416.

Nyirjesy P. Vaginitis in the adolescent patient. *Pediatr Clin North Am*. 1999;46:733-745.

Pollack W. *Real Boys: Rescuing Our Sons From the Myths of Boyhood.* New York, NY: Random House; 1998.

Risin LI, Koss MP. The sexual abuse of boys: prevalence and descriptive characteristics of childhood victimiza-

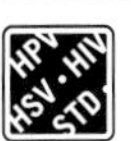

tions. *J Interpers Violence.* 1987;2:309-323.

Schwarcz SK, Whittington WL. Sexual assault and sexually transmitted diseases: detection and management in adults and children. *Rev Infect Dis.* 1990;12:s682-s690.

Shapiro RA, Schubert CJ, Myers PA. Vaginal discharge as an indicator of gonorrhea and Chlamydia infection in girls under 12 years old. *Pediatr Emerg Care.* 1993;9:341-345.

Siegel JM, Sorenson SB, Golding JM, Burnam MA, Stein JA. The prevalence of childhood sexual assault: The Los Angeles Epidemiologic Catchment Area Project. *Am J Epidemiol.* 1987;126:1141-1153.

Siegel RM, Schubert CJ, Myers PA, Shapiro RA. The prevalence of sexually transmitted diseases in children and adolescents evaluated for sexual abuse in Cincinnati: rationale of limited STD testing in prepubertal girls. *Pediatrics.* 1995;96:1090-1094.

Sirotnak AP. Testing sexually abused children for sexually transmitted diseasses: who to test, when to test and why. *Pediatr Ann.* 1994;23:370-374.

Sorenson DD. The invisible victims. *Impact.* Minneapolis, Minn: University of Minnesota, Institute on Community Integration (UAP)/Research and Training Center on Community Living; 1997.

Starling SP. Syphilis in infants and young children. *Pediatr Ann.* 1994;23:334-340.

Tharinger D, Horton B, Millea S. Sexual abuse and exploitation of children and adults with mental retardation. *Child Abuse Negl.* 1990;14:371-383.

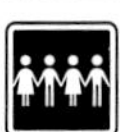

Chapter

Multidisciplinary Teamwork Issues

Angelo P. Giardino, MD, PhD
Eileen R. Giardino, PhD, RN, CRNP

The healthcare provider who conducts the evaluation is responsible for identifying and reporting suspected child sexual abuse and completing an accurate medical evaluation, including history, physical examination, and collection of laboratory specimens. A multidisciplinary team is involved; collaboration is required to provide medical treatment and make appropriate referrals for the child and family for services such as mental health counseling and social services.

- Benefits of teamwork:

1. Improved information sharing among clinicians
2. Joint decision making and planning
3. Collaborative educational approaches
4. Mutual support

- Interdisciplinary team shares responsibility for collecting and processing components of child and family evaluations. Formal protocols at the state, local, or organizational level are helpful in addressing specific details of these shared responsibilities and how they are to be carried out. Important aspects are as follows:

1. Clarity in the roles and responsibilities of each agency
2. Delineation of steps that must be accomplished at each stage of the process

Table 7-1. Dealing With Team Conflict
— Look forward to opportunity, not backward to blame. — Be respectful and consider all points of view. Listen to one another and make sure each position is understood. Restate each position in your own words. — Find something positive in each view and avoid defending your point of view until you clearly understand the opposing view. — State your position clearly and firmly but without excessive emotion. — Once you have been heard, do not continue to restate your position. — Avoid personalizing your position and stay focused on the issue. — Offer suggestions rather than mere criticism of other points of view. — Remember that conflict within a team is natural and work toward mutually agreeable resolutions. — Base resolutions on consensus, not abdication of responsibility or integrity. — Stay focused on the team's agreed-upon purpose and refer to your protocol for guidance.

3. Explicit declaration of time frames essential for completing each stage
4. Assignment of responsibility for each step
5. Practical advice for handling both routine and special circumstances

- Handling conflict among individuals and agencies

1. Be aware that team success is measured by the effectiveness with which conflict is resolved rather than the amount of conflict produced.
2. Quickly address the less important, peripheral issues and move to focus attention on more important, central issues that require discussion and resolution.

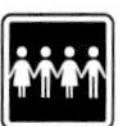

3. Deal with conflict constructively keeping the focus on the purpose outlined in the group's mission statement (**Table 7-1**).

Reporting

Healthcare providers are responsible for reporting all cases of suspected sexual abuse. State laws have been passed to remove the barriers that keep people from reporting, as follows:

- Immunity for good faith reporting (a person can still be sued in civil court but can claim immunity under this statute in the case)
- Standards to guide reasonable suspicion (concern over possible maltreatment need not be absolutely diagnosed before reporting)
- Rules regarding anonymity of the reporter
- Relaxation of privileged communication rights, such as the doctor-patient privilege, that would apply in a setting other than child maltreatment
- Procedures for reporting and how the information is processed
- Guidelines regarding protective custody for the child if deemed necessary for the child's safety
- Penalties for failure to report

State statutes may employ various wordings to describe the level of suspicion that requires reporting. Cause to believe, reasonable cause to believe, known or suspected abuse, reason to suspect, and observation or examination that discloses evidence of abuse are among the phrases employed. The overarching intent remains to ensure that healthcare professionals report suspicions of possible maltreatment when clinical interactions would lead a competent professional to consider child abuse or neglect as a reasonably likely diagnosis or cause to explain the case before them. The primary motivation is to stop further maltreatment and obtain help for the family.

COLLABORATIVE INVESTIGATION AND INTERVENTION (Table 7-2)

CHILD PROTECTIVE SERVICES

- At state or county level, is usually designated as the responsible governmental entity because of legal mandate; central to reporting, investigation, and treatment related to alleged child sexual abuse.
- Lead agency in assessing child and family social service needs, developing intervention strategy that includes treatment for child and family, and ongoing follow-up and monitoring of cases of child maltreatment until they are closed.
- Works with law enforcement to investigate.
- Works with the courts to determine issues involving custody and parental rights.
- Child Protective Services (CPS) Process Phases **(Table 7-3)**:

1. Intake
2. Initial assessment/investigation
3. Family assessment
4. Case planning
5. Service provision
6. Evaluation of family progress and case closure

LAW ENFORCEMENT AGENCIES

- Become involved because sexual abuse is a crime.

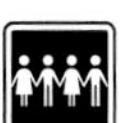

Table 7-2. Typical Case Progression in Joint Investigation

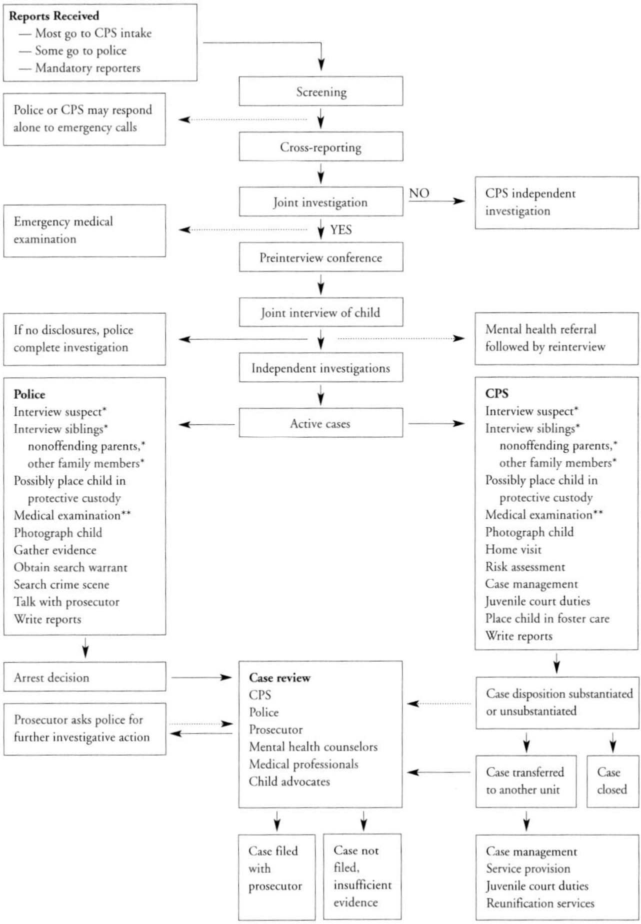

Reports Received
— Most go to CPS intake
— Some go to police
— Mandatory reporters

→ Screening

Police or CPS may respond alone to emergency calls

↓ Cross-reporting

↓ Joint investigation — NO → CPS independent investigation

Emergency medical examination

↓ YES Preinterview conference

↓ Joint interview of child

If no disclosures, police complete investigation

Mental health referral followed by reinterview

↓ Independent investigations

↓ Active cases

Police
Interview suspect*
Interview siblings*
nonoffending parents,*
other family members*
Possibly place child in protective custody
Medical examination**
Photograph child
Gather evidence
Obtain search warrant
Search crime scene
Talk with prosecutor
Write reports

CPS
Interview suspect*
Interview siblings*
nonoffending parents,*
other family members*
Possibly place child in protective custody
Medical examination**
Photograph child
Home visit
Risk assessment
Case management
Juvenile court duties
Place child in foster care
Write reports

Arrest decision

Prosecutor asks police for further investigative action

Case review
CPS
Police
Prosecutor
Mental health counselors
Medical professionals
Child advocates

Case disposition substantiated or unsubstantiated

Case transferred to another unit

Case closed

Case filed with prosecutor

Case not filed, insufficient evidence

Case management
Service provision
Juvenile court duties
Reunification services

**May be joint activity*
***Either agency performs*

Adapted from Sheppard DI, Zangrillo PA. Coordinating investigations of child abuse. Public Welf. *1996;54:21-31.*

Table 7-3. Child Protective Services Process

Phase	Description
Intake	— Receive reports of suspected child sexual abuse — Evaluate reports against statutory and agency guidelines — Determine urgency of response — Educate reporters on state laws, agency guidelines, and CPS functions
Initial assessment/ investigation	Gather sufficient evidence to decide: — If child sexual abuse has occurred — Level of risk for future maltreatment — If child is safe at home — Types of services needed to reduce risk
Family assessment	— Obtain information about nature, extent, and causes of risk — Gain deeper understanding of how abuse occurred — Analyze personal and environmental factors that contributed to abuse
Case planning	— Determine strategies to change conditions and behaviors that resulted in child sexual abuse — Collaborative planning is best when possible — Court often involved
Service provision	— Care plans implemented — CPS arranges, provides, and/or coordinates the delivery of services to child and family

(continued)

Table 7-3. *(continued)*

PHASE	DESCRIPTION
Evaluation of family progress and case closure	Ongoing assessment directed at: — Child's safety — Achievement of treatment goals — Risk reduction — Success in child's and family's needs

Adapted from DePanfilis D, Salus MK. Child Protective Services: A Guide for Caseworkers. *Washington, DC: US Dept of Health and Human Services, National Center on Child Abuse and Neglect; 1992a.*

- Take responsibility for the criminal investigation and are specially trained in conducting interviews, collecting crime scene evidence, and interrogating suspects.
- Work with healthcare providers to interpret information uncovered during the investigation.
- Conduct a series of interviews with multiple people who may be able to shed light on details related to the abuse situation.
- Gather physical evidence and search the crime scene when indicated.
- Support CPS, accompanying them to isolated, potentially dangerous locations.
- Provide immediate response to emergency situations.
- Enforce standing court orders and may assist in removing children from the home when danger is imminent.
- Arrest suspects.

Mental Health Professionals

• Help the child deal with the short- and long-term impact of maltreatment.

• Assist in the initial evaluation and provide treatment after the assessment.

• May be asked to assess the risk to the child of further abuse.

• May provide services in the home.

• Develop a treatment plan to outline supports beneficial to the long-term outcome of child abuse.

• Collaborate with the educational system to encourage early intervention, special education, after-school activities, and recreational enrichment activities.

Court and Judicial Proceedings

Children become involved with the court system through possible maltreatment, contested custody arrangements within divorce proceedings, adoption issues, suspected offenses (delinquency offenses), or traffic offenses. Rarely is a child called as a witness in a nonabuse-related criminal or civil case. Children require handling that differs from that accorded adults, possibly involving a modification of the court environment to make it more child sensitive (eg, using less complex language, downsizing furniture, talking directly to the judge).

Juvenile Court

• Exercises power over minors brought into the system because of all forms of child abuse, neglect, abandonment, unwillingness to submit to parental control (incorrigibility), and delinquency.

• May ask a child witness to provide factual information that may result in taking the child into state custody.

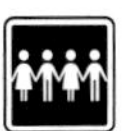

• Two legal doctrines underlie the role of the juvenile court:

1. *Parens patriae:* government has the authority to step in and limit the parents' authority over their child when the court perceives a danger to the child's physical or mental health.
2. Best interests of the child: government must consider what is reasonably in the child's best interest when deciding if the child should be removed from the parents' care or be allowed to remain in their care.

• Purpose of the juvenile court with respect to child maltreatment is as follows:

1. Protect the child from further maltreatment and harm
2. Provide services and treatment to the child and family
3. Terminate parental rights
4. Provide permanent placement for the maltreated child
5. Order mental health evaluation of children and parents when needed

• Has broad discretion in addressing issues and invokes judicial authority to facilitate the social welfare system's goal of rehabilitating and treating the abusive family when possible.

• Guiding principles are as follows:

1. Children are presumed to lack the mental competency and maturity possessed by adults.
2. The child's caregivers must be shown to be unfit, unable, unwilling, or unavailable to care

adequately for the child before the court intervenes.

3. Court intervention may be taken to promote the best interests of the child.

• Judges in juvenile court usually welcome information from CPS caseworkers, psychiatrists, private agency social workers, physiologists, and physicians because their decisions can only be as good as the information at their disposal.

• The 2 roles that the health professional may be asked to assume in the court process are as follows:

1. Provide direct knowledge of information pertinent to the specific case at hand.
2. Provide the court with an interpretation of the information that has been offered (expert witness).

Criminal Court

• Although child abuse is a crime in all states, full criminal prosecution may not be possible for various reasons, as follows:

1. Juvenile courts were viewed traditionally as the ideal place for handling child abuse and neglect cases because they focus on family needs and the provision of services to the child and family.
2. Proving child maltreatment in the criminal court is difficult because of constitutional rights regarding evidence afforded defendants.
3. Criminal court is seen as especially threatening and potentially damaging to children secondary to its nature, specifically:

   Multiple interviews required

   Inevitable delays that extend over years

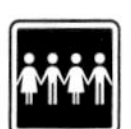

Insensitive questioning

Defendant's rights to face-to-face confrontation with the accuser in court

• The court's proceedings may lead to consequences affecting the home, caregivers, and the child, including the following:

1. Loss of employment
2. Loss of income
3. Disruption or dissolution of the family
4. Incarceration of a parent and potential feeling of guilt on the child's part
5. If there is an acquittal, designation of the child by the family as disruptive and the diminishment of the child's value within the home

• Reasons for carrying out prosecution include the following:

1. Establishes the perpetrator as solely responsible for the maltreatment.
2. Helps vindicate the victim and establish a sense of fairness while recognizing the innocence of the victim.
3. Reduces the risk of further episodes of maltreatment if the perpetrator is found guilty.
4. Establishes a criminal record for the offender.
5. Ensures that the offender is treated.

• Healthcare providers may be asked to participate in 2 ways:

1. Provide direct knowledge of information surrounding the specific case at hand (a fact witness).

2. Provide the court with an interpretation of the information being discussed (an expert witness); this is permitted when the expert is felt to have a broad base of knowledge and expertise in the details concerning child sexual abuse situations.

• Testifying requires that the healthcare provider become familiar with the facts of the case as documented in medical records and meet with the attorneys involved to understand the types of questions that may be posed.

• Support for the child in judicial proceedings includes the following:

1. Child advocacy centers: help the child work through what to expect in court and how to deal with the questioning process.
2. Provision of a supportive person to accompany the child to the court and explain what is happening in the proceedings.
3. Clarification that the child is not judged by his or her performance in the courtroom.
4. Court schools: help the child deal with fears of what to expect in court by role-playing types of questions and appropriate answers.

• It is important to schedule a follow-up visit with the healthcare provider to identify how the child is dealing with the stress and anxiety surrounding court preparation and appearance. Evaluation should focus on acute stress manifestations, adjustment problems, and daily functional status (school performance or social functioning).

Impact on the Child

• No universal set of responses or uniform impact

• Mental and physical health issues are generally

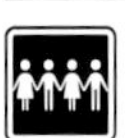

found in long-term assessments of adults with a history of sexual assault.

- Physical health effects:

1. Generally limited impact and treated with standard medical therapies
2. Gastrointestinal disorders, usually functional, include irritable bowel syndrome, nonulcer dyspepsia, and chronic abdominal pain
3. Gynecologic and urologic disorders include chronic pelvic pain, dysmenorrhea, and menstrual irregularities
4. Somatization

- Mental health effects:

1. Symptoms range in severity from mild to severe.
2. Course ranges from relatively short-term effects to those which are long-term or even lifelong.
3. Internalization versus externalization: some respond by internalizing and suffer depression and withdrawal, while others respond by externalizing and manifest aggression and disruptive behaviors.
4. Possible impacts include behavioral problems, posttraumatic stress disorder (PTSD), interpersonal difficulties, and cognitive and emotional distortions.
5. Adult survivors often have difficulties related to early damaging sexual experiences, including depression, low self-esteem, suicide attempts, multiple personality disorder, school failure, regressive behavior, PTSD, drug and alcohol abuse, running away, sexual promiscuity, prostitution, and delinquent behavior.

References

Baglow LJ. A multidimensional model for treatment of child abuse: a framework for cooperation. *Child Abuse Negl.* 1990;14:387-395.

Berkowitz CD. Medical consequences of child sexual abuse. *Child Abuse Negl.* 1998;22:541-550.

Berliner L, Elliott DM. Sexual abuse of children. In: Myers JEB, Berliner L, Briere J, Hendrix CT, Jenny C, Reid TA, eds. *The APSAC Handbook on Child Maltreatment.* 2nd ed. Thousand Oaks, Calif: Sage Publications; 2002:55-78.

Bond JR. The psychologist's evaluation. In: Schmitt BD, ed. *The Child Protection Team Handbook.* New York, NY: Garland Publishing, Inc; 1978:121-133.

Bulkley JA, Feller JN, Stern P, Roe F. Child abuse and neglect: laws and legal proceedings. In: Briere J, Berliner L, Bulkley JA, Jenny C, Reid T, eds. *The APSAC Handbook on Child Maltreatment.* Thousand Oaks, Calif: Sage Publications; 1996:271-296.

Cage RL, Pence DM. *Criminal Investigation of Child Sexual Abuse: Portable Guide to Investigating Child Abuse.* Washington, DC: US Dept of Justice; 1997. Report NCJ-162426.

DePanfilis D, Salus MK. *Child Protective Services: A Guide for Caseworkers.* Washington, DC: US Dept of Health and Human Services, National Center on Child Abuse and Neglect; 1992a.

Dubowitz H, DePanfilis D, eds. *Handbook for Child Protection Practice.* Thousand Oaks, Calif: Sage Publications; 2000.

Ells M. *Forming a Multidisciplinary Team to Investigate Child Abuse: Portable Guide to*

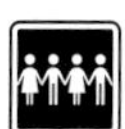

Investigating Child Abuse. Washington, DC: US Dept of Justice; 1998. Report NCJ-170020.

Fargason CA, Barnes D, Schneider D, Galloway BW. Enhancing multi-agency collaboration in the management of child sexual abuse. *Child Abuse Negl.* 1994;18:859-869.

Finkel MA, Ricci LR. Documentation and preservation of visual evidence in child abuse. *Child Maltreat.* 1997;2:322-330.

Golding J. Long-term physical health problems associated with sexual assault history. *The APSAC Advisor.* 2000;13:16-20.

Goldner JA, Dolgin CK, Manske SH. Legal issues. In: Monteleone J, ed. *Recognition of Child Abuse for the Mandated Reporter.* 2nd ed. St. Louis, Mo: GW Medical Publishing Inc; 1996:191-210.

Hibbard RA. Triage and referrals for child sexual abuse medical examinations from the sociolegal system. *Child Abuse Negl.* 1998;22:503-513.

Jenny C. *Medical Evaluation of Physically and Sexually Abused Children: The APSAC Study Guide.* Vol 3. Thousand Oaks, Calif: Sage Publications; 1996a.

Jenny C. Medical issues in sexual abuse. In: Briere J, Berliner L, Bulkley JA, Jenny C, Reid T, eds. *The APSAC Handbook on Child Maltreatment.* Thousand Oaks, Calif: Sage Publications; 1996b:195-226.

Jenny C. Medical issues in sexual abuse. In: Myers JEB, Berliner L, Briere J, Hendrix CT, Jenny C, Reid TA, eds. *The APSAC Handbook on Child Maltreatment.* 2nd ed. Thousand Oaks, Calif: Sage Publications; 2002:235-247.

Jenny C, Sutherland SE, Sandahl BB. Developmental approach to preventing the sexual abuse of children. *Pediatrics*. 1986;78:1034-1038.

Katner D, Plum HJ. Legal issues. In: Giardino AP, ed. *Recognition of Child Abuse for the Mandated Reporter*. 3rd ed. St. Louis, Mo: GW Medical Publishing Inc; 2002:309-350.

Kempe CH. Sexual abuse, another hidden pediatric problem: the 1977 C. Anderson Aldrich Lecture. *Pediatrics*. 1978;62:382-389.

Lanning KV. Criminal investigation of sexual victimization of children. In: Myers JEB, Berliner L, Briere J, Hendrix CT, Jenny C, Reid TA, eds. *The APSAC Handbook on Child Maltreatment.* 2nd ed. Thousand Oaks, Calif: Sage Publications; 2002:329-347.

Lanning KV, Walsh B. Criminal investigation of suspected child abuse. In: Briere J, Berliner L, Bulkley JA, Jenny C, Reid T, eds. *The APSAC Handbook on Child Maltreatment*. Thousand Oaks, Calif: Sage Publications; 1996:246-270.

Ludwig S. A multidisciplinary approach to child abuse. *Nurs Clin North Am*. 1981;16:161-165.

Myers JEB. Expert testimony. In: Briere J, Berliner L, Bulkley JA, Jenny C, Reid T, eds. *The APSAC Handbook on Child Maltreatment*. Thousand Oaks, Calif: Sage Publications; 1996:319-342.

Pence D, Wilson C. *Team Investigation of Child Sexual Abuse: The Uneasy Alliance*. Thousand Oaks, Calif: Sage Publications; 1994.

Runyan DK, Toth PA. Child sexual abuse. In: Krugman RD, Leventhal JM, eds. *Report of the Twenty-Second Ross Roundtable on Critical*

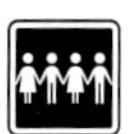

Approaches to Common Pediatric Problems. Columbus, Ohio: Ross Laboratories; 1991:57-75.

Sands RG, Stafford J, McClelland M. "I beg to differ": conflict in the interdisciplinary team. *Soc Work Health Care.* 1990;14:55-72.

Sgroi SM, ed. *Handbook of Clinical Intervention in Child Sexual Abuse.* Lexington, Mass: Lexington; 1982.

Sgroi SM, Bunk BS. A clinical approach to adult survivors of child sexual abuse. In: Sgroi SM, ed. *Vulnerable Populations.* Vol 1. Lexington, Mass: Lexington; 1988:137-186.

Sheppard DI, Zangrillo PA. Coordinating investigations of child abuse. *Public Welf.* 1996;54:21-31.

Siegler EL, Whitney FW, eds. *Nurse-Physician Collaboration.* New York, NY: Springer Publishing Co; 1994.

Stern HC. The psychiatrist's evaluation of the parents. In: Schmitt BD, ed. *The Child Protection Team Handbook.* New York, NY: Garland Publishing Inc; 1978:109-120.

Whitman BY, Munkel W. Multiple personality disorder: a risk indicator, diagnostic marker, and psychiatric outcome for severe child abuse. *Clin Pediatr.* 1991;30:422-428.

Wilson EP. Multidisciplinary approach to child protection. In: Ludwig S, Kornberg AE, eds. *Child Abuse: A Medical Reference.* 2nd ed. New York, NY: Churchill Livingstone; 1992:79-84.

Wolraich ML, Aceves J, Feldman HM, et al. American Academy of Pediatrics. Committee on Psychosocial Aspects of Child and Family Health.

The child in court: a subject review. *Pediatrics.* 1999;104(5:1):1145-1148.

Zellman GL, Faller KC. Reporting of child maltreatment. In: Briere J, Berliner L, Bulkley JA, Jenny C, Reid T, eds. *The APSAC Handbook on Child Maltreatment.* Thousand Oaks, Calif: Sage Publications; 1996:359-384.

Chapter 8

Documentation and Reporting

Martin A. Finkel, DO, FACOP, FAAP
Randell Alexander, MD, PhD
J.M. Whitworth, MD

The medical record for children suspected of having experienced inappropriate sexual contact shares most of the core elements of the standard medical record/consultation format found at either office-based or hospital-based practices. Acceptable medical practice dictates that clinicians follow the standard set of assessment parameters used in evaluating any medical condition. In suspected child abuse examinations, the examiner should assume that child protective services (CPS), law enforcement, and defense counsel will review the record. Therefore, it must be constructed with exacting attention to detail in anticipation of legal scrutiny. It must:

- Be legible
- Be well constructed
- Be educational
- Contain defensible conclusions
- Contain carefully documented medical history and visual findings
- Articulate a diagnosis and treatment recommendations

Principles for Documenting the Clinical Evaluation

Documentation runs the gamut from precise language reflecting historical details of the medical history to a synthesis of the information gathered.

It is not appropriate to present a synthesis of information where "irrelevant" points are deleted; the medical history should have verbatim the questions asked and the responses provided by the child and/or caregiver. Questions should be crafted to be developmentally appropriate and not leading or suggestive but rather open ended.

The Medical Record

• Serves as the vehicle to formalize a diagnostic assessment for the clinician

• Serves as a tool to inform caseworkers, law enforcement, and the courts

• Is generally reviewed in the context of case management discussions in a multidisciplinary team review

Purpose of the Medical Examination

Although the examination and medical report may have investigative value, the purpose for examining a child suspected of being abused is to diagnose and treat any residual consequences of the alleged sexual contact. The medical professional's primary concern is the patient's well-being.

Establishing the Diagnosing and Treating Physician Relationship

• Explain in a developmentally appropriate way that the examination is designed to diagnose and treat the patient.

1. Enhances the potential admissibility of the child's medical history under the diagnosing and treating physician's exception to hearsay
2. Allows the clinician to explain fully the basis on which the diagnostic assessment was made

- Allow the child to express any special concerns; encourage the child to tell the truth.
- Educate parents, colleagues in child protection, mental health professionals, and law enforcement personnel as to the potential medical consequences of sexual abuse and the need to make referrals to diagnostic and treatment services for children suspected of having been abused sexually.

Medical History Documentation

- Do not rely on an independent recollection of an interaction with a patient or limited notations when assessing children for possible maltreatment. The medical record must accurately reflect the evaluation and stand on its own.
- The physician's diagnosis rests on interpretation and integration of the following:

1. The medical history
2. Physical examination findings
3. Laboratory test results

- Record all information verbatim.
- The treatment exception for hearsay allows for admissibility of the child's description of symptoms, sensations, or pain associated with the presenting concern.
- The child's description of the cause of the injury or "illness" may provide idiosyncratic details that would be difficult to explain if the child had not experienced a particular causal event.
- If the child states that the injury or contact was at the hands of a certain individual, explain why the identity of that individual would be important to the diagnosis at hand.

• If the child is too young to verbalize the experience or emotionally unavailable to do so, observe and record behavioral changes and emotional state.

• Do not rely on information provided by CPS, law enforcement personnel, or a nonoffending parent as the sole data when formulating a diagnosis.

• Clinicians have been discouraged from speaking to the child on the presumption that the telling will be traumatic for the child or there may be discrepancies between the new information and the initial disclosure, presenting difficulties in prosecution. If discrepancies arise, they should be addressed.

Components of the Medical Record

• Birth history

• Family history

• Social history

• Developmental history

• Hospitalizations/emergency room visits

• Surgery

• Medications/allergies

• Review of body systems with particular attention to genitourinary (GU) and gastrointestinal (GI) systems

• History obtained from the caregiver regarding the presenting concern

• History obtained from the child

Review of the Genitourinary and Gastrointestinal Systems

In reviewing the GU system, you should include questions concerning the following:

• History of urinary tract infections, vaginal

discharges, vaginal odor, vaginal bleeding, diaper dermatitis, or urinary incontinence

- Use of bubble baths
- Treatment for any sexually transmitted diseases (STDs)
- Menstrual history
- Use of tampons
- Abortions
- Accidental genital injuries
- Vaginal foreign bodies
- Prior examination of the genitalia for any reason other than routine health care
- Self-exploratory activities/masturbation

The review of GI systems should cover the following concerns:

- Age of toilet training and whether there were any difficulties
- Use of rectal suppositories, enemas, or medications for inducing bowel movements
- History of constipation or painful bowel movements
- Frequency and character of stools
- History of recurrent vomiting, diarrhea, blood stools, hemorrhoids, fecal incontinence, rectal itching, or pinworm infestations

The Legally Defensible Medical Record

Key steps in compiling a legally defensible medical record are as follows:

- Document the child's age at the time of the statements.

• Note the duration of elapsed time between the suspected abuse and the child's statements.

• Specify who was present when the child made the statement, where the statement was made, and to whom it was made.

• Document whether specific statements were made in response to questions or were spontaneous.

• Note whether the child's responses were made to leading or nonleading questions.

• Note if the child's statement was made at the first opportunity that the child felt safe to talk.

• Document the child's emotional state. Note if the child was excited or distressed when the statement was made and, if so, what signs or symptoms of excitement or distress were observed.

• Document whether the child was calm, placid, or sleeping before making the statement or soon thereafter.

• Use the exact words that the child used to describe the characteristics of the event.

• Document the child's physical condition at the time of the statement.

• Note any suspected incentives for the child to fabricate or distort the truth.

Recording the Physical Examination Findings

• The record should include introductory statements to reflect the purpose for which the examination was undertaken and background information regarding how the child came for an examination.

• Include the overall medical condition of the child,

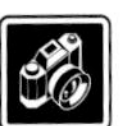

offer general physical examination findings, and describe in meticulous detail the appearance of all genital and anal structures and any relevant extragenital findings.

- Include photographic, colposcopic, or videocolposcopic methods of visual documentation in presenting the case.
- Avoid ambiguous conclusions when integrating the physical examination findings, laboratory results, and medical history in a diagnostic assessment.

Putting It All Together: Formulating a Diagnosis

- Consider and incorporate the salient aspects of each of the following when formulating a diagnosis:

1. Historical details and behavioral indicators reflective of the contact
2. Symptoms that can be directly associated with the contact
3. Acute and healed genital/anal injuries
4. Extragenital trauma
5. Forensic evidence
6. STDs

- Throughout the diagnostic and treatment process and report writing, remain objective, know the limitations of the clinical observation, incorporate differential diagnostic considerations, and formulate a diagnosis in an unbiased manner.

Networks

Formal networks link child abuse physicians to other advanced medical providers and can accomplish the following functions:

• Enhance the education of practitioners regarding child abuse and process issues, such as reporting, investigation, and court procedures

• Create peer review mechanisms, which allow:

1. Improved accuracy and increasing uniformity of conclusions
2. Avoidance of "conclusion creep," which is a gradual change in how findings are interpreted when not periodically contrasted against the interpretations of others
3. Quality assurance
4. Additional weight to the solidity of conclusions as they are perceived by others

• Incorporate interdisciplinary decision making more regularly

• Provide greater consultation opportunities between members of the network and professionals in the community

• Improve the opportunities for research by creating a larger database than individual practitioners or clinics could maintain alone

• Establish a larger, more organized coalition for child abuse advocacy

• Allow an opportunity for reduction of professional stress by providing professional and personal support for clinicians

Telemedicine

• In general, pediatricians have been slow to embrace virtual assessment because of the importance of the interaction between the physician and the parent-child dyad.

• A successful telemedicine program begins with a detailed needs assessment that focuses early on profiling the target consumer of the program. If the people are unwilling or unable to use the electronic equipment or service, the program will languish.

• Use of telemedicine technology for real-time evaluations is new and offers challenges as well as these 5 significant rewards for clinicians and children:

1. It is an effective tool to extend expertise to rural communities.
2. It can increase the accuracy of diagnosis.
3. Unnecessary investigations can be reduced.
4. The range of multidisciplinary teams can be increased.
5. Careful preplanning is required.

• In deploying a new telemedicine program, the following 2 elements are critical:

1. The community must know about the program in detail and key players in abuse evaluations must have a sense of participation or partial ownership.
2. All users must receive detailed training and support from the center to develop and maintain a sense of partnership in doing good things for abused children.

• Distance learning is teaching beyond the range of one's voice and has come to infer the use of television and/or computers as a means of education.

• Systems specific to child abuse education are generally part of larger telemedicine networks and use the "store and forward" technology in 4 ways:

1. An image is posted to other members of the network, perhaps asking an opinion or functioning as a test.
2. Users log onto a secure Web site or respond to an e-mail at a time of their own convenience.
3. If using the Internet, additional encryption is desirable for the highly sensitive photographs that are part of sexual abuse cases.
4. Images sent digitally can be altered by each party to add arrows, question marks, and other notations to aid in the learning process.

• Videoconferencing allows users to connect over the Internet with a video camera, monitor, computer, and sound system.

• The equipment used for effective electronic communications depends on the needs of the group and the funding provided. The recruitment of partners for the project is essential.

Technologies

• The most important component in any technologic apparatus is the expertise of the examiner. Without using a visual aid, there is no ability to provide visual documentation for later review or a second opinion. Visual documentation is helpful for teaching purposes, peer review, and courtroom testimony.

• Colposcopy

1. Uses a low-power microscope with a light source and camera and is designed for gynecologists to evaluate and document lesions of the cervix in adult patients.

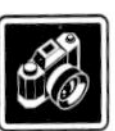

2. Offers the ability to standardize documentation, preserve evidence of what the examiner sees, and provide magnification of small lesions.
3. If colposcopy is not available, macrophotography can be substituted.

• Store and forward examinations are done by an independent examiner in one location capturing images and a medical record, then transmitting them electronically or physically to another independent examiner for consultation, interpretation, or review.

• The 4 limitations of store and forward communications are as follows:

1. Focus and clarity of the photographs
2. Selection of photographs for transmission
3. Sometimes incomplete historical information
4. Timeliness of feedback

• Standard photographs are hampered by delays in store and forward formats due to the need to have them processed, printed, and then scanned into a format suitable for transmission.

• Digital imaging can be stored on a computer and printed whenever needed, maintain original quality over time, and be transmitted electronically as often as required. The digital equipment now used produces images equal to analog images.

• The concern that these digital images may be altered can be answered by the use of software that ensures the integrity of the image.

• Synchronous or real-time evaluation of children with allegations of abuse may also be available.

The Electronic Record

• Records of sexual abuse examinations can be kept in the following 4 formats:

1. Paper hardcopy is the traditional medical record, is easy to read, but has considerable storage requirements and labor in copying a record.
2. Conventional 35-mm photographs or slides can be kept as part of or separated from the medical record; may be dislodged from the rest of the written record and have the disadvantages listed above.
3. Videotape of the forensic genital examination provides more perceptual information than a photograph alone, but requires storage space.
4. Digital photographs or short digital video clips have a quality comparable to standard photographs. They require considerable memory, with video clips taking large amounts of space. Several 10- to 15-second clips are required to capture the examination without exhausting the computer's memory capacity. A back-up copy should be available on a rewriteable CD, or storage on a server should be considered.

• The entire medical record may be electronic, which has the following 4 advantages:

1. Reduces or eliminates storage problems
2. Allows easy access
3. Has the ability to combine text and photographs in a seamless record
4. Allows tailoring specific formats for dissemination to others

- All electronic records should be backed up, with consideration given to using a separate location so that a disaster in one location will not wipe out the child's record.

References

Finkel MA, Ricci LR. Documentation and preservation of visual evidence in child abuse. *Child Maltreat.* 1997;2:322-330.

Myers JEB. *Evidence in Child Abuse and Neglect Cases.* 3rd ed. New York, NY: Wiley Law Publications; 1997.

Myers JEB. *Legal Issues in Child Abuse and Neglect Practice.* 2nd ed. Thousand Oaks, Calif: Sage Publications; 1998.

Teixeira WR. Hymenal colposcopic examination in sexual offenses. *Am J Forensic Med Pathol.* 1981;3:209-214.

Whitworth JM, Wood B, Morse K, Rogers H, Haney M. The Florida Child Protection Team Telemedicine Program. In: Oakley AMM, Woulten R, eds. *Teledermatology.* London, England: Royal Society of Medicine Press, Ltd; 2002:35-149.

Woodling B, Heger A. The use of the colposcope in the diagnosis of sexual abuse in the pediatric age group. *Child Abuse Negl.* 1986;10:111-114.

Chapter 9

Physical Evaluation of Adolescents and Adults

Donna Gaffney, RN, DNSc, FAAN
Iris Reyes, MD, FACEP
Elizabeth M. Datner, MD

The following review of a sexual assault victim focuses primarily on a female victim. Refer to Chapter 6 for information specific to male sexual assault and to Chapter 13 for specifics regarding sexual assault of the elderly. Ideally, the sexual assault evaluation is done at a rape crisis center, where the focus is on providing a compassionate setting for the victim and skilled medical and forensic evidence collection.

Obtaining the History of a Sexual Assault

Role of the Healthcare Provider

- Pay close attention to detail.
- Maintain a caring, nonjudgmental approach.
- Clearly convey to each victim the following points:

1. No one ever deserves to be raped.
2. The perpetrator, not the victim, is responsible for the assault.
3. The victim made the best choices possible for survival under the circumstances.

- With adolescent rape victims, make efforts to establish a trusting relationship and to make the victims aware that regardless of their activity, they are not at fault and no one had the right to force them to participate in sexual activity against their will.

• Make victims aware of clinician mandatory reporting requirements before they disclose information.

• Encourage victims to report the assault to police.

• Make the victim aware that physical evidence can rarely be recovered more than 48 to 72 hours after an incident; therefore, attempts should be made to collect physical evidence early whether or not the victim has decided to pursue the case.

• Most states have crime-victim compensation programs that cover the financial costs of the evaluation and evidence collection.

• Responsibilities of the healthcare provider include the following:

1. Treat physical injuries.
2. Perform a careful physical examination. Rule out any life-threatening conditions, with assessment of the victim's airway, breathing, and circulation (ABCs) as a priority. Treating these vital functions supercedes any data collection or gathering of forensic evidence.
3. Collect legal evidence.
4. Document all pertinent aspects of the history.
5. Provide care in terms of pregnancy and sexually transmitted disease (STD) prophylaxis and psychologic support.
6. Arrange for follow-up care and counseling for the victim.
7. Inform the victim that refusal of any or all of the procedures or questions is up to the victim and that refusal will not affect care.

• Provide a private, quiet environment so that the victim feels safe and in control of what is happening

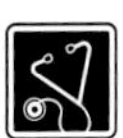

to him or her. However, do not leave the victim alone. In addition, if the person accompanying the victim is suspected of being the perpetrator, isolate the victim from that person until you have explored this possibility and the victim has requested the presence of the other person.

- Limit the victim's exposure to repetitive questioning.
- Inform the victim before beginning the physical examination that it will take about 30 to 60 minutes.
- During the examination, be sure to listen carefully, speak quietly, and perform the evaluation in an unhurried manner.

History of the Adult Victim

- The purpose is to record the events that occurred and guide the clinician in collecting evidence and caring for injuries.
- Elements of a general history include the following:

1. Past history of medical illness
2. Recent surgery
3. Medications
4. Allergies
5. Tetanus immunization
6. History of STDs
7. Contraception use
8. Last consensual sexual experience, tampon use, or douching
9. Illicit drug use or alcohol ingestion
10. Last menstrual period
11. Obstetric history

- For elements of a forensic evaluation see Chapter 10.

The Physical Examination

• The purpose of the physical examination is to identify any injuries requiring medical attention and to collect forensic evidence. Be prepared to perform only one physical examination, but be aware that you may need to also collect forensic evidence.

1. Be prepared to use a rape kit and have one available **(Table 9-1)**.
2. If a rape crisis center is available, transfer the victim in a timely fashion once it has been ascertained that he or she is medically stable.
3. If no center is available, perform a rape examination and gather forensic evidence.

• Make sure that a chaperone is present during the gynecologic examination of any female victim.

• Perform a thorough physical examination, including evidence of nongenital physical trauma.

• Patients should remove all clothing as outlined in Chapters 3 and 4.

• The examination should move from head to foot, paying particular attention to signs of injury **(Table 9-2 and Figures 9-1 and 9-2)**.

1. A method for remembering the types of injuries is to use the acronym TEARS, as follows:

   T: Tear (laceration) or tenderness

   E: Ecchymosis (bruising)

   A: Abrasion

   R: Redness (erythema)

   S: Swelling (edema)

2. Tears or lacerations: occur when the continuity of the skin is broken and disrupted by blunt

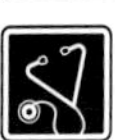

Table 9-1. Rape Kit
RECOMMENDED CONTENTS
1. Instructions
2. Checklist
3. History and physical documentation forms
4. Equipment for specimen collection:
— Paper bags (plastic may produce mildew which contaminates evidence)
— Large paper or cloth sheet
— Cotton-tipped swabs and tubes for their placement
— Comb
— Envelopes
— Patient discharge information
— Red- and purple-topped tubes for blood sampling
— Filter paper
— Cardboard box
— Forceps
— Scissors
— Labels for clinical samples

force, usually applied in a vertical manner, perpendicular to the plane of the skin. Tearing, ripping, crushing, overly stretching, or pulling apart result in this tear, which is often over a bony surface, contributes to the severity of this injury. The laceration's edges are irregular and can be aligned to fit together. This is not the same as a cut, which is made with a sharp instrument. The margins of the laceration may be bruised or crushed, and connective tissue

Table 9-2. Male and Female Genital Structures and Characteristics

FEMALE
(Figure 9-1)

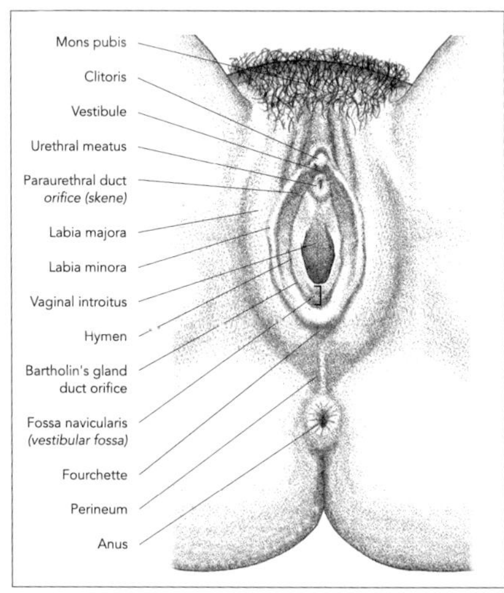

Figure 9-1. *The external genitalia of the adult female.*

Anus: The terminal opening of the digestive tract, which serves as the opening of the rectum. This area has a concentration of nerve endings. Anal folds, or wrinkles of perianal skin radiating from the anus, are caused by the closure of the external anal sphincter.

Cervix: The lower portion of the uterus that protrudes into the vagina.

Clitoris: A small cylindrical body of erectile tissue situated at the most anterior portion of the vulva. A fold of tissue, called the "hood" or prepuce, covers the clitoris. During arousal, the clitoris enlarges and protrudes from the hood. The clitoris is the most sensitive part of the female anatomy.

Fossa navicularis: The area of the vaginal vestibule located between the posterior attachment of the hymen and the posterior fourchette. It presents as a shallow depression at the base of the vulva.

(continued)

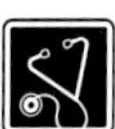

Table 9-2. *(continued)*

Hymen: The circular band of tissue that surrounds (completely or partially) the opening of the vagina. The physical appearance and elasticity of the hymen change over a woman's life span because of hormonal fluctuation (primarily estrogen).

Hymen Morphology

Annular: Circumferential hymen tissue presents 360 degrees around vaginal opening.

Bump: Solid elevation of hymenal tissue.

Crescentic: Posterior rim of hymen, with attachments at the 10 to 1 o'clock and 1 to 2 o'clock positions.

Cribiform: Hymen with multiple small hymenal openings.

External ridge: Longitudinal ridge (raised area) on the external surface of the hymen from the rim to the fossa navicularis or urethra.

Fimbriated: A hymen with a ruffled, and/or fringed edge.

Hymenal cleft: Division or split in the rim of the hymen that does not cross the base of the hymen.

Longitudinal vaginal ridge: A longitudinal ridge extending from the hymenal rim into the vagina, usually on the posterior or posterolateral walls, and parallel to the vaginal axis.

Redundant: Hymen of any type that is folded on itself and does not "open" to reveal the orifice, even when multiple positions and methods are used.

Septate hymen: Two hymenal openings with a band of hymenal tissue in between.

Imperforate: No hymenal opening.

(continued)

Table 9-2. *(continued)*

Labia majora: Latin for "larger lips." These are rounded folds of skin forming the lateral boundaries of the vulva. These outer folds of skin protect the more delicate structures underneath.

Labia minora: Latin for "smaller lips." The longitudinal folds of tissue enclosed within the labia majora that are located on either side of the vaginal orifice. These folds of tissue cover the vaginal orifice and urethral meatus.

Mons pubis: The rounded eminence in front of the pubic symphysis formed by a collection of fatty tissue beneath the integument. It becomes covered with hair at the time of puberty.

Os: The opening located at the center of the cervix, leading to the uterus.

Perineum: The area between the vaginal introitus and anus.

Posterior fourchette: A fold of mucous membrane that connects the labia minora at the base of the vulva.

Rectum: Terminal portion of the lower intestine.

Uterus: A hollow muscular organ, pear-shaped, with a small internal cavity. It is where the fetus grows before birth.

Urethral meatus: The opening to the urethra. Its major purpose is the release of urine from the bladder.

Vagina: The structure that opens to the outside of the body at the vaginal introitus and extends 3 to 5 inches inside the body, ending at the cervix.

Vaginal introitus: Located below the urethral meatus and situated behind the labia minora; the entrance to the vagina.

(continued)

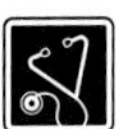

Table 9-2. *(continued)*

Vaginal vestibule: The space posterior to the clitoris, between the labia minora.

Vulva: The external genitalia of the female, or pudendum. Includes the clitoris, labia majora, labia minora, vaginal vestibule, urethral orifice, vaginal orifice, hymen, fourchette, and posterior commissure.

MALE
(Figure 9-2)

Coronal ridge: The widest portion around the glans.

Ejaculation: The release of reproductive fluid via the male urethra. The ejaculate may or may not contain spermatozoa.

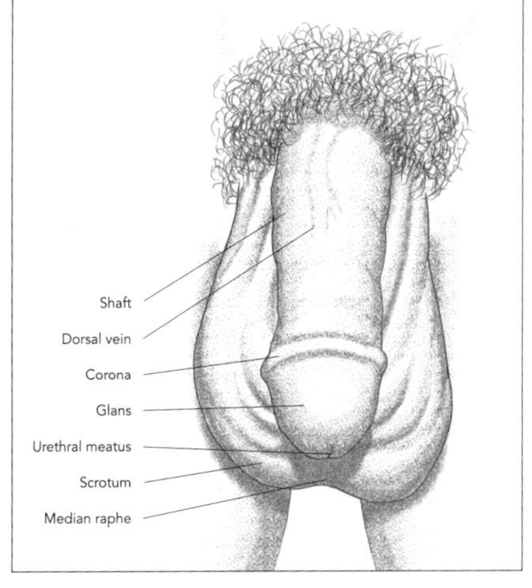

Figure 9-2. *Frontal view of the external male genitalia.*

Foreskin (prepuce): The movable hood of skin covering the glans of the penis. During erection, the foreskin rolls back just below the coronal ridge. In circumcised men, the foreskin has been removed.

Frenulum: On the underside of the penis, with a different texture to its skin, this area is often highly responsive to stimulation.

(continued)

Table 9-2. *(continued)*

Glans: The cone-shaped head of the penis. This fleshy "head" of the penis is most sensitive to stimulation. Usually larger in diameter than the shaft, the glans is responsible for the greatest sensation during intercourse.

Penis: The male organ of reproduction and urination.

Perineum: The area between the base of the scrotum and the anus. Beneath the skin are more chambers that fill with blood during arousal, just as the penis does.

Scrotum: The sac encasing the testicles just below the penis.

Semen: A thick fluid released by the male during ejaculation. It consists of fluids from various glands plus the spermatozoa.

Shaft: The cylindrical part of the penis located between the glans and the body, which is filled with vascular chambers. During arousal these chambers fill with blood, causing the shaft to stiffen and producing an erection. Unlike many other animals, the human has no bone or gristle to ensure stiffness.

Testicles: Two spherical glands within the scrotum that produce sperm. The sperm are carried through spermatic cords, joining fluids produced by the prostate gland and seminal vesicles to produce semen, which is then ejaculated. One of the cords is called the epididymis, and the difference in the length of the two epididymides is responsible for one testicle being slightly lower than the other.

Urethral opening: At the end of the penis, this opening serves as the duct through which both urine and ejaculate (semen) flow.

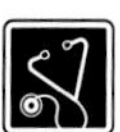

strands may "bridge" across the interior of the wound. Lacerations often contain foreign material, including trace evidence.

3. Ecchymosis (bruising) and contusions: bruises lie below the intact epidermis and consist of an extravascular collection of blood that has leaked from ruptured capillaries or blood vessels. It is not possible to specifically identify the exact "age" of a bruise using color as a guideline because other factors influence the color changes that a bruise undergoes (impaired blood clotting, compromised immune status, certain malignant diseases, diabetes, alcoholism, malnutrition, age). Contusions may cause far more serious injuries and can occur anywhere in the body. Both result from blood vessel leakage when blunt force is applied to a tissue. Petechiae are tiny red or purple spots on the skin or other tissue. Petechiae less than 3 mm in diameter are pinpoint-size hemorrhages of small capillaries in the skin or mucous membranes. Bruises, contusions, and petechiae do not blanch when pressure is applied.
4. Abrasions: superficial injuries to the skin, limited to the epidermis and superficial dermis, are normally caused by rubbing, sliding, or compressive forces against the skin in a parallel manner rather than vertical force.
5. Redness or erythema: should not be mistaken for bleeding under the skin. Erythema blanches under gentle pressure and is usually diffuse and does not exhibit a pattern. The cause can be a forceful slap or increased pressure to the skin, causing blood to be momentarily forced out of the capillaries in the area of contact, then, when pressure is withdrawn, the blood returns to the

capillaries, which may dilate. The result is redness or flushing of the skin.

• Obtain diagrams or photographs of identified injuries.

• Collect forensic evidence as the examination progresses. (See Chapter 10.)

Laboratory Tests

• Perform laboratory studies as needed for the medical treatment of the victim in addition to what is forwarded to law enforcement under the guidelines of the rape kit.

• Use only water or saline solution during the speculum and rectal examinations; do not use standard lubricants, which can interfere with forensic testing.

• Recommended laboratory evaluations are as follows:

1. Pregnancy testing (either urine or serum testing)
2. Rapid plasma reagin (RPR) or Venereal Disease Research Laboratory (VDRL) (test for syphilis at initial visit and again at 3 months)
3. Hepatitis serology (test for hepatitis B recommended; hepatitis C testing not generally required)
4. Gonorrhea/Chlamydia testing (swab sites potentially exposed during the assault, including the mouth, throat, vagina, and rectum)
5. Human immunodeficiency virus (HIV) testing (at initial visit with locally mandated counseling and again at 3, 5, and 12 months; the site best suited to perform appropriate posttest counseling should perform these studies)
6. Blood sample for typing to differentiate victim from perpetrator

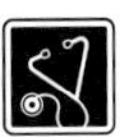

Interpreting Injuries

The clinician must recognize that physical findings for women who have had consensual intercourse can be different from those for victims of sexual assault. Vigorous or intense intercourse ("rough sex") has been suggested as an explanation for a victim's injuries. Patients may hesitate to seek medical services when they have sustained injury to the genitalia after episodes of intense sex, unusual positions during sex, or prolonged sexual contact. The clinician will note during the history that, although the individual may be embarrassed or hesitant to discuss details of the sexual encounter, she is able to recall both her partner's and her own actions that may have led to the injury. Sexual assault victims may not be able to recall the specific actions of the assailant.

A complex relationship exists among the variables that can influence injury type and location. A comprehensive history is critical to understanding the presence or absence of injury. The variables influencing injury can be grouped as factors related to the victim, the perpetrator, the circumstances, or the environment **(Table 9-3)**.

Follow-up Care

- Arrange for follow-up medical care for the victim at 1 to 2 weeks and at 2 to 4 months after the initial evaluation.
- The most significant sequelae after sexual assault are psychologic.
- All patients should receive counseling and referral for ongoing follow-up either during their initial evaluation or within the next 1 to 2 days.

Table 9-3. Variables Influencing Injury Type and Location

Factors Related to the Victim
Anatomy and physiology of the reproductive structures
Health and developmental status
Condition of the genital structures
Previous sexual experience
Lubrication of the vaginal vault (natural or artificial)
Partner participation
Positioning and pelvic tilt
Psychologic response
Factors Related to the Assailant
Object of penetration
Lubrication
Male sexual dysfunction
Force of penetration
Factors Related to Circumstances
Previous history with assailant
Lack of communication
Factors Related to the Environment
Location of the assault
Materials and surfaces in surrounding area

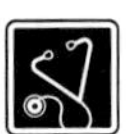

REFERENCES

Besant-Matthews PE. *Blunt Force Trauma.* Unpublished paper. Dallas, Tex: 2001.

Cartwright PS. Factors that correlate with injury sustained by survivors of sexual assault. *Obstet Gynecol.* 1987;70:44-46.

ElSohly MA, Salamone SJ. Prevalence of drugs used in cases of alleged sexual assault. *J Anal Toxicol.* 1999;23:141-146.

Girardin BW, Faugno DK, Seneski PC, Slaughter L, Whelan M. Findings in sexual assault and consensual intercourse. In: *Color Atlas of Sexual Assault.* St. Louis, Mo: Mosby; 1997:19-65.

Kobernick ME, Seiferts S, Sanders AB. Emergency department management of the sexual assault victim. *J Emerg Med.* 1985;2:205-214.

Linden JA. Sexual assault. *Emerg Med Clin North Am.* 1999;17:685-697.

Poirier MP. Care of the female adolescent rape victim. *Pediatr Emerg Care.* 2002;18(1):53-59.

Rabkin M. HIV in primary care. *General Medicine Clinic.* Available at: http://www.columbia.edu/~am430/HIV.htm. Accessed September 21, 2002.

Rambow B, Adkinson C, Frost TH, Peterson GF. Female sexual assault: medical and legal implications. *Ann Emerg Med.* 1992;21:727-731.

Ramin SM, Satin AJ, Stone IC Jr, Wendel GD Jr. Sexual assault in postmenopausal women. *Obstet Gynecol.* 1992;80:860-864.

Slaughter L, Brown CR. Cervical findings in rape victims. *Am J Obstet Gynecol.* 1991;164:528.

Solola A, Scott C, Severs H, Howell J. Rape: management in a noninstitutional setting. *Obstet Gynecol.* 1983;61:373.

Soules MR, Pollard AA, Brown KM, Verma M. The forensic laboratory evaluation of evidence in alleged rape. *Am J Obstet Gynecol.* 1978;130:142.

Tintinalli JE, Hoelzer M. Clinical findings and legal resolution in sexual assault. *Ann Emerg Med.* 1985;14:447-453.

Chapter 10

Forensic Evaluation of Adolescents and Adults

Holly M. Harner, CRNP, PhD, MPH, SANE
Patrick O'Donnell, PhD
Joanne Archambault
Kathy Bell, RN
Kathryn M. Turman

The immediate medical needs after sexual assault, including care of the acutely critical physical needs, are similar to those of victims of any trauma. However, when a violent crime such as rape or domestic violence has been committed, where the victim may know perpetrator, the clinician must ascertain the victim's level of safety.

- If the victim knows the perpetrator, the victim may fear retaliation for seeking medical care.
- It is necessary to seek available hospital or clinic security measures as indicated.
- When the victim may return to the perpetrator, as in marital rape, a safety plan should be reviewed with the victim before discharge.

Health and Assault History

It is important to maintain a professional, sensitive, and nonjudgmental manner throughout the history. Someone from the police department and a local victim advocacy organization should be present during the assault history, which will limit the number of interviews the victim will have to endure. If the treating clinician is a male and the victim a female, the presence of a female chaperone is recommended.

Health History

• Conduct an abbreviated history of acute and chronic illnesses, current medications, and allergies to medications.

• Include a gynecologic history to document the victim's first day of her last menstrual period, contraceptive method, current pregnancy status, and last consensual coitus within the past 72 hours.

• Ask the victim about any chronic psychiatric conditions, including major depression, anxiety disorders, and schizophrenia.

Assault History

• The elements of a forensic interview or focused assault history include the following:

1. Brief description of the incident
2. Number and identity of the attacker(s), if known
3. Time of the attack
4. Location where the assault took place
5. Type of sexual acts that occurred, that is, kissing, fondling, vaginal and/or anal penetration, oral penetration **(Table 10-1)**
6. Contact with ejaculate, urine, or vaginal secretions
7. Use of weapons, restraints, contraceptives, condoms by the perpetrator
8. Use of objects to penetrate or coerce the victim

• For evidentiary purposes, document whether the patient has changed clothing, bathed, urinated, defecated, or douched since the assault.

• Denote all direct quotes made by the patient with quotation marks when recorded.

• Note whether the victim used any alcohol or drugs.

1. Drugs used to facilitate nonconsensual sexual intercourse (date rape drugs) may be present.
2. Most often these are gamma hydroxybutyrate (GHB) or flunitrazepam (Rohypnol).
3. If the victim's recollection of the event is poor, consider whether these substances may have been used intentionally or unintentionally to alter the victim's memory.

Acute Care of the Sexual Assault Victim

• Obtain consent to perform a physical examination and to collect evidence. The purpose is to identify and document injuries and collect evidence. The physical examination will be briefly described here; for details, see Chapter 9.

• Assess physical trauma.

1. Nongynecologic injuries commonly include trauma from kicking, choking, and being tied

Table 10-1. Definitions of Sexual Conduct
Fellatio: any mouth to penis contact
Frottage: rubbing for the purpose of sexual gratification
Cunnilingus: mouth to vulva
Sexual intercourse: contact of the penis to the vagina
Anal intercourse or anal sodomy: contact of penis to the anus
Anilingus: mouth to anus
Oral sodomy: mouth to vagina, anus, or penis

or otherwise restrained, as well as human bites. These may be targeted to vulnerable "sexual" body regions, including the breast and genital areas, even though they are considered nongynecologic.

2. Thoroughly describe the injuries noted, including location, size, color, and pattern of injury. Photodocumentation is recommended, taking at least 2 pictures of each injury and using a ruler or other object to indicate size.
3. Gynecologic injuries often include vulvar, vaginal, perianal, and cervical lacerations, contusions, and hematomas.
4. Begin by visually inspecting the external genitalia and other surrounding areas, including the inner thighs. Use a handheld magnifying lens if needed, document injuries, and take photographs.
5. Thoroughly inspect the vaginal introitus, noting introital tears, abrasions, swelling, or ecchymoses.
6. If foreign bodies are found, remove them, place them in an envelope, and seal them with a description of where on the body they were found and your initials.
7. If pooled secretions in the posterior vaginal fornix are present, aspirate with a syringe without a needle or collect with a cotton swab and include in the evidence kit.
8. Carefully examine the buttocks and anus for evidence of trauma, including fissures, small lacerations, and bruises. If anal penetration is reported, check for rectal bleeding; take rectal swabs for gonococcus and *Chlamydia*.

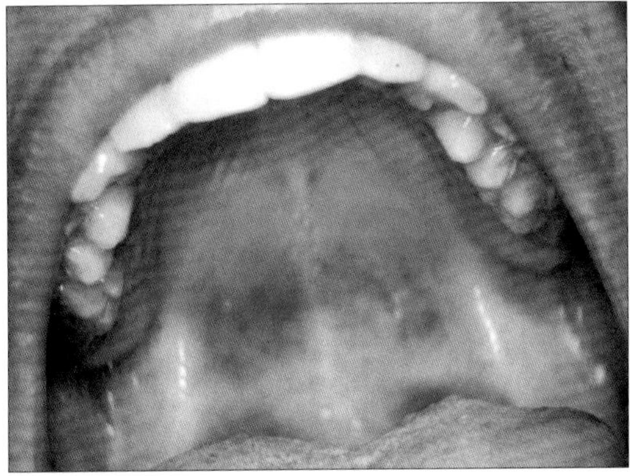

Figure 10-1. *Submucosal hemorrhages at the junction of hard and soft palates, termed fellatio syndrome.*

9. Comb hair over a paper towel and collect debris and loose hair. This applies to pubic hair as well.
10. Examine the oral cavity carefully, looking for fellatio syndrome **(Figure 10-1)**. Use a cotton swab to obtain a sample of fluid between the gum and lips; collect several samples and air dry them before packaging them for evidence. Use slides to make wet mounts, and note any findings on the chart. Also take a swab for *Neisseria gonorrhoeae*. Finally, have the victim rinse his or her mouth with water, wait 5 minutes, and place a filter paper in the victim's mouth to saturate it with saliva to be used for victim blood antigen determination.
11. Scrape stains on the skin with a tongue blade or moist cotton-tipped applicator. Use Wood's lamp to illuminate semen. Inspect fingernails closely for evidence of foreign material or dirt.
12. Speculum examination follows the complete external examination of the perineum, vaginal area, and anus. Look for evidence of trauma

to the cervix and cul-de-sac (perforation may indicate bowel injury). Take samples from the external cervical os. Obtain vaginal swabs for antigen determination, seminal factors, and DNA testing.

13. Be sure to obtain the victim's consent and prepare him or her for every phase of the examination.

- Be aware that while evidence is best collected within 72 hours of the assault, valid evidence can be collected up to 5 days after the event.
- Even if the victim has no complaints of pelvic trauma or discomfort, proceed with a pelvic examination, since up to one third of victims have evidence of traumatic genital injuries after a sexual assault without any symptoms.
- Indicate the time the examination was performed and document all findings.
- Be aware that genital trauma is more likely to occur in postmenopausal female victims and will require surgical repair. Colposcopy or toluidine blue staining can be used to identify microlacerations not apparent initially.

Chain of Evidence

Chain of evidence or chain of custody refers to the direct line of custody of the evidence from time of collection until presentation at court. If this direct line is not established between the clinician and the court, the evidence could be considered inadmissible.

- Place all evidence gathered in separate envelopes or containers, seal them, and initial **(Table 10-2)**.
- Label all specimens with the victim's name, date, examiner's name, and specimen source.

- Seal all containers and envelopes so that it is clear if someone attempts to tamper with the evidence **(Figure 10-2)**.
- Once all specimens are collected and other evidence is separately packaged, package them together, seal them, and label them. Turn the completed package over to the police or place it in a locked cabinet.
- Obtain a receipt for the evidence; have the person handing over the evidence and the person receiving it sign and date the receipt.
- For further documentation principles, see Chapter 8.

Pharmacologic Needs

Prevention of Pregnancy

As many as 25 000 rape-related pregnancies occur annually, so standard of care practice for the rape

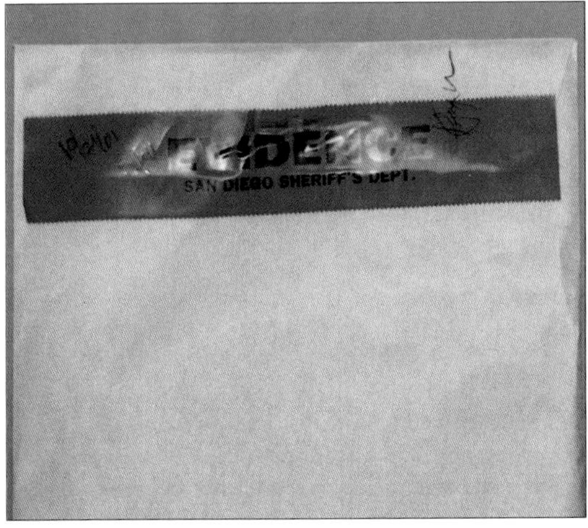

Figure 10-2. *Properly sealed evidence envelope; seal covers entire opening. Date and examiner's name are indicated. Signature crosses envelope and seal.*

Table 10-2. Guidelines for Evidence Collection Following Sexual Assault

CLOTHING COLLECTION

Materials Needed:

- — 2 paper sheets
- — 5-10 paper bags
- — Labels
- — Pieces of paper

Instructions:

Collect all clothing worn at the time of the attack, including shoes. Victim should undress over 2 sheets placed on the floor, handing each clothing item to the nurse. Each piece of clothing should be placed in separately labeled paper bags and sealed. Do not shake out clothing or cut through preexisting rips or tears. If any stains are present on the clothing, place a piece of paper over the stain prior to folding. If clothing is wet/damp, allow to air dry before placing in labeled paper bag. After collecting the clothing, the top paper sheet should be carefully folded and placed in a labeled paper bag and sealed.

PHYSICAL EXAMINATION AND EVIDENCE COLLECTION

Skin

Materials Needed:

- — Wood's lamp
- — Cotton-tipped swabs
- — Normal sterile saline (NSS)
- — Labels
- — Sterile water
- — Paper or cardboard containers

Instructions:

Scan the skin with the Wood's lamp. Areas that react to ultraviolet light may provide biologic evidence. Swab these areas with 2 cotton swabs moistened with NSS, air dry, and place in labeled paper or cardboard container. Collect debris from skin and put in labeled container.

(continued)

Table 10-2. *(continued)*

Fingernails

Materials Needed:

— 2 plastic fingernail scrapers
— Paper towels
— Labels
— Envelopes

Instructions:

Obtain trace evidence from fingernails by scraping nails over a paper towel. Fold evidence in paper towel with fingernail scraper, place in labeled envelope, and seal. Evidence from each hand should be gathered and stored in separate envelopes, labeled "right" or "left" hand.

Oropharynx

Materials Needed:

— 2 red-topped tubes
— Gonorrhea/*Chlamydia* culture
— Cotton-tipped swabs
— Labels
— Paper or cardboard containers

Instructions:

Swab buccal mucosa and along the gingiva with cotton swab, air dry, and place in labeled cardboard or paper container. Salivary samples should be collected at least 25 minutes after the victim last ate, drank, or smoked. Collect gonorrhea/*Chlamydia* oropharyngeal cultures per guidelines. Oropharyngeal evidence may be collected if oral-genital contact occured.

Genitalia

Materials Needed:

— 2 red-topped tubes
— 2 gonnorrhea/*Chlamydia* culture
— 6 cotton swabs
— 3 4x4 gauze pads
— 2 envelopes

(continued)

Table 10-2. *(continued)*

— Comb
— Scissors
— Labels
— Sterile water
— Containers
— Paper towels

Instructions:
Swab external genitalia and inner thighs with 4x4 gauze pads moistened with sterile water. Allow to air dry and place in labeled container.

Swab the vaginal walls and vault with 2 cotton swabs, allow to air dry, and place in labeled container. Repeat with one swab each for cervical and anal specimen.

Place paper towel under victim's buttocks. Comb through pubic hair in downward motion, catching loose hairs in paper towel. Fold paper towel and place in labeled envelope and seal.

Obtain gonorrhea/*Chlamydia* cultures from vagina and rectum when indicated. Label tubes.

Head Hair
Materials Needed:

— Paper towels
— Envelope
— Labels

Instructions:
Pull 15 full-length head hairs, as permitted by patient and by jurisdiction, from back, center, and right and left side of the head, catching the loose hairs in a paper towel. Place paper towel in labeled envelope and seal.

(continued)

Table 10-2. *(continued)*

BLOOD SAMPLE COLLECTION
Materials Needed: — 1 purple-topped tube — 3 red-topped tubes — Labels *Instructions:* Collect 3 mL of blood in labeled purple-topped tube. Blood work for sexually transmitted disease (STD) testing (HIV, Rapid Plasma Reagin [RPR], and hepatitis B) may be collected in labeled red-topped tubes if indicated. Some states use buccal swabs rather than blood for reference DNA.

Adapted from Sexual Assault Evidence Collection Kit Cat. No. VEC100. Youngsville, NC: Sirchie Finger Print Laboratories, Inc; 2002. Suspected Sexual Abuse Form. *Philadelphia, Pa: St. Christopher's Hospital; 2002.*

victim of childbearing age is making available emergency contraception, also referred to as the "morning-after pill," up to 72 hours after a sexual assault **(Table 10-3)**. This should be offered to any woman of childbearing age when there was any vaginal-penile contact, however slight. Even when a male condom was used, this added measure of pregnancy prevention may be reassuring to the victim.

- Determine if the victim is already pregnant before giving medication.
- Give the woman a combination of oral contraceptive pills twice at a 12-hour interval **(Table 10-3)**.
- Offer anti-nausea medications.
- Stress to the woman the importance of eating before each dose of hormones.

Table 10-3. Emergency Contraceptive Guidelines

Brand	Pills per Dose
Alesse	5 pink pills
Levlen	4 light-orange pills
Levlite	5 pink pills
Levora	4 white pills
Lo/Ogestrel	4 white pills
Lo/Ovral	4 white pills
Nordette	4 light-orange pills
Ogestrel	2 white pills
Ovral	2 white pills
Preven	2 blue pills
Tri-levlen	4 yellow pills
Triphasil	4 yellow pills
Trivora	4 pink pills

(continued)

Table 10-3. *(continued)*

PROGESTERONE-ONLY PREPARATIONS	
Ovrette	20 yellow pills
Plan B	1 white pill

Adapted from Trussell J, Koenig J, Ellertson C, Stewart F. Preventing unintended pregnancy: the cost-effeciveness of three methods of emergency contraception. Am J Public Health. *1997;87(6):932-937.*

Drug dosage recommendations listed herein are those of the authors and are not endorsed by the US Public Health Service or the US Department of Health and Human Services.

- For the woman who is already taking contraceptive medications, if she has missed a dose, offer emergency contraception in place of one day of her own hormonal pills.
- The overall effectiveness of emergency contraception is 75%.

PREVENTION OF SEXUALLY TRANSMITTED DISEASES: SEE CHAPTER 11.

FORENSIC EVIDENCE COLLECTION

Table 10-2 offers general guidelines for collecting evidence. Only trained healthcare professionals should undertake evidence collection after sexual assault. Improperly collected and poorly handled evidence may damage the victim's criminal case.

DNA Evidence in Sexual Assault

Importance of DNA Evidence

DNA evidence, in conjunction with the development of the Combined DNA Index System (CODIS) and other DNA databases containing convicted offender profiles and DNA profiles obtained from biologic evidence recovered from sexual assault victims and crime scenes, has given new value to the thousands of unanalyzed rape kits sitting in evidence storage facilities around the country.

• With the recent reexamination of evidence using newer DNA methods, sexual assault victims whose credibility was challenged in court during trial and who believed the conviction was an affirmation of their credibility might resent having their credibility questioned again. Some victims may feel guilty about their part in convicting an innocent person.

• Reassure victims that they did the best they could at the time and that memory can be fallible. Victim services providers and criminal justice officials should emphasize the importance of knowing the truth and identifying the right perpetrator. Victim assistance providers and criminal justice officials must be prepared to help victims understand and cope when DNA evidence points to an individual other than the person the victim identified or investigators suspected.

• Provide victims with a simple but thorough explanation of how DNA testing may be used in their case, the process and procedures followed, and the potential outcomes of test results.

• Provide this information orally and in writing if possible.

Forensic DNA Testing

Serologic Tests

Before the late 1980s and the introduction of DNA testing, forensic examination of biologic crime scene evidence involved serologic tests of 2 broad categories:

1. Tests used to identify specific body fluids
2. Tests used to individualize or type biologic evidence

Identifying a body fluid involves first determining whether a substance is blood or semen, for example. Then a second serologic test is often run to demonstrate that the fluid is of human origin. These methods have changed little over the past 30 years. Serologic tests to type or individualize biologic fluid have been discarded for the most part. Only a few useful serologic markers exist but they are expressed in various body fluids. Drawbacks to typing body fluids are as follows:

- Markers are expressed in components of body fluids that cannot be separated, creating complications when analyzing mixtures from 2 or more individuals.
- Some individuals (nonsecretors) do not express their ABO type in their semen or saliva.
- Because 2 individuals often share the same pattern of types for serologic markers, it is difficult to identify the actual source for the markers. This is illustrated by the ABO system, wherein individuals are grouped into 4 broad categories (A, B, O, and AB), with type A, for example, found in 25% to 40% of individuals of Caucasian, African American, and Hispanic populations.

• Thus, the use of serologic markers has proved inconclusive. Because of the low discrimination power of serologic testing, almost no forensic work was conducted on sexual assault cases for which there was no suspect.

DNA Testing

Two tragic sexual assaults/homicides in a small village in England led to a revolution in forensic evaluation. Separated by 3 years, 2 raped, strangled bodies were found within a short distance of each other. Dr. Alec Jeffreys, an academic scientist working at nearby Leicester University, was studying a repetitive DNA sequence found in the human myoglobin gene and discovered that when this repetitive sequence was used as a probe to analyze human DNA, it revealed an amazing level of variability and individuality. Termed the multi-locus probe, its potential use in analyzing human pedigrees was quickly recognized. There was an extremely remote chance that 2 individuals would share the same multi-locus DNA pattern, and it was incorporated into a technique known as restriction fragment length polymorphism (RFLP), birthing the first generation forensic DNA test. Analyzing sperm evidence from the 2 homicide cases, a single individual was found to be responsible for both crimes, and he was eventually tried and convicted for both murders.

Restriction Fragment Length Polymorphism Analysis

• It was calculated how common a particular RFLP pattern would be among the major racial groups.

• DNA is purified, then specifically dissected using restriction enzymes, which recognize a specific sequence in the DNA molecule and cleave the molecule wherever they encounter this sequence. The

DNA molecules of a forensic sample are thus cleaved into a collection of fragments of many different sizes, which are then separated by size under electrophoresis and transferred to a nylon membrane.

• DNA is fixed to the membrane by heating and a panel of single-locus probes is applied sequentially to the membrane. Each recognizes a unique site in the human genome.

• An image is developed on X-ray film that has a series of bands, each of which differs in position because each represents a different DNA fragment size.

• Using 4 different single-locus probes in RFLP testing makes it extremely unlikely that DNA samples collected from 2 different individuals would exhibit the same DNA banding pattern (except for identical twins).

• RFLP testing rapidly replaced serologic testing, but still had 2 problems, as follows:

1. Required a relatively large sample to obtain the DNA test result
2. Required that a biologic sample be relatively fresh so that undegraded DNA could be obtained

Polymerase Chain Reaction Analysis

• The polymerase chain reaction (PCR) process was invented by Dr. Kary Mullis et al. in the 1980s and revolutionized the analysis of small quantities of DNA as well as profoundly changed molecular biology, medical diagnostics, and forensic science. Before PCR, scientists needed to clone a piece of DNA in a labor-intensive process and then replicate it in order to analyze a DNA sequence; this required weeks and was not a guaranteed process. PCR allows a scientist to create millions of copies of a specific DNA sequence in hours, which can then easily be isolated and analyzed.

• The process is like photocopying, except that each copy is of the same quality as the original.

• First, a primer that is a short, chemically synthesized segment of DNA, typically 15 to 40 nucleotides long, is created. Primers may correspond to unique DNA sequences in the human genome, and a pair of primers is used to flank the designated region of interest.

• An enzyme involved in replicating DNA from bacteria found in thermal hot springs is then used along with a thermocycler (an instrument capable of cyclically altering the temperature of a DNA reaction mix, creating denaturation, annealing, and elongation phases for PCR) to replicate the specific DNA sequence.

• Because the copies are multiplied exponentially in the process, extremely small quantities of DNA can be analyzed routinely.

• PCR testing only consumes DNA from the sample after it has been duplicated millions of times, so PCR is typically 50 to 100 times more sensitive than traditional RFLP testing.

• Segments of DNA that are analyzed tend to be relatively short, so the technique works well even with degraded DNA.

• The PCR process can be used to analyze single hairs, cigarette butts, and as few as 50 to 100 sperm; biologic samples recovered from buried human remains, fire victims, and plane crash victims.

• Types of PCR-based forensic tests

1. DQA1 test kit: allowed forensic scientists to characterize a single genetic marker in the human genome.

2. DQA1/Polymarker test kit: added 5 additional genetic markers and provided a means of analyzing a wide variety of biologic samples.
3. D1S80 test kit: used as a complement to the DQA1/Polymarker kit to provide additional discrimination.
4. Forensic test kit based on short tandem repeats (STRs): the discrimination power of STR testing is comparable to that offered by RFLP testing and is used by most crime laboratories in the United States. (Forensic RFLP testing remains in existence largely because convicted offender databases were constructed using the technology; as states reanalyze their convicted offenders with STRs, RFLP testing will become obsolete.)

Convicted Offender Databases

• As of 1998, all 50 states have authorized legislation requiring certain convicted offenders to provide biologic samples for analysis and entry into the CODIS database.

• Legislation in the states varies widely concerning collection, analysis, sample storage, and maintenance of the databases.

Combined DNA Index System

• The DNA Identification Act of 1994 formalized the authority of the Federal Bureau of Investigation (FBI) to establish a national DNA index system for law enforcement purposes. This index, known as CODIS, consists of 3 hierarchic levels, as follows:

1. All DNA profiles originate at the local level (LDIS).
2. They then flow to the state level (SDIS). SDIS allows laboratories within a state to exchange DNA profiles.

3. They finally reach the national level (NDIS). NDIS is the highest level and allows the participating laboratories to exchange and compare DNA profiles among states.
4. The tiered approach allows state and local laboratories to operate their databases in accordance with specific legislative and legal requirements.

- The 2 parts of the CODIS system are as follows:

1. The Forensic Index contains DNA profiles from crime scene evidence, often referred to as forensic unknowns. Matches made among the DNA profiles in the Forensic Index can link evidence from crime scenes, suggesting a serial offender.
2. The Offender Index contains DNA profiles of individuals convicted of crimes that require a biologic sample be provided to law enforcement for DNA profiling.

Table 10-4. Guidelines for Collecting Samples From the Human Body
— Patients have the right to decline collection of samples.
— Use only paper to package evidence.
— Air dry all evidence 30 to 60 minutes, or until dry, before packaging. (Refer to your state or community protocol.)
— Use only one drop of water to moisten swabs.
— Use only cotton-tipped swabs.
— Do not lick sticky seals on evidence envelopes.
— Maintain chain of custody at all times.

Important Biologic Evidence in Sexual Assaults (Table 10-4)

- Investigators working sexual assault cases must examine the entire range of possible biologic evidence that may prove useful in solving a particular case.

1. Make certain that a complete sexual assault kit is collected from the victim, including swabbings from possible bite marks; collection of breast swabs and body swabs when a history of kissing, licking, or sucking is involved; fingernail scrapings or swabbings; the collection of clothing worn directly after the assault; and the collection of clothing worn to the hospital.
2. When several days have elapsed since the incident, cervical swabs from the postpubescent victim should be collected, as well as any loose hairs from the victim or the victim's clothing, and preserved for future testing.

- Collecting biologic evidence from the suspect

1. If they were in custody within a day of the assault, collect penile swabs from male suspects, including the glans, shaft, and scrotum areas.
2. Routinely collect fingernail scrapings or swabbings during a suspect examination because they often prove valuable in alleged digital penetration.
3. Collect clothing from the suspect. Body fluids from the victim may be transferred to the suspect.
4. If the suspect is not apprehended wearing the same clothing believed to have been worn during the assault, obtain a warrant or consent to search any premise where investigators believe the clothing may be found.

5. Document genital abnormalities, tattoos, and venereal warts, which may help corroborate the identity of the suspect.
6. Note evidence of scratches, bites, and abrasions to counter a consent defense by corroborating the use of force by the suspect and/or resistance by the victim.
7. Be aware that some jurisdictions require a search warrant or court order before authorizing a suspect examination to obtain forensic evidence. A template to facilitate this step of the sexual assault investigation can be invaluable.

• Examination of the environment where the assault took place

1. Examine vehicles, apartments, and houses under appropriate conditions with an alternate light source to detect the presence of possible biologic fluids.
2. Look for condoms, tissues, and hairs at the scene.

• Collecting reference samples

1. Reference standards must be collected from the victim, suspect, and all consensual partners.
2. Failure to collect these reference standards delays DNA testing and can make interpretation of test results incomplete.

Collection Procedures

Unknown Specimens

• DNA on clothing: remove clothing one item at a time and place in separate paper sacks. Take care not to fold through an observed stain. Photograph stains before packaging. Examine clothing for signs of force and relay information to police officers.

Ask whether clothing from the assault is available at another site and relay this information to police officers. Document using an appropriate clothing documentation form.

- Oral swabs in cases of oral copulation: take 2 cotton swabs and carefully swab between the cheek and gums, upper and lower lip and gums, where the gum meets the palate, and behind the incisors. Place these 2 swabs into a labeled holder and air dry before packaging, labeling, and documenting.
- Dental floss in cases of oral copulation: have the victim floss her teeth and collect the floss in a small envelope or paper bindle.
- Biologic material in hair: cut out the suspected area and place it in a paper bindle. Cut out only what is needed to obtain an adequate sample and be sensitive to how the collection process will affect the victim's appearance.
- Biologic material on skin:

1. Semen: moisten a swab with one drop of water and roll it over the area to collect the specimen. Then place the swab in a labeled holder and allow to air dry before packaging.
2. Saliva and bite marks: use a double swab technique. Moisten a cotton swab with one drop of sterile water and roll over the area, then set this swab aside in a labeled swab holder. Roll another nonmoistened swab over the same area. Label, dry, and package both swabs; it is not necessary to identify which was the moistened swab.

- DNA on miscellaneous items and surfaces:

1. Condoms: the condom may be found in the vagina when performing a pelvic examination.

Photograph it where it is found, then carefully remove it and place it in multiple paper bags. Store it frozen as soon as possible. The crime laboratory will later collect swabs from the inside and outside surfaces of the condom.

2. Shoes: photograph any stained areas with the shoes on the person, then remove the shoes and photograph again from different angles. Collect the shoes in a paper bag.

• DNA from an unknown hair: if a loose hair is observed on the person being examined, photograph it and collect it using clean gloved fingers. Sticky-surface note paper works well to pick it up, depending on what type of surface it is located. Alternatively, a swab may be used and placed in a paper bindle. Never use forceps or tweezers to collect unknown hair evidence because you may pluck the victim's or suspect's own hair.

Known Reference Specimens

• Either a buccal swab or a blood specimen is collected from the person being examined.

1. An oral swab is collected by rolling a cotton swab on the inside of the cheeks, drying it, and then packaging it in a labeled holder.
2. One purple-topped tube of blood is collected for the known blood DNA sample. Different methods of preservation are available, but the entire tube is submitted with the identifying information by placing it in a bubble pack and then sealing it in the rape kit. Refrigerate the kit to ensure preservation of the blood sample. Alternatively, blood may be placed onto a blood preservation card, which has quarter-size circles

that are saturated with the sample blood and then dried, labeled, packaged, and sealed in the kit.

- All samples are transported to the police property room or forensic laboratory by law enforcement, maintaining the chain of custody at all times, where they may be analyzed later by crime laboratory personnel.
- Meticulous and thorough evidence collection is important because collected evidence may prove crucial not only to implicate the guilty but also to exonerate the innocent.

References

American College of Emergency Physicians (ACEP). *Evaluation and Management of the Sexually Assaulted or Sexually Abused Patient.* Washington, DC: US Dept of Health and Human Services, Health Resources and Services Administration, Maternal and Child Health Bureau; 1999.

Bechtel K, Podrazik M. Evaluation of the adolescent rape victim. *Pediatr Clin North Am.* 1999;46:809-823, xii.

Budowle B, Chakraborty R, Giusti AM, Eisenberg AJ, Allen RC. Analysis of the VNTR locus D1S80 by the PCR followed by high-resolution PAGE. *Am J Hum Genet.* 1991;48:137-144.

Federal Bureau of Investigation (FBI). *The FBI's Combined DNA Index System (CODIS) Program Brochure.* Washington, DC: US Dept of Justice; 2000.

Fregeau CJ, Fourney RM. DNA typing with fluorescently tagged short tandem repeats: a sensitive and accurate approach to human identification. *Biotechniques.* 1993;15:100-119.

Gaensslen RE. *Sourcebook in Forensic Serology, Immunology, and Biochemistry*. Washington, DC: National Institute of Justice; 1983.

Hampton HL. Care of the woman who has been raped. *N Engl J Med*. 1995;332(4):234-237.

Inman K, Rudin N. *An Introduction to Forensic DNA Analysis*. New York, NY: CRC Press; 1997.

Jeffreys AJ, Wilson V, Thein SL. Individual specific fingerprints of human DNA. *Nature*. 1985;316:76-79.

Lenahan LC, Ernst A, Johnson B. Colposcopy in evaluation of the adult sexual assault victim. *Am J Emerg Med*. 1998;16:183-184.

Linden JA. Sexual assault. *Emerg Med Clin North Am*. 1999;17:685-697, vii.

Mullis KB, Faloona F, Scharf S, Saiki R, Horn G, Erlich H. Specific enzymatic amplification of DNA in vitro: the polymerase chain reaction. *Cold Spring Harb Symp Quant Biol*. 1986;51:263-273.

National Research Council (NRC). *DNA Technology in Forensic Science*. Washington, DC: National Academy Press; 1992.

National Research Council (NRC). *The Evaluation of Forensic DNA Evidence*. Washington, DC: National Academy Press; 1996.

Public Health Service guidelines for the management of healthcare worker exposures to HIV and recommendations for postexposure prophylaxis. *MMWR* [document online]. 1998. Available at: http://www.cdc.gov/mmwr/preview/mmwrhtml/00052722.htm. Accessed April 13, 2001.

Reynolds R, Sensabaugh G, Blake E. Analysis of genetic markers in forensic DNA samples using the polymerase chain reaction. *Anal Chem*. 1991;63:2-15.

Saferstein R, ed. *Forensic Science Handbook*. Englewood Cliffs, NJ: Prentice-Hall Inc; 1982.

Saferstein R, ed. *Forensic Science Handbook*. Vol 2. Englewood Cliffs, NJ: Prentice-Hall Inc; 1988.

Schwarcz S, Whittington W. Sexual assault and sexually transmitted diseases: detection and management in adults and children. *Rev Infect Dis*. 1990;12:682-690.

Sexual Assault Evidence Collection Kit Cat. No. VEC100.Youngsville, NC: Sirchie Finger Print Laboratories, Inc; 2002.

Sexually Transmitted Diseases treatment guidelines 2002. *MMWR* [document online]. 2002. Available at: http://www.cdc.gov/mmwr/PDF/rr/rr5106.pdf. Accessed July 3, 2002.

Stewart F, Trussell J. Prevention of pregnancy resulting from rape: a neglected preventive health measure. *Am J Prev Med*. 2000;19:228-229.

Sweet D, Lorente M, Lorente JA, Valenzuela A, Villanueva E. An improved method to recover saliva from human skin: the double swab technique. *J Forensic Sci*. 1997;42:320-322.

Trussell J, Koenig J, Ellertson C, Stewart F. Preventing unintended pregnancy: the cost-effectiveness of three methods of emergency contraception. *Am J Public Health*. 1997;87:932-937.

Wambaugh J. *The Blooding*. New York, NY: Bantam Doubleday Dell Publishing Group; 1989.

Sexually Transmitted Diseases and Pregnancy

Margot Schwartz, MD
Jeanne Marrazzo, MD, MPH
Janice B. Asher, MD
Elizabeth M. Datner, MD

Male and female victims of sexual assault often fear acquiring sexually transmitted diseases (STDs), including human immunodeficiency virus (HIV) infection. In addition, women who are sexually assaulted may fear becoming pregnant as a result of the attack. STDs in child victims are discussed in Chapter 6.

Sexually Transmitted Diseases

- If the victim comes for medical care within 72 hours of the assault, many STDs will not have had sufficient time to incubate and thus will not be detected.
- If *Chlamydia trachomatis* is present in the semen of the assailant, it may be detected in a female assault victim immediately after the assault.
- It is rarely possible to determine whether an STD was present before the assault. Proving that an STD was acquired as the result of an assault may carry important legal or emotional ramifications.
- Factors that predict the risk of acquiring an STD include the following:

1. Whether or not penile penetration and ejaculation occurred
2. The type of sexual assault that occurred (vaginal, anal, or oral)

3. The number of assailants
4. The victim's susceptibility to infection
5. The size of the inoculum for a given pathogen
6. The organism's infectivity

• Preventive therapy after sexual assault for viral STDs is not routinely offered.

• If recognized at the postassault examination, gonorrhea, chlamydia, and trichomoniasis can be treated.

• Vaccination for preventable STDs such as hepatitis B should be considered.

Recognition and Treatment of Common Sexually Transmitted Diseases and Associated Syndromes

STDs can be caused by bacteria, viruses, protozoa, or treponemes. In addition, ectoparasites such as lice or scabies are parasites that live on skin or hair and may be transmitted during an assault. Chapter 6 summarizes the clinical characteristics of the most common STDs; those not listed there are included here. **Table 11-1** summarizes the treatment options for STDs commonly diagnosed after sexual assault.

Chancroid

• Caused by the bacteria *Haemophilus ducreyi*

• An uncommon cause of genital ulcer in most areas of the United States

• Signs/symptoms: ulcers that are often painful (differentiating them from ulcers of syphilis); tender regional lymphadenopathy

• Diagnosed only by culture; if suspected, consult an expert

Table 11-1. Antibiotic Regimens Used to Treat Common STDs Found After Sexual Assault

GONORRHEA* (uncomplicated urethritis, cervicitis, or proctitis)

Antibiotic	Dose and Route	Duration
Ceftriaxone	125 mg IM†	Single dose
Cefixime	400 mg PO	Single dose
Ciprofloxacin	500 mg PO	Single dose
Levofloxacin	250 mg PO	Single dose

CHLAMYDIA (uncomplicated cervicitis, or proctitis)

Antibiotic	Dose and Route	Duration
Azithromycin	1 g PO	Single dose
Doxycycline	100 mg PO bid**	7 days
Alternatives:		
— Levofloxacin	500 mg qd	7 days
— Ofloxacin	300 mg bid	7 days
— Erythromycin base	500 mg qd	7 days

TRICHOMONIASIS

Antibiotic	Dose and Route	Duration
Metronidazole	2 g PO	Single dose
Metronidazole	500 mg bid	7 days

BACTERIAL VAGINOSIS

Antibiotic	Dose and Route	Duration
Metronidazole	500 mg PO bid	7 days
Metronidazole gel (0.75%)	5 g intravaginally qd	7 days
Clindamycin cream (2%)	5 g intravaginally qhs	7 days
Clindamycin	300 mg PO bid	7 days

(continued)

Table 11-1. *(continued)*

PRIMARY HERPES SIMPLEX VIRUS INFECTION
(first clinical episode)

Antibiotic	Dose and Route	Duration
Acyclovir	400 mg PO tid	7-10 days
Acyclovir	200 mg PO 5 times daily	7-10 days
Famciclovir	250 mg PO tid	7-10 days
Valacyclovir	1 g PO bid	7-10 days

**When treating for gonorrhea, also treat empirically for* Chlamydia.
†IM=intramuscularly, PO=orally, mg=milligrams, g=gram.
***qd=once daily, bid=twice daily, tid=three times daily, qid=four times daily, qhs=at night.*

Drug dosage recommendations listed herein are those of the authors and are not endorsed by the US Public Health Service or the US Department of Health and Human Services.

Mucopurulent Cervicitis

• Characterized by the presence of mucopurulent endocervical exudate, with easily induced cervical bleeding and edematous cervical ectopy possible.

• Over half of cases have no known etiology.

• Controversial criteria for diagnosis; in women under age 25 years, presence of at least 30 polymorphonuclear lymphocytes per 1000 hpf on examination of endocervical exudate suggests but does not offer definitive evidence of infection; many experts recommend that this test not be performed.

• If mucopurulent cervicitis is noted, woman should be tested for gonorrhea and *Chlamydia*.

• Preventive regimens are listed in **Table 11-2**.

Pelvic Inflammatory Disease

- Refers to any combination of endometritis, salpingitis, tubo-ovarian abscess, and pelvic peritonitis
- Associated with sexually transmitted pathogens as well as bacteria that normally colonize the vagina
- Must recognize and treat early to avoid sequelae such as infertility, chronic pelvic pain, and ectopic pregnancy
- Increased risk with vaginal douching
- Signs/symptoms: lower abdominal pain, nausea and/or vomiting, fever, vaginal discharge, sometimes a change in menstrual pattern, abdominal tenderness, adnexal tenderness, cervical motion tenderness
- Hospitalization may be needed for patients who are pregnant, unable to take oral therapy, with suspected tubo-ovarian abscess, or who have severe illness with nausea, vomiting, or higher fever, or another surgical diagnosis

Proctitis and Proctocolitis

- At-risk individuals are all those having anal penetration by the assailant's penis
- Signs/symptoms of proctitis: inflammation of the rectum with anorectal pain or itching, tenesmus (a sensation that one must defecate when stool is not passed), or rectal discharge; caused by *Neisseria gonorrhoeae*, *C. trachomatis*, *Treponema pallidum*, and herpes simplex virus
- Signs/symptoms of proctocolitis: inflammation of the colon and rectum; those listed for proctitis plus diarrhea and/or abdominal cramping; caused by enteric pathogens transmitted by fecal-oral contact (*Campylobacter* sp., *Shigella* sp., *Entamoeba histolytica*, or *C. trachomatis* serovars)

Table 11-2. Recommended Treatment for Pelvic Inflammatory Disease

OUTPATIENT

— Levofloxacin 500 mg once daily or ofloxacin 400 mg twice daily
PLUS
Metronidazole 500 mg twice daily for 14 days

OR

— Ceftriaxone 250 mg or probenecid 1 g with cefoxitin 2 g intramuscularly (once)
PLUS
Doxycycline 100 mg orally twice daily for 14 days, with or without metronidazole 500 mg twice daily for 14 days

INPATIENT

— Intravenous cefoxitin or cefotetan
PLUS
Doxycycline 100 mg intravenously or orally twice daily for 14 days

OR

— Intravenous clindamycin plus gentamicin initially, followed by clindamycin 450 mg orally 4 times daily or doxycycline 100 mg orally twice daily to complete 14 days of therapy

Drug dosage recommendations listed herein are those of the authors and are not endorsed by the US Public Health Service or the US Department of Health and Human Services.

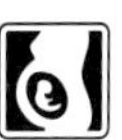

• Diagnosed on anoscopy, abdominal examination, Gram stain of exudate or mucus obtained, rectal cultures and cultures for herpes simplex virus, dark-field examination, and RPR; obtain stool samples for evaluation of enteric pathogens

Pubic Lice

• Caused by *Phthirus pubis*

• Signs/symptoms: itching and/or visible lice or nits in the pubic hair; may also affect other areas of the body with hair, including the thighs, eyelashes, eyebrows, and trunk

• Treatments (NOTE: none of these should be used around the eyes)

1. Permethrin 1% cream rinse (Nix)
2. Pyrethrin lotion (Rid, etc.)
3. Lindane 1% shampoo (Kwell, Scabene); should not be used in pregnant or lactating women, young children, individuals with severe dermatitis or open skin lesions, or those with seizure disorders or after a bath
4. All clothing and bedding must be washed and dried at high temperatures to prevent reinfection

Scabies

• Caused by *Sarcoptes scabiei*

• Signs/symptoms: itching and a papular erythematous rash, often with excoriation; commonly affects the finger webs and arms, trunk, inguinal area, labia majora, penis, scrotum, or buttocks

• Diagnosis confirmed by microscopic examination of a scraping from a fresh papule; examination under oil or potassium hydroxide (KOH) may reveal the mite, eggs, or feces of *S. scabiei*

- Treatments

1. Permethrin 5% cream (Elimite) recommended
2. Lindane 1% lotion or cream an alternative; observe the precautions listed above
3. All clothing and bedding must be washed and dried at high temperatures to prevent reinfection

Viral Hepatitis

- Hepatitis A and hepatitis B viruses can be transmitted by sexual contact.

- Hepatitis A

1. Shed in the feces; transmission is fecal-oral.
2. Men who have sex with men are at higher risk of sexually acquired hepatitis A.
3. Infection is self-limited; treatment is supportive.
4. Preventive vaccination after sexual assault should be considered if a high-risk exposure occurred.

- Hepatitis B

1. From 30% to 60% of new cases in the United States are transmitted sexually.
2. May become chronic in 1% to 6% of cases.
3. Preventive vaccination after sexual assault recommended; for the highest risk exposures from an assailant believed to be a carrier of hepatitis B, hepatitis B immunoglobulin can be given to the nonimmune victim.

History and Physical Examination

- **Table 11-3** lists important information to obtain from the sexual assault victim regarding the sexual history.

Table 11-3. Important Info to Assess STD Risk for Sexual Assault Victims

1. Date and time of the assault
2. Interval between the assault and the initial medical evaluation
3. Number of assailants
4. Description and identification, if possible, of the assailant(s)
5. If the assailant is known, is his/her HIV status known?
6. Are the assailant's history of STD and risk behaviors, such as intravenous drug use known?
7. Description of the assault, including type of sexual contact (vaginal, anal, and oral), penetration by a body part or other object, ejaculation, condom use, extragenital contact (vaginal, anal, and oral), trauma or threats that occurred, use of weapons by the assailant. Include a description of any contact with the assailant's blood or bodily fluid (especially on mucosal surfaces or breaks in the skin).
8. History of consensual sexual intercourse (ever, most recent, including any voluntary sexual intercourse that occurred between the assault and the initial evaluation, or between the initial evaluation and follow-up examination)
9. Last menstrual period and pregnancy status (for female victims)
10. Use of contraception (for female victims)
11. History of bathing, urinating, defecating, douching, changing clothes, or brushing teeth between the assault and the initial examination
12. History of STD in the victim
13. History of previous sexual assault
14. Any symptoms including vaginal or rectal discharge; pelvic or rectal pain; genital, perianal, or oral lesions
15. History of prior or chronic medical conditions, including thrombosis, liver disease, or hypertension, which are theoretical contraindications to pregnancy prophylaxis
16. Medication allergy

• Perform a targeted examination for STDs along with collection of specimens for STD testing.

1. Examine the genitals, mouth, throat, and anus.
2. Inspect the lower abdomen, inguinal areas, thighs, hands, palms, and soles for rashes or lesions.
3. Examine the inguinal and femoral areas for lymphadenopathy.
4. In women, perform a speculum examination of the vagina and cervix and a bimanual pelvic examination; colposcopy to evaluate internal genital trauma.
5. In men and women, evaluate the anus for seminal fluid and signs of trauma (eg, relaxed external sphincter, fissures, hemorrhoids).
6. If anorectal injury is suspected, perform proctoscopy or anoscopy.
7. In men, inspect the penis, including retraction of the foreskin and visualization of the urethral meatus; examine the prostate gland during a digital rectal examination.

Diagnostic Evaluation

• Perform a microscopic analysis of a cervical Gram stain for evidence of gram-negative intracellular diplococci (indicating gonorrhea) and a saline preparation and *Trichomonas* culture (if available) of vaginal fluid **(Table 11-4)**.

• Culture for *Trichomonas vaginalis.*

• Perform saline microscopy to look for clue cells or yeast.

• Perform the "whiff test" to detect fishy odor indicative of bacterial vaginosis.

Table 11-4. Recommended Evaluation for STDs in Adult and Adolescent Victims of Sexual Assault

WOMEN

— Saline preparation of vaginal fluid to examine for motile trichomonads, clue cells, and yeast
— Culture of vaginal fluid for *T. vaginalis*
— Culture or NAA tests for *N. gonorrhoeae* and *C. trachomatis*
— Serum testing for HIV, hepatitis B (surface antigen and antibody), and syphilis
— Culture of suspicious lesions for herpes simplex virus if diagnosis was not established
— Optional: pH of vaginal fluid and whiff test for evidence of bacterial vaginosis: cervical Gram stain for evidence of gram-negative intracellular diplococci and PMNs

MEN

— Culture or NAA tests for *N. gonorrhoeae* and *C. trachomatis* from any site of penetration or attempted penetration
— Gram stain of any rectal or urethral discharge for evidence of gram-negative intracellular diplococci and PMNs
— Serum testing for HIV, hepatitis B, and syphilis

FOLLOW-UP EXAMINATIONS

— 2 weeks after the assault or sooner (1 week) if no prophylactic therapy was provided
— Repeat tests as above, unless prophylactic treatment was provided or if symptoms are reported
— Follow-up serologic testing for HIV, hepatitis B, and syphilis 6, 12, and 24 weeks after the assault if initial results were negative

- If rectal or urethral discharge is present, perform a Gram stain to look for PMNs and gram-negative intraceullar diplococci.
- Culture a cervical, urethral, pharyngeal, or rectal specimen for *N. gonorrhoeae* when penetration or attempted penetration has occurred.
- Obtain a Dacron-tipped swab of the areas listed above (except the throat) to detect *C. trachomatis.*
- NAA tests are sensitive in detecting *C. trachomatis* and *N. gonorrhoeae*; while false-positive results occur rarely, in a sexual assault evaluation it may be necessary to confirm nonculture tests by a second FDA-approved nucleic amplification test that targets a different molecule from the initial test; LCR and PCR tests are approved using specimens only from the cervix, urethra, and urine. Other nonculture tests for *C. trachomatis* are the DNA probe, fluorescent antibody, and enzyme immunoassay (EIA) tests. Culture for gonorrhea and *Chlamydia* are the gold standard for legal evidence.
- If prophylactic treatment was used after nonculture techniques during the initial evaluation, retesting for legal evidence is problematic.
- Male victims are at higher risk for syphilis, HIV, and enteropathogens; they should be tested and treated for these illnesses if symptomatic.
- Perform baseline serologic tests for hepatitis B (in a victim not previously vaccinated) and syphilis; offer serologic testing for HIV; perform serum or urine pregnancy tests for women.
- Perform a follow-up examination in 2 weeks to detect newly acquired infections and continue efforts to counsel and treat victims of sexual assault.

1. Include repeat testing for gonorrhea and *Chlamydia*.
2. Include saline microscopy of vaginal fluid in women if they did not receive prophylactic therapy against specific STDs or if they have new symptoms of STDs.

• Perform follow-up serologic testing for syphilis and HIV 6, 12, and 24 weeks after the assault if the test results were negative at the initial examination and offer follow-up pregnancy tests to women at these points.

Treatment and Prophylaxis of STDs

• Offer treatment for any STDs diagnosed at the initial follow-up examination; be aware that follow-up rates for victims of sexual assault are poor and encourage the victim to come for care.

• Offer routine prophylaxis at the initial examination **(Table 11-5)**.

Human Immunodeficiency Virus Exposure Prophylaxis

• The risk of acquiring HIV infection through sexual assault is low, but HIV seroconversion has occurred after sexual assault. The highest rate of HIV acquisition is with receptive anal intercourse among men who have sex with men and with receptive vaginal intercourse.

• Individuals with high viral loads of HIV in the blood are more likely to transmit HIV through sexual intercourse than are those with low viral loads.

• Serum levels are generally highest immediately after seroconversion during the acute or primary HIV illness or in the late stages of acquired immunodeficiency syndrome (AIDS).

Table 11-5. STD Prophylaxis in the Adult Victim of Sexual Assault
— Ceftriaxone 125 mg intramuscularly once PLUS Azithromycin 1 g orally once, or doxycycline 100 mg twice daily for 7 days PLUS Metronidazole 2 g once (for women or men who were assaulted by women)
— Hepatitis B vaccine if no prior history of vaccination or natural immunity; first dose at initial examination, second dose at 1 to 2 months, and third dose at 4 to 6 months after the initial dose
— HIV prophylaxis (optional): see **Table 11-6**.
Drug dosage recommendations listed herein are those of the authors and are not endorsed by the US Public Health Service or the US Department of Health and Human Services.

- If the HIV status of the assailant is not known, determine if the assailant has any known risk factors for HIV (intravenous drug use or a male who has male sex partners) and note the type of contact that occurred during the assault and to which body fluids the victim may have been exposed; the number of assailants may also be a factor, as may the type and severity of physical trauma.
- Be aware that STDs are cofactors for HIV transmission, so the presence of an STD, especially a genital ulcer, may increase the likelihood that HIV transmission will occur.
- If the victim did not know the assailant, so that risk cannot be established, consider the length of time since the exposure, the health and reproductive

status of the victim, the local epidemiology of HIV, and the victim's attitude toward postexposure prophylaxis. Clearly discuss the risks versus benefits of postexposure prophylaxis before it is given.

- Beginning postexposure prophylaxis within 4 hours of a blood exposure is the most effective method.
- The choice of antiretroviral agents used for postexposure prophylaxis is based on guidelines for occupationally exposed individuals and for treating patients with known HIV infection.

1. Once antiretroviral agents are initiated, continue for 4 weeks unless the assailant was confirmed to be HIV negative and is not likely to be in the process of seroconversion or a prohibitive side effect develops.
2. Side effects to antiretroviral agents are common. Counsel the victim about what to expect; encourage the victim to call if side effects develop.
3. Make a follow-up appointment within 2 weeks. Perform a complete blood count and liver function test. If a protease inhibitor is used, assess serum glucose levels; if indinavir is used, do an amylase evaluation and urinalysis; and if didanosine is used, perform an amylase test.
4. Obtain a baseline HIV test in 6 weeks, 3 months, and 6 months.
5. **Table 11-6** lists the suggested regimens for HIV postexposure prophylaxis.

- Educate the victim regarding the symptoms of primary HIV infection: prolonged febrile or flu-like illness, fatigue, lymphadenopathy, rash, and pharyngitis.

- Cost factors

1. For high-risk exposures, postexposure prophylaxis should be offered regardless of cost.
2. For a 2-drug antiviral regimen, the cost is about $500 for a 4-week supply; the cost is roughly doubled if a protease inhibitor is added.

Emergency Oral Contraception

- Five percent of women of reproductive age who are raped in the United States will become pregnant; approximately 32 000 rape-related pregnancies occur annually.

- Immediate access to emergency oral contraception should be made available to all female victims of sexual assault who seek medical care.

- A common regimen is 2 doses of oral contraceptives 12 hours apart. **Table 11-7** lists recommended regimens.

- The most common side effects of emergency oral contraception are nausea and vomiting. Other effects include delayed return of menses, fatigue, headaches, breast tenderness, and abdominal pain.

- Counsel all women who receive emergency oral contraception regarding the predicted efficacy and potential side effects. Also remind them that oral contraception or hormonal contraceptives do not prevent STDs.

- Instruct the victim to seek pregnancy testing if menses does not resume within a week of the expected date.

Table 11-6. Recommended Regimens for Postexposure Initiated Within 72 Hours of Sexual Exposure to HIV

Treatment Regimen (4 weeks)

Zidovudine (ZDV) 300 mg orally twice daily or 200 mg orally 3 times daily
PLUS
Lamivudine (3TC) 150 mg orally twice daily (Zidovudine 300 mg/lamivudine 150 mg are available in a combination pill)

OR

Stavudine (D4T) 40 mg orally twice daily
PLUS
Lamivudine (3TC) 150 mg orally twice daily

OR

Stavudine (D4T) 40 mg orally twice daily
PLUS
Didanosine (ddI) 200 mg orally twice daily

Consider adding to either regimen for highest risk exposures (assailant with a viral load >50 000 copies/mL or suspected advanced HIV disease or has suspected resistance to the one or both nucleoside analogue medications in the regimen):

Nelfinavir 1250 mg orally every 12 hours or 750 mg every 8 hours
OR
Indinavir 800 mg orally every 8 hours
OR
Alternatives: efavirenz, abacavir, lopinavir/ritonavir

Drug dosage recommendations listed herein are those of the authors and are not endorsed by the US Public Health Service or the US Department of Health and Human Services.

Table 11-7. Recommended Regimens for Emergency Oral Contraception
Levonorgestrel Regimen — Levonorgestrel 0.75 mg within 72 hours of assault, and repeated 12 hours later
Yuzpe Regimen — 100 µg of ethinyl estradiol and 1 mg of norgestrel (2 Ovral) within 72 hours of assault, and repeated 12 hours later
Drug dosage recommendations listed herein are those of the authors and are not endorsed by the US Public Health Service or the US Department of Health and Human Services.

Pregnancy

Violence in pregnancy represents a unique challenge in that there are 2 victims: mother and fetus.

Domestic Violence During Pregnancy

• An abuser employs many tactics to maintain power over his partner, including physical violence, emotional abuse, intimidation, and isolation. Sexual assault and/or coercion is yet another tactic for exerting control over a partner.

• More pregnant women die as a direct result of domestic violence than of any medical complication of pregnancy, yet more than 60% of obstetrician-gynecologists do not routinely screen pregnant patients for violence. Domestic violence during pregnancy is more common than preeclampsia, gestational diabetes, and placenta previa, with an incidence of 4% to 20%.

• The single greatest risk factor for partner violence in pregnancy and postpartum is a history

of violence by that partner within the year before pregnancy. Of women abused in the year before pregnancy, 40% to 60% are abused during pregnancy as well.

• Domestic violence tends to escalate in frequency and intensity during pregnancy.

1. Pregnancy represents a new opportunity for the maintenance of power and control.
2. The partner may be jealous toward the baby.
3. The abuser may feel anger toward the baby if the pregnancy was unintended or unwanted.
4. Other stresses may be present (eg, obstetric complications, financial concerns). Stress does not cause violence, but increased stress may be a precipitating factor in the escalation of violence.

Pregnancy as a Window of Opportunity for Intervention

• The numerous visits with clinicians that pregnancy affords and the common goal of delivering a healthy baby provide the opportunity for a trusting relationship to develop between patient and provider.

• During pregnancy, an abused woman may do on behalf of her baby what she would not otherwise do for herself.

• Social, economic, and community support systems are in place for the pregnant woman and can be used to a greater advantage.

Domestic Violence and Child Abuse

• Child abuse and maternal abuse are inextricably linked. Nearly 60% of abused children have mothers who are also abused.

• Women who were abused as children have earlier first pregnancies than women without such a history.

• Women who were sexually abused as children are almost 5 times as likely to be sexually abused as adults.

• Unintended pregnancy is a common outcome in abusive relationships because abused women may not be able to negotiate sexual activity or contraceptive use.

• Barriers to addressing domestic violence in pregnancy are as follows:

1. Pregnant women may feel more vulnerable emotionally and financially, including being dependent on her partner's health insurance.
2. Women may also be particularly anxious to try to keep the family together.
3. A woman may hope that the situation will improve after the baby is born and that her most intense fears are groundless.

Sexual Assault and Abuse of Pregnant Women

• Pregnant women who are abused may be at increased risk for various obstetric, medical, and psychosocial complications.

1. Sexual assault of the pregnant woman who has a placenta previa places her and the fetus at risk for potentially fatal hemorrhage.
2. Genital trauma in the pregnant woman may be much more severe than in the nonpregnant woman because of the area's increased vascularity during pregnancy.

- Clinical manifestations include inadequate prenatal care, abdominal and genital trauma, adverse outcome for the pregnancy, unintended pregnancy and STDs, depression, drug and alcohol abuse, and pregnancy termination.
- Red flags in identifying abuse and assault are as follows:

1. History of abuse in year prior to pregnancy
2. Unintended pregnancy
3. Late entry into prenatal care
4. Poor compliance with appointments, medical recommendations
5. Maternal trauma, particularly of the breast, abdomen, or genitals
6. Fetal trauma, particularly fractures
7. Poor weight gain
8. STDs
9. Depression
10. Substance abuse
11. Partner refuses to leave or answers questions for woman
12. Adolescent pregnancy

Clinician Response to Abuse During Pregnancy

- First, identify the abuse through your assessment; this is a powerful form of intervention.
- Take a history about the nature and severity of abuse to assess danger and potential lethality.
- Be aware that the pelvic examination and the experience of labor may be particularly traumatic for women who have been sexually abused or assaulted.

• When a woman seems especially frightened while being examined, make the examination as patient-driven as possible.

• As with all victims of abuse, it is vital to assist the pregnant patient to take necessary steps to ensure her safety and that of her baby, as follows:

1. Offer assistance at each prenatal appointment.
2. Make safety assessment and planning a part of every prenatal visit for women who are being abused.
3. Provide safety information and lists of local resources, hotlines, and shelters. Because women may not feel safe taking such information or deny needing it, place it in all lavatory areas, where it can be read in private.
4. Document the patient's statements concerning abuse, including the perpetrator's name and weapons used.
5. Document the physical findings associated with battering and sexual assault, ideally using photographs.

Role of Pediatricians in Preventing Child Abuse and Domestic Violence

• Perform a domestic violence assessment.

• Ask questions about domestic violence in the child's presence as long as the child is sufficiently young that he or she will not report the content of the discussion back to the abusive parent.

• Incorporate the topics of child and domestic abuse in the context of discussions about discipline, or into general home safety questioning.

• When maternal and child abuse are suspected, the pediatric practitioner is legally obligated to report

the abuse and take steps to ensure the safety of mother and child. Interdisciplinary, collaborative approaches are important in this regard.

Abuse and Assault in Adolescent Pregnancy

- Adolescents are overrepresented among abused pregnant women, with as many as 29% of pregnant adolescents experiencing abuse, including sexual abuse and assault.
- Pregnant teens, compared to those who are not pregnant, have a much greater likelihood of having a history of being sexually abused as children.
- Teen parenthood is associated with particularly painful outcomes for mother and baby.

1. Teen mothers display more aggressive, inappropriate, and abusive behavior toward their babies.
2. Two major risk factors for infanticide are maternal age under 15 years and short interpregnancy interval among cases where the maternal age is under 17 years.
3. School-age children of adolescent mothers have more cognitive and behavior problems than do children of adult mothers.

- Abused teens are more likely to smoke cigarettes and abuse drugs and alcohol during pregnancy.
- Their school drop-out rate is twice that of nonabused teens.
- They have a much higher rate of STDs.
- They enter into prenatal care much later than nonabused mothers.
- They are less likely than adult women to have long-term emotional, financial, and familial attachments to their partners.

• They may feel less compelled or threatened to remain in abusive relationships.

• If they are in school, systems and social supports are in place to assist them and their children.

Sexual Assault Resulting in Pregnancy

Most women who have been raped do not seek medical care and, therefore, do not have access to emergency contraception or STD prophylaxis. An estimated 22 000 pregnancies in the United States could be prevented if all women who had been raped had emergency contraception available to them within 72 hours of the assault.

Prophylaxis and Treatment of STDs in Pregnancy

• Because of the effects of certain antibiotics and other medications on the fetus, the treatment of pregnant women with STDs may differ from that of nonpregnant women.

• Genital herpes (herpes simplex virus type II [HSV 2]): acyclovir has not been approved for routine use for recurrent herpes or herpes prophylaxis in pregnancy but may be used to treat a primary outbreak and for any outbreak at term.

• Human papillomavirus (HPV; condyloma accuminata, or genital warts): podophyllin is contraindicated in pregnancy but cryotherapy and acid preparations can be safely used.

• *Trichomonas:* pregnant women may be treated with a 2 g single-dose regimen of metronidazole.

• *Chlamydia:* erythromycin and amoxicillin are listed as drugs of choice for treating chlamydia in pregnant women, but azithromycin appears to be safe and is

linked with markedly improved compliance because it is a single-dose treatment. Doxycycline and all other tetracyclines are contraindicated in pregnancy because they damage fetal bones and teeth. Erythromycin estolate is contraindicated because of its association with drug-induced hepatotoxicity.

• Gonorrhea: treat with an appropriate cephalosporin (eg, cefixime or ceftriaxone) unless the woman cannot take cephalosporins; in that case spectinomycin is used. Quinolones are contraindicated.

• Syphilis: penicillin is the drug of choice, but pregnant women who are allergic to penicillin cannot take tetracycline, the alternative given to nonpregnant women who are allergic to penicillin. Erythromycin cannot be used because it does not adequately treat fetal syphilis, which can cause fetal and neonatal death along with other potentially devastating complications. Penicillin-allergic pregnant women should undergo penicillin desensitization in a hospital setting, then receive a therapeutic course of penicillin. Jarisch-Herxheimer reaction occurs rarely in pregnant women, causing uterine contractions. Thus, patients receiving penicillin should remain in the clinic or physician's office when they receive their first dose of penicillin.

• Hepatitis B: use of hepatitis B and hepatitis B immunoglobulin vaccines is not contraindicated in pregnancy.

• HIV infection: HIV-positive women should be offered treatment with zidovudine (ZDV) to reduce the risk of HIV transmission to the fetus. HIV-positive mothers should not breastfeed because HIV crosses into breast milk.

References

American Academy of Pediatrics Committee on Child Abuse and Neglect. The role of the pediatrician in recognizing and intervening on behalf of abused women. *Pediatrics.* 1998;101:1091-1092.

Amsel R, Totten PA, Spiegel CA, Chen KC, Eschenbach D, Holmes KK. Nonspecific vaginitis. Diagnostic criteria and microbial and epidemiologic associations. *Am J Med.* 1983;74:14-22.

Asher J, Berlin M, Petty V. Abuse of pregnant adolescents: what have we learned? *Obstet Gynecol.* 2000;95:41S.

Bamberger JD, Waldo CR, Gerberding JL, Katz MH. Postexposure prophylaxis for human immunodeficiency virus (HIV) infection following sexual assault. *Am J Med.* 1999;106:323-326.

Berenson A, SanMiguel VV, Wilkinson GS. Prevalence of physical and sexual assault in pregnant adolescents. *J Adolesc Health.* 1992;13:466-469.

Boyer D, Fine D. Sexual abuse as a factor in adolescent pregnancy and child maltreatment. *Fam Plann Perspect.* 1992;24(4):4-19.

Campbell JC, Alford P. The dark consequences of marital rape. *Am J Nurs.* 1989;89:946-949.

Campbell JC, Oliver C, Bullock L. Why battering during pregnancy? *AWHONNS Clin Issues Perinat Womens Health Nurs.* 1993;4:343-349.

Centers for Disease Control and Prevention (CDC). Updated US Public Health Service guidelines for the management of occupational exposures to HBV, HCV, and HIV and recommendations for postexposure prophylaxis. *MMWR Recomm Rep.* June 29, 2001;50(RR11);1-42.

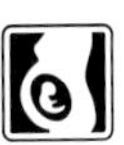

Centers for Disease Control and Prevention (CDC). Sexually transmitted diseases treatment guidelines 2002. *MMWR Recomm Rep*. 2002;51(RR-6):1-78.

Dietz PM, Spitz AM, Anda RF, et al. Unintended pregnancy among adult women exposed to abuse or household dysfunction during their childhood. *JAMA*. 1999;282:1359-1366.

Duffy SJ, McGrath ME, Becker BM, Linakis JG. Mothers with histories of domestic violence in a pediatric emergency department. *Pediatrics*. 1999;103:1007-1013.

Elster AB, Ketterlinus R, Lamb ME. Association between parenthood and problem behavior in a national sample of adolescents. *Pediatrics*. 1990;85:1044-1050.

Fauci AS, Pantaleo G, Stanley S, Weissman D. Immunopathogenic mechanisms of HIV infection. *Ann Intern Med*. 1996;124:654-663.

Fildes J, Reed L, Jones N, Martin M, Barrett J. Trauma: the leading cause of maternal death. *J Trauma*. 1992;32:643-645.

Fiscella K, Kitzman JH, Cole RE, Sidora KJ, Olds D. Does child abuse predict adolescent pregnancy? *Pediatrics*. 1998;101:620-624.

Flanagan P, Coll CG, Andreozzi L, Riggs S. Predicting maltreatment of children of teenage mothers. *Arch Pediatr Adolesc Med*. 1995;149: 451-455.

Fleming DT, Wasserheit JN. From epidemiological synergy to public health policy and practice: the contribution of other sexually transmitted diseases to sexual transmission of HIV infection. *Sex Transm Infect*. 1999;75:3-17.

Gazmararian JA, Adams MM, Saltzman LE, et al. The relationship between pregnancy intendedness and physical violence in mothers of newborns. *Obstet Gynecol.* 1995;85:1031-1038.

Gazmararian JA, Lazorick S, Spitz AM, Ballard TJ, Saltzman LE, Marks JS. Prevalence of violence against pregnant women. *JAMA.* 1996; 275:1915-1920.

Glaser JB, Hammerschlag MR, McCormack WM. Sexually transmitted diseases in victims of sexual assault. *N Engl J Med.* 1986;315:625-627.

Glaser JB, Hammerschlag MR, McCormack WM. Epidemiology of sexually transmitted diseases in rape victims. *Rev Infect Dis.* 1989;11:246-254.

Glaser JB, Schachter J, Benes S, Cummings M, Frances CA, McCormack WM. Sexually transmitted diseases in postpubertal female rape victims. *J Infect Dis.* 1991;164:726-730.

Grant LJ. Effects of childhood sexual abuse: issues for obstetric caregivers. *Birth.* 1992;19:220-221.

Gray RH, Wawer MJ, Brookmeyer R, et al. Probability of HIV-1 transmission per coital act in monogamous, heterosexual, HIV-1-discordant couples in Rakai, Uganda. *Lancet.* 2001;357: 1149-1153.

Greenblatt RM, Lukehart SA, Plummer FA, et al. Genital ulceration as a risk factor for human immunodeficiency virus infection. *AIDS.* 1988;2:47-50.

Hawes SE, Hillier SL, Benedetti J, et al. Hydrogen peroxide-producing lactobacilli and acquisition of vaginal infections. *J Infect Dis.* 1996;174:1058-1063.

Holmes MM, Resnick HS, Kilpatrick DG, Best CL. Rape-related pregnancy: estimates and descriptive characteristics from a national sample of women. *Am J Obstet Gynecol.* 1996;175:320-325.

Horon IL, Cheng D. Enhanced surveillance for pregnancy-associated mortality—Maryland, 1993-1998. *JAMA.* 2001;285:1455-1459.

Jenny C, Hooton TM, Bowers A, et al. Sexually transmitted diseases in victims of rape. *N Engl J Med.* 1990;322:713-716.

Katz MH, Gerberding JL. Postexposure treatment of people exposed to the human immunodeficiency virus through sexual contact or injection-drug use. *N Engl J Med.* 1997;336:1097-1100.

Kreiss JK, Coombs R, Plummer R, et al. Isolation of human immunodeficiency virus from genital ulcers in Nairobi prostitutes. *J Infect Dis.* 1989;160:380-384.

Martin SL, Mackie L, Kupper LL, Buescher PA, Moracco KE. Physical abuse of women before, during, and after pregnancy. *JAMA.* 2001; 285:1581-1584.

Mayer L. The severely abused women in obstetric and gynecologic care: guidelines for recognition and management. *J Reprod Med.* 1995;40:13-18.

Mayer L, Liebschutz J. Domestic violence in the pregnant patient: obstetric and behavioral interventions. *Obstet Gynecol Surv.* 1998;53:627-635.

McCauley J, Kern DE, Kolodner K, et al. Clinical characteristics of women with a history of childhood abuse: unhealed wounds. *JAMA.* 1997;277:1362-1368.

McFarlane J. Abuse during pregnancy: the horror and the hope. *AWHONNS Clin Issues Perinat Womens Health Nurs.* 1993;4:350-362.

McFarlane J, Parker B. Preventing abuse during pregnancy: an assessment and intervention protocol. *MCN Am J Matern Child Nurs.* 1994:19:321-324.

McKibben L, De Vos E, Newberger E. Victimization of mothers of abused children: a controlled study. *Pediatrics.* 1989;84:321-325.

Overpeck MD, Brenner RA, Trumble AD, Trifletti LB, Berendes HW. Risk factors for infant homicide in the United States. *N Engl J Med.* 1998;339: 1211-1216.

Peterman TA, Stoneburner FL, Allen JR, Jaffe HW, Curran JW. Risk of human immunodeficiency virus transmission from heterosexual adults with transfusion-associated infections. *JAMA.* 1988;259:55-58.

Quinn TC, Wawer MJ, Sewankambo N, et al. Viral load and heterosexual transmission of human immunodeficiency virus type 1. Rakai Project Study Group. *N Engl J Med.* 2000;324:921-929.

Raj A, Silverman JG, Amaro H. The relationship between sexual abuse and sexual risk among high school students: findings from the 1997 Massachusetts youth risk behavior survey. *Matern Child Health J.* 2000;4:125-134.

Rhodes H, Hutchinson S. Labor experiences of childhood sexual abuse survivors. *Birth.* 1994; 21:213-220.

Schacker T, Collier AC, Hughes J, Shea T, Corey L. Clinical and epidemiologic features of primary HIV infection. *Ann Intern Med.* 1996;125:257-264.

Schechter S, Gary LT. *Health Care Services for Battered Women and Their Abused Children: A Manual About Advocacy for Women and Kids in Emergencies (AWAKE)*. Boston, Mass: Children's Hospital; 1992.

Sellors J, Howard M, Pickard L, Jang D, Mahony J, Chernesky M. Chlamydial cervicitis: testing the practice guidelines for presumptive diagnosis. *CMAJ*. 1998;158:41-46.

Stevens-Simon C, McAnarney ER. Childhood victimization: relationship to adolescent pregnancy outcome. *Child Abuse Negl*. 1994;18:569-575.

Stewart DE. Incidence of postpartum abuse in women with a history of abuse during pregnancy. *Can Med Assoc J*. 1994;151:1601-1604.

Stier DM, Leventhal JM, Berg AT, Johnson L, Mezger J. Are children born to young mothers at increased risk of maltreatment? *Pediatrics*. 1993;91:642-648.

Telzak EE, Chiasson MA, Bevier PJ, Stoneburner RL, Castro KG, Jaffe HW. HIV-1 seroconversion in patients with and without genital ulcer disease. A prospective study. *Ann Intern Med*. 1993; 119:1181-1186.

Thompson RS, Krugman R. Screening mothers for intimate partner abuse at well-baby care visits: the right thing to do. *JAMA*. 2001;285:1628-1630.

Tsai CC, Emau P, Follis KE, et al. Effectiveness of postinoculation (R)-9-(2-phosphonylmethoxypropyl) adenine treatment for prevention of persistent simian immunodeficiency virus (SIV) infection depends critically on timing of initiation and duration of treatment. *J Virol*. 1998;72:4265-4273.

World Health Organization, Task Force on Postovulatory Methods of Fertility Regulation, Special Programme of Research Development and Research Training in Human Reproduction. Randomised controlled trial of levonorgestrel versus the Yuzpe regimen of combined oral contraceptives for emergency contraception. *Lancet*. 1998; 352:428-433.

Wright RJ. Identification of domestic violence in the community pediatric setting: need to protect mothers and children. *Arch Pediatr Adolesc Med*. 2000;154(5):431-433.

Wright RJ, Wright RO, Isaac NE. Response to battered mothers in the pediatric emergency department: a call for an interdisciplinary approach to family violence. *Pediatrics*. 1997;99:186-192.

Violence and Rape Issues

Janice B. Asher, MD
Christine M. Peterson, MD
Elizabeth M. Datner, MD
Bruce D. Rubin, MD

Dating Violence and Acquaintance Rape

Acquaintance rape is unusual among crimes in that it is often not considered to be a crime by the perpetrator, by the criminal justice system, by society, and sometimes even by the victim. Nonetheless, acquaintance rape is a crime that is common and that may have devastating consequences for the victim.

Epidemiology

- Data about the incidence of acquaintance rape are limited.
- Estimates are that about 1 million sexual assaults take place each year in the United States, two thirds of which are not reported to the police and two thirds of which are committed by a perpetrator known to the victim.
- Adolescents and young adults are 4 times more likely to be victims of sexual assault than are women in all other age groups.
- It is more likely that adolescents rather than adults will be raped in the context of a voluntary social encounter such as a date. Twenty-five percent of college women and 6% of college men have been victims of sexual assaults that meet the legal definition of rape.

Risk Factors

• Dating violence is associated with early sexual activity and prior sexual victimization.

• Increased alcohol and substance abuse, increased suicidality, and increased high-risk sexual behavior are also risk factors.

• Women are at greater risk of sexual assault where rape myths are more widely accepted, where violence toward women is tolerated, and where sex role stereotypes are followed.

• Factors associated with the date itself:

1. The male pays for the date.
2. The date occurs in an isolated location.
3. Alcohol and/or drugs are used.

Role of Drugs and Alcohol in Acquaintance Rape

• As many as 73% of assailants and 55% of victims have used alcohol and/or drugs immediately before the episode of sexual assault.

• Male perpetrators of date rape are held less accountable if they committed the rape while they were intoxicated.

• Conversely, female victims are more likely to be held accountable if they were intoxicated at the time.

• Common misconception is that alcohol causes people to become violent; alcohol is in fact a disinhibitor and is associated with increased violence but is not a cause of violence.

• Other drugs used in sexual assaults:

1. Flunitrazepam (Rohypnol): a fast-acting benzodiazepine

2. Ketamine
3. Gamma hydroxybutyrate (GHB) and its cogeners

• These drugs cause disinhibition and anterograde amnesia, so that the victim does not clearly remember the incident.

Victim's Response to Dating Violence and Acquaintance Rape

• Victim often blames herself.

• She may not want the perpetrator to be charged with a serious crime and be sentenced to prison.

• She may not want to go through the difficult and sometimes humiliating ordeal of a trial.

• Often all that is looked for is an acknowledgment and apology by the perpetrator.

Psychologic Consequences

• Victims may decide to "just forget it ever happened" but the psychologic sequelae of date rape may be evident as long as 15 years after the assault.

• Included in these sequelae are the following:

1. Depression
2. Social isolation
3. Self-blame, which is linked to greater psychologic distress and an even longer recovery period
4. Posttraumatic stress disorder (PTSD)

• Characteristics of PTSD:

1. Involuntary reexperiencing of the traumatic event through thoughts, nightmares, and/or flashbacks
2. Avoidance of activities, including those that were previously pleasurable

3. Avoidance of circumstances in which the rape occurred
4. A state of increased psychomotor arousal, which may be associated with sleep disturbances and panic attacks
5. Depression
6. Difficulty forming emotional attachments
7. Decreased appetite
8. Victims of date rape are 11 times more likely to be clinically depressed and 6 times more likely to experience social phobia than nonvictims

Male Victims

- Five percent of rape victims are male.
- Male victims are more likely than female victims to have had multiple assailants and to have had weapons used against them.
- Males are more likely to blame themselves and to feel more anxious.
- Males are less likely to report their assault because of shame and a paucity of options for support.

Perpetrator's Response to Dating Violence and Acquaintance Rape

- The perpetrator may have grown up in a family, peer group, or culture where manhood is defined as being sexually aggressive.
- He may believe that women are "supposed" to refuse sex and that men are "supposed" to pressure, coerce, or even force them.

Effective Clinician Responses

- Because the victim of acquaintance rape may never even seek medical or forensic evaluation,

clinicians must routinely raise the subject of relationship violence and acquaintance rape with patients.

- Included should be information about sexually transmitted diseases (STDs) and emergency contraception.
- Once an assault has occurred, the clinician's responsibility is as follows:

1. Identification and treatment of injuries
2. Prevention of STDs and pregnancy
3. Psychologic assessment with appropriate referral for counseling
4. Collection of forensic evidence

- Chapters 9 through 11 outline the specifics of these steps.

Preventing Dating Violence and Acquaintance Rape

- School-based and college-based programs endeavor to educate males about their ethical and legal responsibility to be certain they have their sex partner's consent before engaging in intimate activity.
- Young men are being trained to relate in specific empathic and supportive ways to their girlfriends, friends, and acquaintances who have been the victims of assault.
- The message must be conveyed that men must help other men learn to respect a woman's right to determine when, where, and with whom she will engage in sexual activity, essentially redefining "masculine" behavior.
- Young women are being taught that they have a right to refuse sex under any circumstances and that there are ways to increase their safety.

Domestic Violence and Partner Rape

Domestic violence is common in a society that fosters the dominance of males over females. Clinicians must identify and assess victims of domestic violence and help women make self-protective changes in their lives.

Domestic Violence Overview

Domestic violence, including marital rape, is not about "losing control" but about maintaining power and control. Generally, one intimate partner, usually male, uses violence to maintain power and control over the other intimate partner, usually female.

- At the outset, episodes of domestic violence may occur infrequently, but subsequently, they occur with great regularity.
- Severity varies from simple verbal or emotional assaults escalating to intentional infliction of brutal physical injuries.
- Although death is the most serious sequela of domestic violence, many forms of domestic abuse result in significant short- and long-term physical and mental health problems for women.
- Risk factors:

1. Poverty, although marital rape is not limited to any specific socioeconomic or racial group
2. Substance abuse
3. Depression
4. Unintended pregnancy
5. Short interpregnancy intervals

6. History of child abuse of the victim and/or perpetrator
7. Concurrent presence of child abuse in the family

Marital Sexual Assault

• Included are vaginal intercourse against one's will, being forced to imitate acts from pornographic movies or magazines, performing or enduring oral and anal sex, being beaten and insulted during intercourse, being forced to have sexual activity with a third person, and having foreign objects penetrated into the vagina or anus.

• About half of women who are raped by their marital partner report being threatened with a weapon and about half report being forced to have sex immediately after having been beaten.

• Women also report being hit, kicked, or burned during sex; being forced to have homosexual sex or sex with animals; being forced to engage in prostitution; or being forced to involve their children with sex acts.

• Marital rapes occur most often within the context of other types of ongoing battering and are a recurrent event.

• Reported prevalence rates vary significantly, partly because there are no commonly accepted definitions applicable to sexual assaults within marriage and partly because of variations in the populations studied and the method of survey used. It is clear that most cases are never reported.

• Reasons for not reporting marital rape include embarrassment, feelings of guilt, fear of retaliation, lack of faith in the legal system, fear of police involvement, lack of knowledge of rights, and concerns about confidentiality.

Role of Coercion

- Sexual coercion, in the absence of actual physical force or violence, is another method of maintaining power and control over an intimate partner.
- Reasons for acquiescence are listed in **Table 12-1**.

Clinical Presentation and Sequelae

Physical Injuries and Symptoms

- Clinical presentation can vary, ranging from injuries directly resulting from violence to chronic complaints that neither patient nor clinician recognize as a manifestation of domestic violence.
- Somatic complaints include headache, abdominal pain, pelvic pain, fatigue, shortness of breath, gastrointestinal disturbances, and sleep disorders.

Table 12-1. Types of Acquiescence

Unwanted turns to wanted	In these cases, the women did not desire sex initially but were able to enjoy it after a few minutes. This was reported by 10% of women and occurred almost exclusively in relationships that were current, happy, and healthy according to the women.
"It's my duty"	This concept of a "wifely obligation inherent in the marital contract" is a common belief. The unwanted sex was considered an "inconvenience of married life" in an effort to "keep peace" and the wife's inherent "responsibility" or "duty." Seventy-six percent of the respondents participated in sex for this reason, and 34% reported this as the main reason they had unwanted sex.

(continued)

Table 12-1. *(continued)*	
"Easier not to argue"	The respondents described this circumstance as occurring when verbal or nonverbal behavior from a partner became overwhelming and giving in to sex was the easiest way out of the situation. This was frequently associated with other forms of emotional manipulation, pressure, and in some instances, control. Twenty-seven percent of the respondents reported this experience.
"Don't know what might happen if I don't"	In these cases, women acquiesced to unwanted sex due to fear of negative reactions, including threats of violence, from their partners. Verbal threats and elements of emotional control were also present in these relationships. Seven percent of women reported this reason for submitting to unwanted sexual acts.
"Know what will happen if I don't"	These women had experienced physical abuse in their relationships and submitted to unwanted sex in an effort to avoid more physical abuse from their partner. Twenty percent of respondents fit into this category. A statement from one respondent is illuminating: "When you're intimidated by someone and they want to have sex no matter what the reason or what the situation, you do it, otherwise, you get the hell beat out of you, to be quite honest . . .you just let him do it. It's not him actually holding you down and forcing you, but it is being forced because you can't say no."

• Women who experience marital rape suffer more severe physical injuries than do either acquaintance rape victims or victims of domestic violence without concomitant sexual assault. Marital rape victims also report increased physical health symptomatology and mental health problems.

• Physical injuries include gynecologic complaints (including vaginal and anal tearing or pain, bladder infections, dysmenorrhea, dyspareunia, and other forms of sexual dysfunction), pelvic pain, urinary tract infections, increased frequency of STDs, painful intercourse, and vaginal pain.

• Sexually abused domestic violence victims are at increased risk for death. Detecting marital rape in a woman's experience should heighten a practitioner's concern for the safety of that individual.

Psychologic Effects

• Psychologic effects can be significant and include depression, lower self-esteem, and poor body image.

• Depression is frequently associated with relationship violence.

• Abusers often seek custody of children as another tactic to use against their partners.

Health Status and Disease Prevention

• Victims of domestic abuse experience significant negative effects on their health and well-being, including perceived evaluation of their own health.

• The ability to enhance one's health and prevent disease is compromised in abusive relationships. Women are less likely to use condoms, more afraid to ask their partner to use condoms, and more likely to be emotionally abused or threatened with

physical abuse when discussing safe sex than women in nonviolent relationships.

- Women raped by their partners have a significantly higher mean number of somatic symptoms.

Associated Behaviors

- Drug and alcohol abuse are more common in victims and perpetrators of abuse.

1. Victims often use drugs and alcohol as a form of self-medication in response to abuse.
2. A drug-using abusive partner may also coerce or force his partner to use drugs or alcohol to "keep him company."

Identification of Abuse

- It is often difficult for a clinician to discover that a patient has suffered from marital rape unless physical abuse has also taken place.

- Women are more likely to discuss abuse with their healthcare provider than with anyone else, including family members, friends, and clergy, but do so only when asked.

- Victims of partner rape are even less likely than victims of stranger rape to report events or to seek additional services.

- Because abuse crosses all racial, ethnic, religious, and socioeconomic lines, screening must be universal and is most effective when performed by a clinical provider rather than by filling in a self-assessment tool.

- Recommended screening questions:

1. Are you in a relationship in which you have been hit, pushed, or kicked?

2. Are you in a relationship in which you have been forced to have sex?

• Make information about the following available to all female patients: domestic violence, partner rape, and the availability of STD prophylaxis, emergency contraception, and long-term contraception.

• Interview the patient alone. Strategies to separate patient and partner are as follows:

1. Posting a sign stating a policy of having partners leave during the physical examination.
2. Ordering tests and accompanying the patient to the test site while the partner is asked to wait.
3. Having a staff member ask the partner to come outside of the examination room to provide additional insurance information.

• Keep abuse-related materials, particularly safety planning information, in all patient bathrooms.

• If the patient denies abuse but you strongly suspect abuse has occurred, it may be helpful to return to questions about abuse with the following introductory statements:

1. An injury like yours often occurs because of being punched. Is that what happened?
2. Because abuse is so common, we are asking all of our patients about it. Has someone hurt you?

• When there is physical abuse, it is not uncommon to find out that sexual abuse has also occurred. It is vital to ask about the possibility.

• Be familiar with and able to recognize symptoms that may be indicative of spousal rape.

The Clinician's Response to Domestic Violence

• Communicate to the patient a concern for her safety and an appreciation of the complex dynamics of an abusive relationship.

• Recognize that a hallmark of abuse is that the victim, rather than the perpetrator, feels embarrassed, ashamed, and blameworthy for the abuse.

• Support and validate the patient who discloses abuse. Particularly effective statements include the following:

1. I'm glad you've told me about this.
2. I believe what you've told me.
3. The abuse is not your fault.
4. No one deserves to be assaulted.
5. The situation is likely to become worse, not better.
6. If you are not safe, your child cannot be safe.
7. Help is available.

Documentation

• Document the patient's statements regarding abuse as well as the physical findings associated with battering.

• Documentation is critical because it may eventually be useful in a court of law, particularly if custody issues arise.

• Use the patient's own words.

• Include the following information: name of the perpetrator, nature of the weapon used, dated photographs of the injuries or body maps or written descriptions of them, and whether injuries appeared recent or old.

INTERVENTION

• A useful clinical tool for domestic violence assessment is the RADAR model:

R = Routine screening

A = Ask direct questions

D = Document findings

A = Assess safety

R = Review options and refer

• Once a victim of domestic violence is identified, refer the patient to a domestic violence expert. This individual may be a hospital-based or community-based social worker, a colleague who is knowledgeable about domestic violence, a local domestic violence advocacy organization, or the national domestic violence hotline at 1-800-799-SAFE.

• Offer a sexually assaulted woman emergency contraception if she is not currently pregnant. Injectable contraception that can be used surreptitiously may protect the woman by eliminating the need for the partner's consent or cooperation.

• Offer STD screening and sexual assault forensic examinations.

• Use caution in prescribing any sedatives to a domestic abuse victim. These medications can impair the patient's ability to defend herself, escape, or seek immediate help if needed.

• Remember that safety is the paramount goal in abuse intervention.

1. Insisting that an abused women leave her partner

is neither the responsibility nor the right of the clinician.

2. Data show that the most dangerous time for a woman to be seriously injured or killed by her violent partner is when she attempts to leave the relationship.
3. Assist the victim to take the necessary steps to ensure her safety and that of her children.

• Safety assessment includes immediate and long-term aspects.

1. Immediate safety: indicators that it may not be safe to return home that day are finding out that the partner has recently obtained a gun; that the frequency and/or severity of attacks has escalated; that he has made suicidal and/or homicidal threats; that he has threatened the children; that he has displayed violence toward a pet; or that he has escalated drug and/or alcohol abuse.
2. Long-term safety: while the clinician must respect the patient's autonomy if she decides it is safe to go home, you should ask, "What will you do if this happens again?" Thus, you will assist the patient in planning safety and/or exit strategies. Reviewing safety measures or giving out printed material is also helpful.

• In-house social workers and women's advocacy groups in the community can assist in obtaining referral information. Note that routine referral for couples counseling is not recommended.

• For patients who wish to maintain confidentiality regarding abuse, take the same precautions as for other similarly sensitive healthcare issues, such as human immunodeficiency virus (HIV) status.

Societal Reaction to Marital Rape

• Laws have only recently reflected an understanding of marital rape as a crime.

• Rape within a relationship can have the same components of forcible sex that occur in acquaintance rape: coercion, physical force, and physical and mental trauma to the victim.

• Social awareness of the prevalence of marital rape has been accompanied by corresponding legal aid to its victims.

Special Populations

Immigrants

• A woman who is an immigrant may be particularly vulnerable to abusive relationships, possibly as a result of the following:

1. She may have come from a culture in which the subordination of women is the norm.
2. She may be completely dependent economically on her partner.
3. She may be particularly isolated because of an inability to speak English comfortably.
4. There may be disincentives for an abused woman who is unfamiliar with the language, culture, and laws to disclose abuse, such as dependence on her partner economically, little means of supporting herself or her children, lack of opportunity to disclose the abuse if her partner is her translator, or fewer options for escape from the situation.

• Be aware of the importance of cultural sensitivity and knowledge of the woman's culture.

• Become familiar with local resources for women of other countries and cultures.

Women With Disabilities

• Women with disabilities are at increased risk for physical and sexual abuse and assault for the following reasons:

1. Physical vulnerability
2. Dependence on caregivers, including family members, healthcare workers, and attendants
3. Difficulty making and carrying out a safety or escape plan
4. Lack of accessibility to services

• Twenty-five percent of mentally retarded adolescent girls and 31% of adolescent girls with congenital physical disabilities have been sexually abused.

Gay and Lesbian Relationships

• Same-sex physically and/or sexually abusive relationships are filled with the same problems as heterosexual relationships, but additional issues may make terminating a same-sex violent relationship more difficult or dangerous, as follows:

1. The abusive partner may threaten to "out" the victim, that is, disclose his or her status as being homosexual. This threat may have tremendous real or perceived implications for employment and family relationships.
2. Gays and lesbians may live within small social frameworks. Leaving an abusive partner may mean leaving an entire social network, increasing the sense of isolation.
3. In male same-sex relationships, the abusive partner may threaten the victim with exposure to HIV (although this threat is clearly not limited to same-sex relationships).

4. The abusive partner may claim to be the victim. Particularly in relationships in which one member of the couple is larger or appears physically stronger or more "masculine," outsiders may draw erroneous conclusions as to who is the batterer.
5. There is perceived and real lack of resources for abused partners in same-sex relationships, especially for males.

- Physical and sexual violence is more common in heterosexual and homosexual male relationships than in lesbian relationships.

References

Acierno R, Resnick H, Kilpatrick DG, Saunders B, Best CL. Risk factors for rape, physical assault, and posttraumatic stress disorder in women: examination of differential multivariate relationships. *J Anxiety Disord.* 1999;13:541-563.

Avery-Leaf S, Cascardi M, O'Leary KD, Cano A. Efficacy of a dating violence prevention program on attitudes justifying aggression. *J Adolesc Health.* 1997;21:11-17.

Basile KC. Rape by acquiesence: the ways in which women "give in" to unwanted sex with their husbands. *Violence Against Women.* 1999;5:1036-1058.

Beebe DK. Initial assessment of the rape victim. *J Miss State Med Assoc.* 1991;32:403-406.

Bowker L. Marital rape: a distinct syndrome? *Soc Casework.* 1983;64:347-352.

Brown DE. Factors affecting psychosexual development of adults with congenital physical disabilities. *Phys Occup Ther Pediatr.* 1998;8:43-58.

Campbell JC, Alford P. The dark consequences of marital rape. *Am J Nurs.* 1989;89:946-949.

Campbell JC, Soeken KL. Forced sex and intimate partner violence: effects on women's risk and women's health. *Violence Against Women.* 1999; 5:1017-1035.

Chamberlain A, Rauh J, Passer A, McGrath M, Burket R. Issues in fertility control for mentally retarded female adolescents: I. Sexual activity, sexual abuse, and contraception. *Pediatrics.* 1984;73:445-450.

Council on Scientific Affairs, American Medical Association. Violence against women: relevance for medical practitioners. *JAMA.* 1992;267: 3184-3189.

Easteal PW, Easteal S. Attitudes and practices of doctors toward spouse assault victims: an Australian study. *Violence Vict.* 1992 Fall;7:217-228.

Farley R. Homicide trends in the United States. In: Hawkins DR, ed. *Homicide Among Black Americans.* New York, NY: University Press of America; 1986:13-27.

Foshee VA, Bauman KE, Arriga XB, Helms RW, Koch GG, Linder GF. An evaluation of Safe Dates, an adolescent dating violence prevention program. *Am J Public Health.* 1998;88:45-50.

Grevalamus DE, Shaw RD, Kennedy EL. Examination of sexually abused adolescents. *Semin Adolesc Med.* 1987;3:59-66.

Grisso JA, Wishner AR, Schwarz DF, Weene BA, Holmes JH, Sutton RL. A population-based study of injuries in inner-city women. *Am J Epidemiol.* 1991;134:59-86.

Hammock GS, Richardson DR. Perceptions of rape: the influence of closeness of relationship, intoxication and sex of participant. *Violence Vict.* 1997;12:237-246.

Hong L. Toward a transformed approach to prevention: breaking the link between masculinity and violence. *J Am Coll Health.* 2000;48:269-279.

Humphrey JA, White JW. Women's vulnerability to sexual assault from adolescence to young adulthood. *J Adolesc Health.* 2000;27:419-424.

Katz B, Burt M. Self-blame in recovery from rape. In: Burgess AW, ed. *Rape and Sexual Assault II. Garland Reference Library of Social Science.* Vol 361. New York, NY: Garland; 1988:151-190.

Kessler R, McGonagle K, Nelson C, Hughes M, Swartz M, Blazer D. Sex and depression in the National Comorbidity Survey: II. Cohort effects. *J Infect Dis.* 1994;30:15-26.

Kilpatrick DG, Best CL, Saunders BE, Veronen LJ. Rape in marriage and in dating relationships: how bad is it for mental health? *Ann NY Acad Sci.* 1988;528:335-344.

Kilpatrick DG, Edmunds CN, Seymour AK. *Rape in America: A Report to the Nation.* Charleston, SC: Crime Victim Research and Treatment Center; 1992.

Lacey HB, Roberts R. Sexual assault on men. *Int J STD AIDS.* 1991;2:258-260.

Lopez P. He said . . . she said . . . an overview of date rape from commission through prosecution through verdict. *Criminal Justice.* 1992;13:275-302.

Marsh CE. Sexual assault and domestic violence in the African American community. *West J Black Stud.* 1993;17(3):149-155.

McAfee RE. Physicians and domestic violence: can we make a difference? *JAMA*. 1995;273:1790-1791.

Merrill GS, Wolfe VA. Battered gay men: an exploration of abuse, help seeking, and why they stay. *J Homosex*. 2000;39:1-30.

Peipert JF, Domagalski LR. Epidemiology of adolescent sexual assault. *Obstet Gynecol*. 1994; 84:867-871.

Richardson D, Campbell JL. Alcohol and rape: the effect of alcohol on attributions of blame for rape. *Pers Soc Psychol Bull*. 1982;8:468-476.

Rickert VI, Wiemann CM. Date rape among adolescents and young adults. *J Pediatr Adolesc Gynecol*. 1998;11:167-175.

Schuller RA, Stewart A. Police responses to sexual assault complaints: the role of perpetrator/complainant intoxication. *Law Hum Behav*. 2000; 24:535-551.

Schwartz RH, Milteer R, LeBeau MA. Drug-facilitated sexual assault ('date rape'). *South Med J*. 2000;93:558-561.

Smith KM. Drugs used in acquaintance rape. *J Am Pharm Assoc*. 1999;39:442-443.

Sutherland C, Bybee D, Sullivan C. The long-term effects of battering on women's health. *Womens Health*. 1998;4:42-70.

Tjaden P, Thoennes N. *Prevalence, Incidence and Consequences of Violence Against Women: Findings From the National Violence Against Women Survey*. Washington, DC: Research in Brief, US Dept of Justice, National Institute of Justice; 1998. NCJ 172837.

Warshaw R. *I Never Called It Rape: The Ms. Report on Recognizing, Fighting, and Surviving Date and Acquaintance Rape*. New York, NY: Harper & Row; 1998.

Weingourt R. Wife rape in a sample of psychiatric patients. *Image J Nurs Sch*. 1990;22:144-147.

Weissman M, Klerman G. Depression: current understanding and changing trends. *Annu Rev Public Health*. 1992;13:319-339.

Wilson MD, Joffe A. Adolescent medicine. *JAMA*. 1995;273:1657-1659.

Young ME, Nosek MA, Howland CA, Chanpong G, Rintala DH. Prevalence of abuse of women with physical disabilities. *Arch Phys Med Rehabil*. 1998;78(special issue):S34-S38.

Chapter 13

Special Settings

Michael Clark, MSN, CRNP
Hannah Ufberg Rabinowitz, MSN, CRNP
Thomas Ervin, RNC, FN, BSc
Sharon W. Cooper, MD, FAAP

Rape and Sexual Abuse in Older Adults

The true prevalence of rape committed against older adults can only be inferred from the existing literature. Existing social services for sexual assault victims are generally not designed to address the needs presented by older adults, especially their vulnerabilities, exposure patterns, and physical and emotional responses.

Incidence of Sexual Abuse Among Older Adults

- Older adults are less likely to experience violent crime than younger individuals.
- The overall incidence of elder abuse is thought to be significant, with estimates of 10 cases per 100 000 population per year. Thus, those over age 50 years would represent about 3% of sexual assault victims.
- Many incidents of abuse remain undetected either by those intimately involved in the care of older adults or state investigative agencies.

Defining Rape and Sexual Assault of Older Adults

- In the past, the definition of rape focused more exclusively on forced vaginal intercourse by a male with a female who was not his wife.

• Currently, the definitions of the terms rape, sexual assault, and sexual abuse include victims and perpetrators of both genders, and the definition of the nature of the sexual contact includes oral and anal penetration.

• Sexual abuse of older adults is defined as sexual activity that occurs when a person over age 60 years is forced, tricked, coerced, or manipulated into unwanted sexual contact. It also includes situations in which the older adult is incapable of giving consent because of cognitive and other impairments, including impairments associated with aging.

• This definition is not limited to rape but can include other forms of unwanted sexual contact (eg, fondling).

• Seeing older adults as asexual may inhibit the ability to recognize and respond to patterns of sexual victimization.

Exposure to Sexual Abuse

• Older adults differ significantly from younger victims in characteristics that leave them vulnerable and exposed to the threat of sexual assault.

• Sexual abuse in the older adult often implies a violation of a relationship between caregiver and dependent. Older adults must rely on the perpetrator because of physical or cognitive limitations or impairments.

• Older adults may also differ from younger victims in their ability to report and respond to assaults based on their relative degree of isolation and physical or cognitive impairments.

• Many older adults do not know their assailants. These attacks by strangers are more frequently

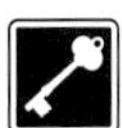

accompanied by higher levels of violence. Generally, the assaults on older women are more violent, brutal, and sadistic.

SEXUAL ABUSE OF OLDER ADULTS RESIDING IN INSTITUTIONAL SETTINGS

- Those residing in nursing homes fall into 2 subpopulations:

1. Those admitted for short stays from hospitals to undergo rehabilitation associated with acute illness
2. Those staying much longer because of disabilities that cannot be managed in the community; these individuals may be more vulnerable to sexual assault

- Sexual abuse and physical abuse allegations of institutionalized persons are not reported promptly and law enforcement personnel are rarely summoned to investigate. Even when allegations are substantiated, minimal disciplinary action occurs, with cases rarely leading to criminal prosecution despite severe abuse.
- Often the incidents are witnessed but not reported, or residents inform a family member who does not follow through.
- Indicators of sexual abuse include psychologic manifestations (sleep disorders, irritability, mood swings, depression) that may also accompany menopausal changes or other psychosocial problems and are, thus, nonspecific for abuse.
- Psychologic warning signs that may alert healthcare providers that the patient may be a victim of a sexual assault are as follows:

1. Aggressive/regressive behavior
2. Mistrust in others
3. Disturbed peer interactions
4. Nightmares

• Some incidents are discovered by physical findings such as signs of trauma to genital or surrounding tissue.

• Some cases have been detected through signs and diagnostic findings that confirmed the presence of sexually transmitted infections.

• Nursing home residents are often immunocompromised and may have had minimal sexual experiences. The onset of symptoms (fever, malaise, changes in blood pressure, skin rashes) in a patient suspected to have been abused or assaulted requires a thorough medical assessment.

Perpetrators in Nursing Homes

• Three approaches are used by perpetrators in assaulting frail older adults:

1. The "confidence" approach is used with mobile, more highly functional victims and involves gaining the victim's confidence through verbal manipulation or coercion.
2. A "blitz" approach involves overtaking the victim through injurious force.
3. A "surprise" approach employs the use of threats but no force when the victim is either unsuspecting or incapacitated.

Reporting and Investigating Suspected Abuse

• Nursing homes are obligated to investigate suspected abuse within 5 days of a report to the nursing home administration.

• If sexual abuse is suspected, it is important for the nursing home staff and administration to take care to avoid subjecting the victim to unnecessary further trauma during the investigation process.

• Carefully consider the location of the interview, taking special care to establish that the interview process is as safe as possible for the resident.

• Be aware that it may be problematic to perform a thorough physical assessment for the following reasons:

1. Joint contractures
2. Victim resistance because of the pain of the assault
3. Difficulty communicating with a patient who has dementia and cognitive impairment

• Forensic evidence may be difficult to obtain if the incident is discovered in a delayed manner.

• It should be clear that the nursing home can be held liable when foreseeable risks may have contributed to a sexual assault.

Sexual Assault of Older Adults Residing in Noninstitutional Settings

• Family members perpetrate the majority of abuse and violence inflicted on older adults outside of an institutional setting.

• Five types of offenders commit violence against family members, with sexual abuse rarely occurring among the first 2 types:

1. The otherwise competent but overwhelmed caregiver
2. The willing but physically or cognitively impaired caregiver

3. The caregiver with a "user mentality" who expects to gain something from the caregiving relationship
4. The unstable, angry, and volatile caregiver who "lashes out" toward those less powerful than himself or herself
5. The sadistic caregiver who gains pleasure by harming or intimidating others

• The 2 distinct phases of sexual abuse are covert sexual abuse and overt sexual abuse.

1. Covert sexual abuse: sexual interest may be expressed or sexual activity discussed. The perpetrator treats the victim as a sex object or potential sexual partner.
2. Overt abuse: activities such as voyeurism and inflicting pornography on the victim may escalate to various degrees of sexual contact ranging from kissing and fondling to oral-genital contact to various forms of oral, vaginal, or anal penetration.

Immediate and Long-term Responses of Older Sexual Assault Victims

• Rape trauma syndrome

1. Acute phase: marked by disorganization and fear; somatic symptoms may be seen in all survivors of sexual abuse and include tension headaches, fatigue, sleep disturbances, and gastrointestinal irritability.
2. Reorganization phase: involves the process of stabilization and begins 4 to 8 weeks after the assault; symptoms are often consistent with those of posttraumatic stress disorder (PTSD). Criteria include a stressor of significant magnitude such that it would likely evoke distinguishable symp-

toms in most individuals; the victim reexperiencing the trauma through recurrent and sometimes intrusive recollection of the event; and the victim developing a constricted view of and reduced involvement with the environment.

• Other symptoms of rape trauma syndrome include exaggerated startle response or hyperarousal state, guilt, impaired memory surrounding the event, and problems with concentration and attention.

Framework for Working With Older Sexual Assault Victims

• As mentioned, existing services for those experiencing sexual victimization are generally not designed to meet the needs of older adults.

• The concepts, theories, and practices characteristic of victimology and those related to gerontology must be integrated to address the needs of older victims of sexual assault.

1. Victimology addresses selected aspects of sexual victimization, including the vulnerability patterns of the victim, the exposure patterns of the incident, and factors that influence the degree of adaptation on the victim's part after the traumatic event.
2. Gerontology addresses selected aspects of the aging process, defining age in terms of the ability of an individual to respond to stressors and looking at the older adult more holistically. The focus is on the quality of life of the individual as measured by how well day-to-day functioning is in accord with the values and expectations of the older adult. It also takes into account the coping strategies and supports that help the older adult maintain optimal functioning.

- Older adults differ in their ability to adapt successfully to stress, which is termed homeostenosis.
- Gerontologists attempt to view aspects of successful aging, specifically selective optimization with compensation. The individual optimizes the adaptation process by employing successfully chosen and practiced behaviors to respond to stressors and accommodates by modifying conditions to meet ability level.
- Healthcare providers often frame their interactions with older adult patients using a problem-oriented perspective. The common endpoint in considering the adaptive capabilities of an older adult revolves around an assessment of the overall frailty of the individual.
- Appreciation of the altered responses to stress and the need to look at contextual factors in supporting the quality of life for older adults are central to providing effective care for the older victim of sexual assault.

Effective Clinical Response to Elder Sexual Abuse

Effective clinical care responses include the following:

- Prompt detection of sexual abuse
- An understanding of the cognitive, physical, and emotional issues unique to elder victims of sexual abuse
- A nonjudgmental and caring approach to interviews, examinations, and other caregiving activities
- Support for the adaptation and optimal return of functioning

Screening

- The initial evaluation of geriatric patients should

include a social history and assessment, screening for indicators of all types of abuse even in the absence of any suspicion of abuse.

• Because many older adults come to the emergency department for evaluation through an emergency medical system, EMTs, paramedics, and other transport personnel should be trained in the needs of older adult victims of sexual abuse or assault. Be alert to and make note of residential conditions, physical signs, and verbal or other behaviors indicative of sexual assault or abuse and be aware of the need to preserve evidence that may be important to a forensic investigation.

1. Generally, do not wash the patient or change her or his clothing.
2. If clothing is removed, keep it in a paper bag to prevent bacterial overgrowth.
3. See Chapter 10 for the details of forensic evidence collection.

Interview

• Before conducting the interview of a sexual assault patient, consider the following details:

1. Who should conduct the interview? Generally, the interviewer should be of the same gender as the victim.
2. Where should the interview take place? Usually, holding the interview away from the site of the suspected assault is preferable. Interviews may be conducted in the victim's residence as long as the interviewer provides a sense of safety and privacy. The victim should be assured that the assailant will not overhear the interview or be privy to what was said.

3. How should the interview be conducted?

   Build rapport with the victim.

   Address the victim by her or his last name unless otherwise directed by the patient.

   Avoid caretaker speech, in which the patient is addressed in familiar terms.

   Have a family member or other trusted individual present.

   Allow the older adult as much control as possible.

   Make sure the interviewee knows that he or she has the right to terminate the interview at any point.

   Initiate questions in an open-ended manner and provide sufficient time for the older adult to answer.

   Be alert to any subtle sensory impairments the victim may have but also ask directly if he or she has any difficulty seeing or hearing.

   Perform a brief minimental status examination if there is any question regarding cognitive impairment that could hinder the interview.

   Speak in a well-modulated, slower-paced, and lower-pitched voice to counter the effects of age-related hearing loss. You may also place earpieces of a stethoscope in the ears of the older patient and speak through the diaphragm or employ a small portable amplifying device.

   Ask one question at a time.

   Be alert to indirect verbal references to sexual assault or cues that indicate fear, guilt, shame, or inappropriate sexual references.

4. What actions need to be taken as a result of information gathered during the interview? If action must be taken, provide emotional support of the victim as the top priority.
5. What information should the interviewer share and with whom?

Examination

• Only people with training and expertise along with compassion and exceptional communication skills should examine the sexual assault victim.

• Older adult female sexual assault victims have an increased incidence and degree of genital trauma, mostly because of normal postmenopausal changes, as follows:

1. Menopause generally occurs between ages 45 and 55 years.
2. Structural changes result from a decline in the hormone levels after ovulation ceases.
3. Estrogen levels fall, resulting in smaller labia and clitoris.
4. The uterus and ovaries diminish in size and breast tissue loses elasticity.
5. There is loss of fatty tissue deposits and elastic tissue of the labia majora.
6. Pubic hair thins.
7. Bartholin's glands produce lesser amounts of vaginal secretions, causing a decrease in lubrication during intercourse and resulting dyspareunia (painful intercourse).
8. Vaginal walls may be light pink or pale and appear tissue-paper thin and dry. They also lose some capacity for expansion.

9. Some older women also develop urinary frequency or urgency, or stress incontinence.

• Be aware that less serious injuries have more serious consequences in terms of morbidity and mortality among older adult patients, so that seemingly minor injuries may require greater attention.

• When sexual assault is considered, evidence of bruising to the perineum, pain with micturition, vaginal bleeding, and discharge are all ominous signs.

• Proceed carefully and slowly with the pelvic and rectal examination, reassuring the patient and realizing that it may take longer than with a younger woman.

• Be alert to difficulty walking or sitting and torn, stained, or bloody clothing.

• Red flags for suspecting sexual assault are as follows:

1. Pain or itching of the genital area
2. Recurrent vaginal infections
3. Bruising or bleeding of the external genitalia, vaginal or anal area
4. Unexpected or unreported reluctance to cooperate with toileting or the physical examination of the genitalia

Provision of Care and Resources

• Offer explanations and instructions that are clear and unambiguous.

• Provide written instructions using large bold lettering.

• Take the time to thoroughly discuss everything and encourage questions.

• Relate new information and tasks to previous experiences.

- Use language that is familiar to the patient.
- Make a follow-up phone call within 24 hours.
- Plan for follow-up referrals and communicate the plans clearly to the patient.
- Include the patient's family whenever possible in any educative effort.

Reporting Requirements

- Be familiar with state elder abuse reporting laws.
- Provide training to staff regarding the detection and management of elder abuse.

Sexual Assault in Correctional Settings

Overview of the Problem

- Poor systems surveillance with resultant inaccurate epidemiology reports of the incidence and prevalence of prison rape
- Inadequate laws to protect prisoners or to provide adequate reporting abilities by victims
- Indifference of correctional staff to the victim impact of such sexual assaults
- Insufficient facility capability to provide isolation and, therefore, protection for vulnerable inmates
- High incidence of mentally impaired victims, for whom no special provisions are made and investigation of complaints is inadequate
- Problem of mixing juveniles into the adult prison population, placing them at extreme risk of exploitation, victimization, and subsequent mental health injury
- Unavailability of counseling for victims of prisoner-on-prisoner sexual assault

- Inadequate medical services for the sexually transmitted disease (STD) risk
- Inadequate training programs on male and female prisoner-on-prisoner sexual abuse for both high-level corrections officials and front-line staff
- Nonexistent standard operating procedures for response to prisoner-on-prisoner sexual assault
- Inadequate numbers of guards and monitoring systems to ensure safety of the prison population
- Need to consistently report sexual assault behind bars to local authorities and prosecutorial agencies for investigation and possible criminal prosecution
- Lack of recognition and action to address the problem of racial tensions within prisons, which also contributes to violent sexual assaults of specific minority groups
- Poor attention to the gang dynamics that exist in the prison systems and the need to prevent multiple-perpetrator sexual assaults
- Common practice of merely transferring perpetrators to different units, where further abuse of a different group of potential victims is facilitated instead of taking appropriate disciplinary action
- Practice of placing more than one prisoner per cell (double celling) without consideration of a prior report or suspicion of a sexual assault involving one or more than one of the inmates
- Poor public awareness of the serious and tragic nature of this type of crime, leading to misrepresentations of prison rape as a joke in the media
- Poor recognition that prison rape is a contributing factor to prison homicides, violence against inmates

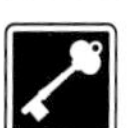

and staff, and institutional riots and insurrections

• Poor attention to the problem of custodial abuse of inmates

• Inadequate federal laws to affect prison funding for the complex problem of prisoner sexual assault

Scope of the Problem

• Twenty-two to twenty-five percent of prisoners are victims of sexual pressuring, attempted sexual assault, or completed rapes.

• Ten percent of prisoners are victims of a completed rape at least one time during the course of their incarceration.

• Two thirds of those reporting sexual victimization have been repeatedly victimized on an average of 9 times during their incarceration, with some male prisoners experiencing up to 100 incidents of sexual assault per year.

Consequences of Attacks

• It is not possible for an individual to undergo forced sex without subsequent trauma, which may be equally physical and emotional, or mostly emotional or psychologic.

• Regardless of the type or extent of trauma sustained, there will be consequences for the individual, society, and those professionals working with these special populations and the aftermath of their experiences.

• Mental health ramifications:

1. Extreme
2. More mentally ill inmates in prison than in psychiatric hospitals; most correctional facilities have minimal mental health capability

3. Include PTSD, anxiety, depression, and the exacerbation of existing mental disorders
4. Inmates at risk for suicide become more unstable and are much more likely to attempt or succeed at committing suicide to avoid continuous trauma
5. May display anger, depression, loss of self-esteem and self-worth, alteration of self-image, and a desire for revenge

• Categories of inmates especially vulnerable to sexual assault:

1. Young and inexperienced
2. Short in stature, with small body habitus and physically weak
3. Mentally ill or with developmental disabilities
4. Not "street-wise" or savvy
5. Not gang affiliated
6. Homosexual, overtly effeminate, or transgendered
7. Violated the "code of silence" or are seen as a snitch
8. Disliked by the staff or other inmates
9. Prior sexual assault victims

Role of Medical Professionals

• Healthcare professionals are obligated to provide unbiased, professional care.

• Clinical guidelines for medical management must address the following **(Table 13-1)**:

1. Viral hepatitis (A, B, C, and D)
2. Human immunodeficiency virus (HIV) infection

3. Tuberculosis (TB)
4. STDs
5. Endocarditis prophylaxis
6. Varicella

Table 13-1. Process of Identification of Infectious Diseases in the Prison Population

Infectious Disease	Screen, Assess, and Test Inmates
Tuberculosis (TB) infection and possible TB disease	— On initial incarceration before placed in general population — Annually — When clinically indicated — To find evidence of spread surrounding a case of contagious TB disease
Human immunodeficiency virus (HIV) infection	— If history of risk behavior — If clinical indications — Before release — For surveillance purposes — After an exposure
Other infections transmittable by casual contact	— On intake and before being placed in the general population — Before assigned to the food service area — If clinical indications — With contact investigators

Adapted from Federal Bureau of Prisons Report on Infectious Disease Management, January 2001:3.

Role of Social Services Professionals and Prison Staff

- Cope with the reality of life behind bars.
- Exercise the necessary caution without developing paranoia or disregard for the humanity of those incarcerated.
- Be aware of gang-related incidents and seek to take preventive action.
- Keep in mind that the overall control of the institution is paramount to the individual's needs.
- Adhere to a high professional and personal ethic.

Sexual Predators and Moving From Victim to Predator

- Sexual predators may be used to intimidate, control, or punish other inmates for real or perceived transgressions of the prison law.
- Individuals who survive the single or multiple sexual assaults, in addition to having a high incidence of PTSD and depression, may become violent themselves as an act of immediate self-defense and to avoid further victimization.
- The transition from victim to predator may follow the individual beyond the penal system confinement, contributing to the over 75% rate of return to incarceration for inmates.

References

Bickley LS. *Bates Guide to Physical Exam and History Taking*. 7th ed. Philadelphia, Pa: Lippincott Williams & Wilkins; 1999.

Bureau of Justice Statistics. *Criminal Victimization in the US 1995*. Washington, DC: US Dept of Justice; May 2000. NCJ171129.

Burgess AW. *Rape and Sexual Assault III: A Research Handbook*. New York, NY: Garland Publishing, Inc; 1991.

Burgess AW, Dowdell EB, Prentky RA. Sexual abuse of nursing home residents. *J Psychosoc Nurs Ment Health Serv*. 2000;38(6):11-17.

Burgess AW, Holmstrom LL. Rape trauma syndrome. *Am J Psychiatry*. 1974;131(9):981-986.

Capezuti EA, Swedlow DJ. Sexual abuse in nursing homes. *Elder's Advisor: J Elder Law and Post-Retirement Planning*. 2000;2(2):51-61.

Cartwright PS, Moore RA. The elderly victim of rape. *South Med J*. 1989;82:988-989.

Chelala C. More mentally ill people reported in US prisons. *BMJ*. 1999;319(7204):210.

Clarke ME, Pierson W. Management of elder abuse in the emergency department. *Emerg Med Clin North Am*. 1999;17(3):631-644.

Corrections in the US—The Picture Today. The Lionheart Foundation Web site. Available at: http://www.lionheart.org/corrections.html. Accessed November 12, 2002.

Cotton DJ, Groth AN. Inmate rape: prevention and intervention. *J Prison Jail Health*. 1982;2(1):47-57.

Cotton DJ, Groth AN. Sexual assault in correctional institutions: prevention and intervention. In: Stuart IR, ed. *Victims of Sexual Aggression: Treatment of Children, Women, and Men*. New York, NY: Van Nostrand Reinhold; 1984:127-155.

Deming JE, Mittleman RE, Wegli CV. Forensic science aspects of fatal sexual assaults on women. *J Forensic Sci*. 1983;28(3):572-576.

Dumond RW. The sexual assault of male inmates in incarcerated settings. *International Journal of Sociology of Law.* 1992;20(2):135-157.

Dumond RW. Inmate sexual assault: the plague which persists. *The Prison Journal.* 2000;80(4):407-414.

Dumond RW, Dumond DA. The treatment of sexual assault victims. In: Hensley C, ed. *Prison Sex: Practice and Policy.* Boulder, Colo: Lynne Rienner Publishers; 2002:67-88.

Federal Bureau of Prisons. *Report on Infectious Disease Management.* January, 2001:3.

Fulmer T, Paveza G, Abraham I, Fairchild S. Elder neglect assessment in the emergency department. *J Emerg Nurs.* 2000;26(5):436-443.

Groth AN. The older rape victim and her assailant. *J Geriatr Psychiatry.* 1978;11:203-215.

Harrington SPM. New Bedlam: jails—not psychiatric hospitals—now care for the indigent mentally ill. *Jail Suicide/Mental Health Update.* 1999;9(2):12-17.

Hazelwood RR, Burgess AW. *Practical Rape Investigation.* Boca Raton, Fla: CRC Press; 1995.

Kane RL, Ouslander JG, Abrass IB. *Essentials of Clinical Geriatrics.* 4th ed. New York, NY: McGraw-Hill; 1999.

Knowles GJ. Male prison rape: a search for causation and prevention. *The Howard Journal.* 1999;38(3):267-282.

Loggins SA. Rape as an intentional tort. *Trial.* Oct 1985;45-55.

Mariner J. *No Escape: Male Rape in US Prisons.* New York, NY: Human Rights Watch; 2001.

National Center on Elder Abuse. *The National Elder Abuse Incidence Study.* Washington, DC: Administration for Children and Families, Administration on Aging; 1998.

Ramsey-Klawsnik H. Elder sexual abuse: preliminary findings. *J Elder Abuse Negl.* 1991;3(3):73-89.

Ramsey-Klawsnik H. Interviewing elders for suspected sexual abuse: guidelines and techniques. *J Elder Abuse Negl.* 1993;5(1):5-18.

Ramsey-Klawsnik H. Speaking the unspeakable: an interview about elder sexual abuse. *Nexus.* 1998;4(1):4-6.

Sanders AB. Care of the elderly in the emergency department: conclusions and recommendations. *Ann Emerg Med.* 1992;21(2):830-834.

Struckman-Johnson CJ, Struckman-Johnson DL. Sexual coercion rates in seven Midwestern prison facilities for men. *The Prison Journal.* 2000;80 (4):379-390.

Struckman-Johnson CJ, Struckman-Johnson DL, Rucker L, Bumby K, Donaldson S. Sexual coercion reported by men and women in prison. *J Sex Res.* 1996;33(1):67-76.

Torrey EF. How did so many mentally ill persons get into America's jails and prisons? *American Jails.* 1999;13(5):9-13.

Yurick AG, Speir BE, Robb SS, Ebert NJ. *The Aged Person and the Nursing Process.* 3rd ed. Norwalk, Conn: McGraw-Hill/Appleton & Lange; 1989.

Chapter 14

Psychological and Social Supports

Sandra L. Bloom, MD
Jeffrey R. Jaeger, MD
Ann E. Gaulin, MS, MFT
Janice B. Asher, MD

Revised Trauma Theory: Understanding the Traumatic Nature of Sexual Assault

Sexual assault has immediate and long-term consequences that can be devastating for the physical, emotional, and relational health of the victim. Exposure to the overwhelming stress of assault alters the psychobiology, personal adjustment, and systems of meaning for the victim, and the consequences of these changes influence physical health, mental health, social adjustment, revictimization experiences, and the ability to parent. Trauma theory presents a comprehensive biopsychosocial and philosophic model within which one can understand these effects. The trauma of sexual assault has an effect on every level of a person's adjustment.

Trauma Theory

• Trauma theory helps us to understand how victims' bodies and minds respond normally to abnormal events and then become stuck, as a "state becomes a trait."

• In work with disaster victims, combat veterans, and Holocaust survivors, trauma is well defined, representing experiences of terror, exposure to atrocities, or the fear of imminent death.

• The formal diagnosis of posttraumatic stress disorder (PTSD), according to the *Diagnostic and Statistical Manual of Mental Disorders, vol 4* (DSM-IV), mandates that the victim must experience, witness, or be confronted with an event or events that involve actual or threatened death or serious injury or threat to physical integrity of self or others.

• Child victims of sexual abuse and many victims of intimate partner rape are not in imminent fear of loss of life or even loss of physical integrity. Yet sexual abuse and non–life-threatening rape are some of the most traumatizing of experiences.

• The discrepancy is explained by the complexity of the interaction of the victim and the traumatic event. Events occurring during and subsequent to the traumatic event can make a profound difference in how the victim experiences and interprets the event.

• Thus, it is not only the trauma itself that does damage to the victim but also how the individual's mind and body react to the traumatic experience combined with the unique response of the individual's social group.

Heredity's Legacy: The Autonomic Nervous System

• The way we think, the way we learn, the way we remember things, the way we feel about ourselves, the way we feel about other people, and the way we make sense of the world are all profoundly altered by traumatic experience.

• Like all mammals, humans are equipped to respond to emergencies with a "fight-or-flight" reaction via the autonomic nervous system, which has 3 purposes:

1. Creates a state of extreme hyperarousal
2. Serves a protective function, preparing the

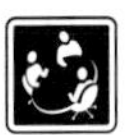

individual to respond automatically and aggressively to a perceived threat

3. Preferentially steers the individual toward action and away from the time-consuming effort of thought and language

• Prolonged hyperarousal leaves people physically and emotionally exhausted, irritable, burdened with hair-trigger tempers, and tending to perpetuate violence.

• When hyperarousal stops being a state and becomes a trait, human beings lose their capacity to assess and predict danger accurately. A consequence may be avoidance and reenactment instead of adaptation and survival.

• Complex brains and powerful memories are unique to humans and indicate extreme intelligence. However, this very intelligence creates a vulnerability to the effects of trauma in the form of flashbacks, body memories, posttraumatic nightmares, and behavioral reenactments.

• Dependence on language is important. Experiences that occurred before the age language was acquired are not integrated into consciousness and a coherent sense of identity. The individual becomes haunted by an unresolved, or even unknown, past.

• Humans are particularly ill-suited to having the people to whom they are attached also be the people doing the violating.

• Trauma profoundly disrupts the ability to manage emotional experience and people tend to either overreact or underreact. An impaired ability to respond with the appropriate emotional signal impairs the capacity to create and maintain healthy relationships.

• Humans are also physiologically designed to function best as an integrated whole, from which emerges meaning, purpose, values, belief, identity, and wisdom. The fragmentation that accompanies traumatic experience degrades this integration and impedes maximum performance.

1. Humans have a need for order, safety, and adequate protection.
2. Without balance between stimulation and soothing, humans cannot reason properly or make sense out of what happened.

Fight-or-Flight Response

• Changes in physiologic function occur that are so dramatic that in many ways, people are not the same when they are terrified as when they are calm.

• Attention becomes riveted on the potential threat, so the capacity for reasoning and exercising judgment is negatively influenced by the rising anxiety and fear.

• People become less attentive to words and more focused on threat-related signals in the environment.

• As fear rises, they may lose language functions entirely.

• People can take in vital information only in nonverbal form at this stage, specifically, through physical, emotional, and sensory experiences.

• As the level of arousal increases, "dissociation" may be triggered as an adaptive response to the hyperarousal, physiologically lowering heart rate and reducing anxiety and pain.

• Each episode of danger connects to every other episode in the human mind, so the greater the

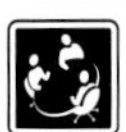

danger exposure, the greater the sensitivity to danger. Even minor threats eventually can trigger an involuntary sequence of physical, emotional, and cognitive responses.

Learned Helplessness

- Repetitive exposure to helplessness is so toxic to emotional and physiologic stability that in the service of continued survival, persons are compelled to adapt to the helplessness itself, a phenomenon termed "learned helplessness."
- If people are subjected to a sufficient number of experiences teaching them that nothing they do will affect the outcome, they give up trying.
- Once the mechanism of learned helplessness is in place, it does not automatically reverse when escape becomes possible.
- Adults in situations of domestic violence may be exposed repetitively to marital rape and experience the same sense of helpless adaptation. Persons exposed to other forms of sexual assault may also freeze up and be unable to protect themselves when similar triggering circumstances are presented.

Thinking Under Stress—Action, Not Thought

- The ability to think clearly is severely impaired when individuals are under extreme stress. Decisions tend to be based on impulse and an experienced need to protect oneself.
- Decisions are characterized by inflexibility, oversimplification, direction toward action, and poor construction, with an intolerance of mistakes, denial of personal difficulties, and anger as a problem-solving strategy.

Remembering Under Stress

• Exposure to trauma alters people's memory, producing extremes of remembering too much and recalling too little. Unlike other memories, traumatic memories appear to become etched in the mind, unaltered by the passage of time or by subsequent experience.

• There may be 2 memory systems that normally work together but are disrupted by extreme stress:

1. One for verbal learning: the "normal" memory, based on language, is particularly vulnerable to high levels of stress.
2. The other largely nonverbal: when a person is overwhelmed by fear, "speechless terror" may result. The mind shifts to a mode of thinking characterized by visual, auditory, olfactory, and kinesthetic images; physical sensations; and strong feelings. Processing of information is more rapid and the possibility of survival is generally greater in the face of threat.

• Problems arise because these powerful images, feelings, and sensations do not just go away once the danger has passed. They are deeply imprinted, in fact, more strongly so than normal everyday memories. This kind of memory may be difficult or impossible to erase although one can learn to override some responses.

• A "flashback" is a sudden, intrusive reexperiencing of a fragment of one of those traumatic unverbalized memories. A flashback has 6 characteristics:

1. Likely to occur when people are stressed or frightened, or when triggered by any association to the traumatic event.

2. One's mind is flooded by images, emotions, and physical sensations.
3. Feels like the traumatic experience is happening again; difficulty separating past from present.
4. Often individuals do not recognize that they are having a flashback but instead feel that they are "losing their mind" or having a panic attack.
5. Flashbacks may occur in the form of physical symptoms, known as a "body memory."
6. As people try to limit situations that promote hyperarousal and flashbacks, limit relationships that trigger emotions, and employ behaviors designed to control emotional responses, they may become progressively numb to all emotions and feel depressed and alienated. In this state, it takes greater and greater stimulation to feel a sense of being alive. Thus, they engage in risk-taking behaviors because it is the only way they feel "inside" themselves once again. This is one of the most devastating aspects of prolonged stress.

- The person may also develop amnesia for the traumatic event. The memory is there but no words are attached to it so it cannot be talked about or even thought about.
- For healing to occur, people must put the experience into a narrative, give it words, and share it with themselves and others. Words allow one to put things into a time sequence that finally allows a flashback to become a true memory instead of a haunting presence.

Emotions and Trauma—Dissociation

- A fundamental reason that few people die from emotional upsets is the built-in "safety valve" called "dissociation."

• Dissociation is defined as a disruption in the usually integrated functions of consciousness, memory, identity, or perception of the environment. It allows one to do more than one thing at a time.

• One common way to dissociate involves splitting off experience from feelings about that experience.

• Cutting off all emotions, or emotional numbing, occurs only in extreme cases of repetitive and almost unendurable trauma.

1. Normal responses and emotional experiences that could lead back to the traumatic memory are increasingly shut off.
2. The person is likely to become increasingly depressed.
3. Slow self-destruction through addictions or fast self-destruction through suicide are often the final outcomes of these syndromes.
4. Rage at others may also occur. People who allow rage to become dominant can become significant threats to other people as well as to themselves.

Endorphins and Stress—Addiction to Trauma

• Endorphins relieve distress, calm anxiety, improve mood, and decrease aggression.

• Endorphins are also analgesics, chemically related to morphine and heroin.

• People exposed to repeated experiences of prolonged stress experience repeatedly high levels of circulating endorphins and are likely to develop "stress-induced analgesia." It is hypothesized that this represents an addiction to their own internal endorphins, so that they feel calm only when they are under stress. Relieving stress for these individuals

can lead to fearfulness, irritability, hyperarousal, or even violence.

Trauma-Bonding

- Trauma-bonding refers to a relationship based on terror and the distortion of normal attachment behavior into something perverse and cruel.
- For victims of repetitive abuse, abusive relationships may become the normative idea of what relationships are all about.

Traumatic Reenactment

- People who have been traumatized develop what may begin as life-saving coping mechanisms, but these mechanisms may lead to compulsive repetition.
- Through reenactment, people are trying repeatedly to "tell their story" in overt or highly disguised ways. They may use the language of physical symptoms or deviant behavior.
- As emotional, physical, or social symptoms of distress pile up, victims try to extricate themselves by using the same protective devices that they used to cope with threat in the first place: dissociation, avoidance, aggression, destructive attachments, damaging behaviors, and substance addiction.

The Consequences of Traumatic Experience

- Adjustment problems
- Psychiatric disturbance, including PTSD, major depression, dysthymia, suicidality, self-mutilation, somatic complaints, poor self-esteem, anxiety disorders, sleep disturbances, substance abuse disorders, learning disabilities, conduct disorders, delinquency, aggression, increased health risk behaviors, and inappropriate sexual behavior

- Substance abuse
- Comorbid problems: panic disorder and social phobia, borderline personality disorder, somatiform disorders, obsessive-compulsive disorder, and anxiety disorders
- Adult survivors of child sexual abuse: poorer social and interpersonal relationship functioning, greater sexual dissatisfaction and dysfunction, and a greater tendency toward revictimization through adult sexual assault and physical partner violence
- Most common clinical presentation, described as "complex PTSD":

1. Includes 7 clusters of symptoms: alterations in regulating affective arousal, alterations in attention and consciousness, somatization, alterations in self-perception, alterations in perception of the perpetrator, alterations in relations to others, and alterations in systems of meaning
2. Differentiates adult victims of childhood interpersonal violence and abuse from adult-onset trauma syndromes associated with disasters

Sexual Assault and Neurobiologic Changes

- Early adverse experiences raise the sensitivity to the effects of stress later in life and make a person more vulnerable to stress-related psychiatric disorders.
- Early abuse affects brain development; the left hemisphere appears to be more vulnerable than the right.
- Women with a history of prior physical or sexual assault show a significantly attenuated cortisol response to the acute stress of rape compared to women without such a history.

• Women who develop PTSD secondary to childhood sexual abuse show a much higher rate of neurologic "soft sign" scores, that is, subtle neurologic changes, than women who were also sexually abused as children but did not develop PTSD. These differences could not be explained by alcoholism or head injury.

Health Consequences of Trauma

• Victims of trauma suffer a multitude of physical disorders not directly related to their injuries.

• PTSD has been connected to fibromyalgia, chronic pain, irritable bowel syndrome, asthma, peptic ulcer, other gastrointestinal illness, and chronic pelvic pain.

Stress, Moods, and Immunity

• Even mild stress has an impact on the immune system.

• Interpersonal stressors have 3 different effects compared to nonsocial stressors:

1. Objective stressful events are related to greater immune changes than subjective self-reports of stress.
2. Immune response varies with the duration of the stressor.
3. Interpersonal events are linked to different immune outcomes than nonsocial events.

• Factors such as stress, negative emotion, clinical depression, lack of social support, and repression or denial can negatively influence cellular and humoral indicators of immune status and function.

• Stress and negative emotion are convincingly linked to disease onset and progression.

Chronic Violence and Health

• Women who have been sexually abused and sexually assaulted routinely visit their gynecologists with a number of complaints.

• Sexual assault and abuse can take a heavy toll on sexual adjustment.

• Associations have been found between childhood maltreatment and adverse adult health outcomes: perceived poor overall health, physical and emotional functional disability, distressing physical symptoms, and health risk behavior.

Sexual Assault and Revictimization

• While victims of sexual assault tend to be revictimized, this risk is especially high among child sexual abuse survivors. Victimization before age 14 years almost doubles the risk of later adolescent victimization.

• Revictimization appears to arise because the childhood and family factors associated with childhood sexual abuse are also associated with increased sexual risks during adolescence.

• Exposure to childhood sexual abuse may encourage early onset of sexual activity, which places the victim at greater risk for sexual problems over the period of adolescence.

• Prostitution is a special case of revictimization, with a marked and dramatic relationship between prostitution and a previous history of sexual abuse.

• Victim-to-victimizer behavior

1. A victim is helpless and powerless, and helplessness is a noxious human experience that people seek to avoid.

2. Once victimized, a possible outcome is to assume the power of the perpetrator by becoming someone who terrorizes and abuses others.
3. Such behavior can reduce anxiety and provide a certain excitement; the combination of these 2 effects can become habit forming.
4. These effects can be culturally influenced. For example, boys may accommodate more easily to the victimizer role and women to the victim role in traditionally focused culture.
5. Childhood victimization is a significant predictor of the number of lifetime symptoms of antisocial personality disorder and of a diagnosis of antisocial personality disorder. However, no one-to-one direct relationship between being victimized and becoming a victimizer exists; most sexually abused people do not go on to victimize others.

Sexual Assault and Parenting

• Violence in one generation often leads to violence in the next. Parenting behavior can be profoundly affected by the impact of trauma.

• Mothers who were abusive to their children have been found to be more dissociative about their own history tending to idealize their own childhoods more, to avoid dealing with the implications of the past, and to be inconsistent in their childhood descriptions as compared to mothers who broke the cycle of abuse.

• Maternal sexual abuse history combined with maternal drug use places daughters at elevated risk.

• PTSD is significantly overexpressed in the children of mothers diagnosed with PTSD. The onset of maltreatment was significantly earlier among children whose mothers met PTSD criteria than among other maltreated children.

• Prolonged hyperarousal accompanies stress in those previously exposed to trauma.

• A close connection exists between child abuse and domestic violence.

• Abused mothers who were able to break the abusive cycle had the following 3 characteristics:

1. Were significantly more likely to have received emotional support from a nonabusive adult during childhood
2. Were more likely to have participated in therapy during some period of their lives
3. Were more likely to have had a nonabusive and more stable, emotionally supportive, and satisfying relationship with a mate

• Abused mothers who reenacted their maltreatment with their own children had the following 6 characteristics:

1. Experienced significantly more life stress
2. Were more anxious, dependent, immature, and depressed
3. Identified with their abuser or with a nonprotective parent
4. Had poor attachment with their own parents
5. Used dissociation or other defensive behaviors to protect themselves from memories of their abuse
6. Had not been able to discuss their abuse with a supportive person

Responding to Sexual Assault: Creating Sanctuary

Creating sanctuary refers to the process involved in creating safe environments that promote healing and sustain human growth, learning, and health. All medical and social institutions must find ways to address the problem by creating environments that promote and sustain better physical, emotional, and relational health.

- Change the presenting question with which we verbally or implicitly confront another human being whose behavior we do not understand from "What's wrong with you?" to "What's happened to you?"

1. Shifts the perspective, moving toward a position of compassion and understanding and away from blame and criticism
2. Provides the survivor with an important ingredient—hope

- Focus on the human need for safety.

1. Includes not just physical safety but psychologic, social, and moral safety as well; an environment cannot be truly safe unless these safety levels are addressed
2. Psychologic safety: the ability to be safe with oneself
3. Social safety: the ability to be safe in groups and with other people
4. Moral safety: the maintenance of a value system that does not contradict itself and is consistent with healthy human development as well as physical, psychologic, and social safety

• Because the individual has been exposed to helplessness, interventions to overcome the traumatizing experience must focus on mastery and empowerment and avoid further experiences of helplessness.

1. Understand that prolonged hyperarousal and loss of ability to manage emotional states appropriately produce many behaviors that are socially objectionable or even destructive but that represent the individual's only method of coping with overwhelming and uncontrollable emotions.
2. Offer better substitutes, specifically, healthy and sustaining human relationships.
3. Reduce stress when good decisions must be made.
4. Reduce memory problems by providing opportunities for individuals to talk about their experiences; this includes programs that focus on nonverbal expression (art, music, movement, and drama as well as sports), which can be vital adjuncts to healing efforts.
5. Develop techniques to help people manage their emotions more effectively and build and reinforce the acquisition of "emotional intelligence."

• For individuals who are addicted to trauma, intervention strategies must focus on helping to "detoxify" them from this behavior in 3 ways:

1. Provide environments that insist on the establishment and maintenance of safety.
2. Provide opportunities to learn how to create relationships not based on terror and the abuse of power, even though abusive power feels "normal" and "right."

3. Provide direct relationship coaching and the experience of engaging in relationships that are not abusive and that do not permit or tolerate abusive and punitive behavior.

• Individuals who have been sexually assaulted or traumatized significantly must be able to grieve.

1. Unresolved grief prevents recovery from the psychologic and physical problems that result from exposure to a traumatic experience.
2. To heal, survivors must open up the old wounds, remember and reconstruct the past, resolve the accompanying painful emotions, and reconnect to their internal world and the world around them.

Social Supports

The rape trauma syndrome is comparable to what was originally described by government researchers as PTSD. Interventions must take into account this syndrome and where the survivor is in his or her recovery. If and when the survivor chooses to reach out and tell his or her story, the nature and extent of the support provided can play a critical role in the survivor's ability to modulate symptoms and recover from the trauma.

Nature of Social Supports

Social Services

• Rape crisis centers are traditionally nonprofit, community-based organizations staffed by paid professional counselors and volunteers.

1. Services are usually free and offered to adult and child survivors of both genders.

2. They traditionally offer a 24-hour hotline, hospital and court accompaniment, short-term crisis counseling services, and a strong advocacy-based organizational system within the community.
3. State coalitions of rape crisis centers have sprung up to distribute state and federal funding, monitor quality of services, and help establish guidelines for community education and training about sexual violence.
4. Collaborative efforts have been made between rape crisis centers and domestic violence agencies.
5. Many rape crisis centers have established partnerships with district attorneys, police, hospitals, and other agencies to provide more comprehensive services to individuals and families with increasingly more complex problems.

• Domestic violence programs are often found to be related to services for survivors of sexual assault.

1. Counseling for survivors of domestic violence has traditionally focused on safety planning, empowerment, and restoration of self-esteem.
2. Counseling for sexual assault survivors treats and prevents the debilitating effects of PTSD.

• Victim assistance programs are often funded through a prosecuting attorney's office and provide services for all victims of violent interpersonal crime.

1. They offer court accompaniment and victim compensation services to survivors who report their assaults to the police department.

2. Much of their funding comes from states' victims compensation funds collected from adjudicated offenders.
3. Assistance in filing monetary claims to the state usually depends on the survivor making a police report about his or her assault.

Healthcare System

- Acute care

1. In the postassault setting, the medical provider's chief role is to assess and treat the victim's acute medical needs and collect evidence.
2. The medical provider can also play an important role as a social support for victims in the acute setting and throughout recovery.
3. Medical personnel can employ strategies that begin the healing process or at least prevent repeat traumatization.
4. Members of the medical team must ensure a safe, private environment for recording the victim's history and the examination.
5. The responsibility for calling a friend, family member, or rape crisis counselor may also belong to the medical acute-care provider.
6. The healthcare provider can also assist with the restoration of a sense of order and predictability.
7. The patient's safety must be emphasized.
8. Take care to inform the patient in advance what will happen during the examination and how long it might last, then ask the patient's permission to begin the examination. This will help restore the victim's sense of control over what is happening to his or her body.

9. Healthcare institutions have a responsibility to their staff and to survivors to train and support staff involved in the care of sexual assault victims.
10. The creation and maintenance of a caring healthcare environment is crucial.

• Sexual assault nurse examiner (SANE) and sexual assault response team (SART) programs

1. SANE programs provide 24-hour availability of personnel who can offer immediate, comprehensive, and compassionate evaluation and treatment of sexual assault victims. Program goals are to lessen the traumatizing nature of the rape examination, reduce repeated questioning and examination of the victim, and increase effective collection and preservation of evidence. SANE practitioners can be nurses, nurse practitioners, physician assistants, or other healthcare providers. These individuals are called immediately when a sexual assault victim is identified, whether by law enforcement personnel, rescue personnel, or emergency department staff. They are responsible for completing the entire evidentiary examination (including leading the team interview); conducting assessments of sexually transmitted disease (STD) and pregnancy as well as their prevention strategies; performing the colposcopy evaluation with photographs; and ensuring appropriate referrals for support and care, which often take lower priority when the responsibility for this is left to busy emergency department personnel.
2. A SART team is activated immediately upon identification of a sexual assault victim. A SART team may include SANE staff, law

enforcement personnel, and rape crisis center staff or volunteers. Early involvement of law enforcement personnel reduces repeated questioning of the victim because the medical history obtained by the SANE practitioner can link with the questioning by law enforcement personnel. A rape crisis center volunteer can establish an early link with the victim should he or she wish to pursue a relationship with the agency later. Many communities have SART partner agencies located at one site, which fosters better interagency cooperation and communication and can further reduce the trauma of survivors.

- Postacute care medical support

1. Nonacute care medical providers are likely to provide postassault care and support for most survivors.
2. The unique confidential relationship between a healthcare provider and the patient makes the patient-provider relationship a natural place for survivors to turn to for support.
3. It is also reasonable to expect all medical providers to have the basic skill set required to assess, evaluate, and treat the psychosocial complications of sexual assault.
4. Healthcare providers should be familiar with the phases of the rape trauma syndrome; be comfortable treating depression; provide a "safe" nonjudgmental setting where survivors can feel comfortable discussing their experience, their feelings, and their fears; and have access to referral information should a patient decide to pursue professional postsexual assault counseling.

- Churches and religious groups

1. Pastors, priests, nuns, and rabbis are now reaching out for special training to counsel members of their congregation who have disclosed sexual abuse issues. They are also learning assessment skills to refer their members to mental healthcare providers as they learn of the longer-term effects of severe trauma.
2. Collaboration of rape crisis centers with community churches can be mutually beneficial, allowing rape crisis centers to access an audience that may not have heard their message and to provide workshops and training to church-sponsored groups, thereby increasing awareness of sexual abuse issues and increasing access to services for survivors. PTSD and its impact on victims and their families are now being taught at many seminaries and pastoral colleges.

- Other social supports

1. Most survivors of sexual assault turn to someone in their informal support network immediately after an assault. This form of social support is important to recovery.
2. Social support reliably moderates psychologic distress after sexual assault, with the extent of informal support determined by the number of people with whom the survivor felt he or she could confide as a moderating factor in the severity of physical symptoms and perceived health up to 1 year after the assault.
3. The reaction of those close to the survivor can affect recovery, with sexual assault traumatizing family members and significant others in addition to the victim. How they cope with

trauma influences how they interact with the victim, as follows:

Maladaptive responses: overprotection, encouraging the victim to keep the assault secret, focusing primarily on their own sense of victimization

Adaptive responses: empathy and allowing the victim to express fears without fear of criticism while responding to his or her own concerns as a secondary issue

4. Girlfriends, husbands or boyfriends, and police have received the highest ratings of supportiveness; physicians were rated the lowest.
5. Victims of "attempted" rapes have just as many problems with adjustment 3 months after the assault as those who identified their assault as "completed," yet they receive much less support in that period, indicating that support is at least partially related to society's perception of the stressfulness of the assault.

Program Development

The steps to establishing or improving a community's response to sexual assault vary according to size of the community, presence and organization of existing victims' rights or advocacy organizations, and level of knowledge of the healthcare community regarding sexual assault. Those outlined here reflect principles to be included.

• Involve the multiple agencies and disciplines necessary to develop effective services. This facilitates communication and cooperation.

1. Develop a task force with clearly defined goals.
2. Members include hospital administrators, emergency department nurses, rape crisis center

leaders, law enforcement representatives, and the judiciary. Special efforts should be made to recruit representatives from underserved minority communities and sexual minorities.

3. Schedule regular meetings and ensure that all voices are heard to maintain continued engagement from all parties.

• Invite respected leaders to participate and lend support to the effort. This ensures community support, with members of administration more willing to promote the needs of the agency or program if their superiors have been publicly and visibly involved from the outset of a project.

• Optimize efforts by using existing personnel and resources as building blocks.

• Provide for coordination of services across multiple disciplines. This has been found to be predictive of a relatively positive victim experience with the social support system. The coordination of services should be prioritized as they unfold and are developed:

1. Look objectively at what attributes of sexual assault support systems have proved successful.
2. Provide for interagency training.
3. Keep the services victim-centered rather than agency- or service-centered.

• Provide education and risk reduction strategies, as follows:

1. Target prevention efforts at the attitudes and stereotypes of men in particular and society as a whole.
2. Target young boys at the elementary and middle school levels.

3. Develop or incorporate innovative prevention strategies for use at high schools and colleges.
4. Develop special programs to change sexual stereotypes and interpersonal violence to attract more men to serve as instructors and male role models.
5. Remember to perform outreach activities for parents to reduce the risk for sexual abuse of children. Services to families of sexual assault survivors greatly increase the chance of successful recovery.

- Address funding issues, exploring private and corporate foundations interested in funding targeted social service projects.

Moving Beyond the Don't-Ask–Don't-Tell Approach to Abuse and Assault

Don't Ask

Interpersonal violence is not detected in the majority of cases because of acknowledged or unacknowledged barriers limiting the effectiveness of clinicians.

Acknowledged Barriers

Clinicians perceive many barriers to routinely screening for or asking relevant questions pertaining to violence, as follows:

I haven't been trained to do this.

I don't have time to do this.

It isn't my job; it isn't a medical problem.

I'm not a domestic violence expert.

This doesn't happen in the patient population I see.

This is a personal problem and isn't my business.

If it's so bad, why doesn't she leave?

What's the point? She'll just go back to him or find another abuser.

Table 14-1. Stages of Behavior Change

STAGE 1: PRECONTEMPLATION

The patient does not perceive a problem. Her partner's violence is "no big deal" or is "no different from what happens in any other family." During this stage, the clinician can provide information: violence is common, it is not the victim's fault, it is dangerous for the victim and for children who witness the violence, and resources exist to help. The patient can be offered written material about violence, safety planning, and local resources. She can be offered a referral to a social worker or domestic violence counselor.

STAGE 2: CONTEMPLATION

The patient perceives a problem and is considering change. However, although she may be more open to information and offers of help, she probably feels intensely ambivalent about the risks versus the rewards of leaving the relationship. As a result, many patients remain in this stage for many years. During this stage, stressing the rewards of leaving, expressing optimism about the possibility of change, and supporting safety measures while the patient is considering change may be of great benefit. Remind the patient that the abuse is not her fault and that help is available. Specifically, in addition to discussing safety strategies, she should be offered referrals to social service and advocacy resources.

STAGE 3: PREPARATION

The patient is actively planning change. She has already taken some measures to prepare for ending the relationship. It is crucial to help her understand the potential danger for herself and her children when she does actually leave and even afterward. At this time, in addition to referrals to other experts, an exit strategy is essential. The patient should be urged to consider a plan that includes identifying people she can stay with, planning ways to save and hide money, making copies of all important papers and documents, etc.

(continued)

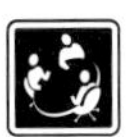

Table 14-1. *(continued)*

STAGE 4: ACTION

The patient has ended the relationship. She needs to appreciate that she is still vulnerable to violent assaults. Safety strategies must be emphasized. The clinician should support her decision while explaining that relapse is common; victims of abuse, for many reasons, often return to the abuser. However, this behavior is not "going around in circles." Instead, it is a return to a prior stage of change and is much more likely to result in a more successful move forward later. This knowledge and attitude are important for the clinician as well. Without this understanding, clinicians can easily feel overwhelmed by frustration and anger with the patient now perceived as "wasting our time."

STAGE 5: MAINTENANCE

The patient has maintained the successful behavior change for several months. Even at this time, she is not free from assaultive and abusive behavior from the partner. He may stalk her; he may engage in a prolonged custody battle to further exhaust, intimidate, and impoverish her; or he may engage the children in spying behavior against her. In addition, many emotional, financial, psychologic, cultural, and familial pressures may occur that do not support the changes she has made. For example, her partner may urge her to come back, promising that he will never hurt her again. She may feel pressure from her children or other family members to keep the family together. She may feel emotionally and financially overwhelmed. The clinician must support her healthy behavioral changes while helping her avoid feeling demoralized if she returns to the relationship.

Unacknowledged Barriers

- The issue of relationship violence is too close for comfort with regard to clinicians' own personal histories as well as their sense of safety in their own communities.
- Medical training itself may be viewed as an abusive experience.
- Victims of abuse may be difficult and unlikable patients.
- Physicians do not want to open a Pandora's box.

Don't Tell: Barriers to Disclosure by the Victim

- Fear of retaliation
- Shame
- Insensitive responses by their healthcare providers

Treating Victims Without Feeling Hopeless

- Viewing chronic lifestyles and behaviors, such as smoking and unhealthy dietary habits, as acute illnesses that need to be "cured" is inappropriate and futile.
- Because a person in an abusive relationship is at greatest risk for being seriously injured or even killed when he or she tries to leave, urging the victim to leave without having thought out a safety plan is irresponsible, and leaves the victim who is not planning to end an abusive relationship feeling even more isolated and worthless.

Stages of Behavior Change

The Transtheoretical Model (TTM) of Change, or Stages of Behavioral Change Model, takes into account stages of attitude that precede behavioral

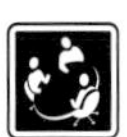

change. By understanding these different stages, clinicians can appreciate how to help patients who are either unwilling or unable to leave violent relationships. The clinician can help the patient and not become frustrated or angry about the patient's noncompliance in leaving an abusive relationship and the patient does not feel like a failure for being unable to comply **(Table 14-1)**.

References

Ackerman PT, Newton JE, McPherson WB, Jones JG, Dykman RA. Prevalence of posttraumatic stress disorder and other psychiatric diagnoses in three groups of abused children (sexual, physical, and both). *Child Abuse Negl.* 1998;22:759-774.

Alford JD, Mahone C, Fielstein EM. Cognitive and behavioral sequelae of combat: conceptualization and implications for treatment. *J Trauma Stress.* 1988;1:489-501.

American Medical Association. *Strategies for the Treatment and Prevention of Sexual Assault.* Chicago, Ill: American Medical Association; 1995.

American Medical Association, Council on Scientific Affairs. Violence against women: relevance for medical practitioners. *JAMA.* 1992; 267:3184-3189.

American Psychiatric Association. *Diagnostic and Statistical Manual of Mental Disorders.* 4th ed. Washington, DC: American Psychiatric Press; 1994.

Amir M, Kaplan Z, Neumann L, Sharabani R, Shani N, Buskila D. Posttraumatic stress disorder, tenderness and fibromyalgia. *J Psychosom Res.* 1997;42:607-613.

Angst J, Degonda M, Ernst C. The Zurich Study: XV. Suicide attempts in a cohort from age 20 to 30. *Eur Arch Psychiatry Clin Neurosci.* 1992;242:135-141.

Bachen EA, Manuck SB, Marsland AL, et al. Lymphocyte subset and cellular immune responses to a brief experimental stressor. *Psychosom Med.* 1992;54:673-679.

Badura AS, Reiter RC, Altmaier EM, Rhomberg A. Dissociation, somatization, substance abuse, and coping in women with chronic pelvic pain. *Obstet Gynecol.* 1997;90:405-410.

Benedikt RA, Kolb LC. Preliminary findings on chronic pain and posttraumatic stress disorder. *Am J Psychiatry.* 1986;143:908-910.

Berliner L, Elliott DM. Sexual abuse of children. In: Briere J, Berliner L, Bulkley JA, Jenny C, Reid T, eds. *The APSAC Handbook on Child Maltreatment.* Thousand Oaks, Calif: Sage Publications; 1996:51-71.

Bloom SL. *Creating Sanctuary: Toward the Evolution of Sane Societies.* New York, NY: Routledge; 1997.

Brosschot JF, Benschop RJ, Godaert GL, et al. Influence of life stress on immunological reactivity to mild psychological stress. *Psychosom Med.* 1994;56:216-224.

Burgess AW, Holmstrom LL. Rape trauma syndrome. *Am J Psychol.* 1974;131:981-986.

Bushnell JA, Wells JE, Oakley-Browne MA. Long-term effects of intrafamilial sexual abuse in childhood. *Acta Psychiatr Scand.* 1992;85: 136-142.

Coe CL. Psychosocial factors and immunity in nonhuman primates: a review. *Psychosom Med.* 1993;55:298-308.

Cohen S, Herbert TB. Health psychology: psychological factors and physical disease from the perspective of human psychoneuroimmunology. *Annu Rev Psychol.* 1996;47:113-142.

Connors ME, Morse W. Sexual abuse and eating disorders: a review. *Int J Eat Disord.* 1993;13:1-11.

Davidson JR, Hughes D, Blazer DG, George LK. Posttraumatic stress disorder in the community: an epidemiological study. *Psychol Med.* 1991; 21:713-721.

DeBellis MD, Lefter L, Trickett PK, Putnam FW. Urinary catecholamine excretion in sexually abused girls. *J Am Acad Child Adolesc Psychiatry.* 1994; 33:320-327.

Drossman DA. Sexual and physical abuse and gastrointestinal illness. *Scand J Gastroenterol Suppl.* 1995;208:90-96.

Egeland B, Jacobvitz D, Sroufe LA. Breaking the cycle of abuse. *Child Dev.* 1988;59:1080-1088.

Egeland B, Susman-Stillman A. Dissociation as a mediator of child abuse across generations. *Child Abuse Negl.* 1996;20:1123-1132.

Famularo R, Fenton T, Kinscherff R, Ayoub C, Barnum R. Maternal and child posttraumatic stress disorder in cases of child maltreatment. *Child Abuse Negl.* 1994;18:27-36.

Fergusson DM, Horwood LJ, Lynskey MT. Childhood sexual abuse, adolescent sexual behaviors and sexual revictimization. *Child Abuse Negl.* 1997;21:789-803.

Geisser ME, Roth RS, Bachman JE, Echert TA. The relationship between symptoms of posttraumatic stress disorder and pain, affective disturbance and disability among patients with accident and nonaccident related pain. *Pain*. 1996;66:207-214.

Glover H. Emotional numbing: a possible endorphinmediated phenomenon associated with posttraumatic stress disorders and other allied psychopathologic states. *J Trauma Stress*. 1992; 5:643-675.

Goleman D. *Working With Emotional Intelligence*. New York, NY: Bantam Books; 1998.

Green AH. Factors contributing to the generational transmission of child maltreatment. *J Am Acad Child Adolesc Psychiatry*. 1998;37:1334-1336.

Hampton HL. Care of the woman who has been raped. *N Engl J Med*. 1995;332:234-237.

Herbert TB, Cohen S. Stress and immunity in humans: a meta-analytic review. *Psychom Med*. 1993;55:364-379.

Herman JL, Perry JC, Van der Kolk BA. Childhood trauma in borderline personality disorder. *Am J Psychiatry*. 1989;146:490-495.

Holmstrom LL, Burgess AW. Rape: husbands' and boyfriends' initial reactions. *Fam Coord*. 1979; 28:321-330.

International Association of Forensic Nurses. *Sexual Assault Nurse Examination Guidelines*. Pittman, NJ: IAFN; 1999.

Irwin C, Falsetti SS, Lydiard RB, Ballenger JC, Brock CD, Brener W. Comorbidity of posttraumatic stress disorder and irritable bowel syndrome. *J Clin Psychiatry*. 1996;57:576-578.

James B. *Handbook for Treatment of Attachment-Trauma Problems in Children.* New York, NY: Lexington Books; 1994.

Janis IL. Decision making under stress. In: Goldberger L, Breznitz S, eds. *Handbook of Stress: Theoretical and Clinical Aspects.* New York, NY: Free Press; 1982:69-87.

Kimerling R, Calhoun KS. Somatic symptoms, social support, and treatment seeking among sexual assault victims. *J Consult Clin Psychol.* 1994;62:333-340.

LeDoux JE. Emotion, memory, and the brain. *Sci Am.* 1994;270:50-57.

Ledray L. *SANE Development and Operation Guide.* Washington, DC: US Dept of Justice, Office for Victims of Crime; 1999.

Leserman J, Drossman DA, Li Z, Toomey TC, Nachman G, Glogau L. Sexual and physical abuse history in gastroenterology practice: how types of abuse impact health status. *Psychosom Med.* 1996;58:4-15.

Luntz BK, Widom CS. Antisocial personality disorder in abused and neglected children grown up. *Am J Psychiatry.* 1994;151:670-674.

McCown W, Galina ZH, Johnson JL, DeSimone PA, Posa J. Borderline personality disorder and laboratory-induced cold pressor pain: evidence of stress-induced analgesia. *J Psychopath Behav Assess.* 1993;15:87-95.

Perry BD. The neurodevelopmental impact of violence in childhood. In: Schetky D, Benedek E, eds. *Textbook of Child and Adolescent Forensic Psychiatry.* Washington, DC: American Psychiatric Press, Inc; 2002:221-238.

Perry BD, Pate JE. Neurodevelopment and the psychobiological roots of posttraumatic stress disorder. In: Koziol LF, Stout CE, eds. *The Neuropsychology of Mental Disorders: A Practical Guide*. Springfield, Ill: Charles C. Thomas; 1993:129-146.

Perry JC, Herman JL, Van der Kolk BA, Hoke LA. Psychotherapy and psychological trauma in borderline personality disorder. *Psychiatr Ann*. 1990;20:33-43.

Petter LM, Whitehill DL. Management of female sexual assault. *Am Fam Physician*. 1998;58:920-926.

Pollack MH, Otto MW, Rosenbaum JF, Sachs GS. Personality disorders in patients with panic disorder: association with childhood anxiety disorders, early trauma, comorbidity, and chronicity. *Compr Psychiatry*. 1992;33:78-83.

Prochaska JA, Redding CA, Harlow LL, Rossi JS, Velicer WF. The transtheoretical model of change and HIV prevention: a review. *Health Educ Q*. 1994;21:471-486.

Rodriguez MA, Quiroga SS, Bauer HM. Breaking the silence: battered women's perspectives on medical care. *Arch Fam Med*. 1996;5:153-158.

Selig C. Sexual assault nurse examiner and sexual assault response team (SANE/SART) program. *Nurs Clin North Am*. 2000;35:311-319.

Silverman D. Sharing the crisis of rape: counseling the mates and families of victims. *Am J Orthopsychiatry*. 1978;48:166-173.

Sisley A, Jacobs LM, Poole G, Campbell S, Esposito T. Violence in America: a public health crisis—domestic violence. *J Trauma*. 1999;46:1105-1112.

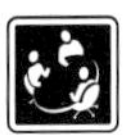

Solomon SD, Davidson JRT. Trauma: prevalence, impairment, service use, and cost. *J Clin Psychiatry*. 1997;58:5-11.

Sugg NK, Inui T. Primary care physicians' response to domestic violence, opening Pandora's box. *JAMA*. 1992;267:65-68.

Teicher MH, Ito Y, Glod CA, Andersen SL, Dumont N, Ackerman E. Preliminary evidence for abnormal cortical development in physically and sexually abused children using EEG coherence and MRI. *Ann N Y Acad Sci*. 1997;821:160-175.

Van der Kolk BA. The body keeps the score: approaches to the psychobiology of posttraumatic stress disorder. In: Van der Kolk BA, McFarlane C, Weisaeth L, eds. *Traumatic Stress: The Effects of Overwhelming Experience on Mind, Body, and Society*. New York, NY: Guilford Press; 1996a:214-241.

Van der Kolk BA. Trauma and memory. In: Van der Kolk BA, McFarlane C, Weisaeth L, eds. *Traumatic Stress: The Effects of Overwhelming Experience on Mind, Body, and Society*. New York, NY: Guilford Press; 1996b:279-302.

Van der Kolk BA, Burbridge JA, Suzuki J. The psychobiology of traumatic memory: clinical implications of neuroimaging studies. In: Yehuda R, McFarlane AC, eds. *Psychobiology of Posttraumatic Stress Disorder*. New York: New York Academy of Sciences; 1997:99-113, 821.

Walker EA, Gelfand AN, Gelfand MD, Green C, Katon WJ. Chronic pelvic pain and gynecological symptoms in women with irritable bowel syndrome. *J Psychosom Obstet Gynaecol*. 1996; 17:39-46.

Walker EA, Katon WJ, Hansom J, et al. Medical and psychiatric symptoms in women with childhood sexual abuse. *Psychosom Med.* 1992;54:658-664.

Walling MK, O'Hara MW, Reiter RC, Milburn AK, Lilly G, Vincent SD. Abuse history and chronic pain in women: II. A multivariate analysis of abuse and psychological morbidity. *Obstet Gynecol.* 1994;84:200-206.

Chapter 15

Caregiver Issues

Sandra L. Bloom, MD
Linda E. Ledray, RN, PhD, SANE-A, FAAN
Rena Rovere, MS, FNP

Caring for the Caregiver: Avoiding and Treating Vicarious Traumatization

Definitions

- Vicarious traumatization: cumulative transformative effect on the helper of working with survivors of traumatic life events, positive and negative; symptoms resemble those of posttraumatic stress disorder (PTSD) but also indicate a disrupted frame of reference, including identity, worldview, and spirituality, and impacts on psychologic need areas.
- Secondary traumatic stress: behavior and emotions that result from knowledge about a traumatizing event experienced by another and the stress resulting from helping or wanting to help a traumatized or suffering person; closely resembles PTSD; includes symptoms of hyperarousal, emotional numbing, avoidance, and intrusive experiences.
- Compassion fatigue: the natural, predictable, treatable, and preventable unwanted consequence of working with suffering people.
- Burnout: a collection of symptoms associated with emotional exhaustion and generally attributed to increased work load and institutional stress, described by a process that includes gradual exposure to job strain, erosion of idealism, and lack of achievement; may result from repetitive or chronic exposure to vicarious traumatization that is unrecognized and unsupported by the organizational setting.

• Countertransference: a broader term that refers to all reactions to a client and the material he or she brings; reactions are specific to the particular client and are tied to interactions with that client; vicarious traumatization is a specific form of countertransference experience, differentiated from other countertransference reactions in that it can continue to affect lives and work long after interactions with the other person have ceased.

Symptoms Specific to Vicarious Traumatization

• Disturbed frame of reference.

• Disrupted beliefs about other people and the world, including beliefs about causality and higher purpose.

1. World is seen as a much more dangerous place.
2. Caregiver may see other people as malevolent and evil, untrustworthy, exploitative, or alienating.
3. Maintaining a sense of hope and belief in the goodness of humanity is increasingly difficult.

• Psychologic areas affected are safety, trust, esteem, intimacy, and control.

1. Loss of secure sense of safety leads to increased fearfulness, heightened sense of personal vulnerability, excessive security concerns, behavior directed at increasing security, and increased fear for the lives and safety of loved ones.
2. Capacity to trust may be so impaired that a belief develops that no one can be trusted. Trust in one's own judgment and perceptions can be negatively altered.
3. It becomes difficult to maintain a sense of self-esteem, particularly around areas of competence.

It may also be difficult to maintain a sense of esteem about others, leading to a pervasive suspiciousness of other people's motivations and behavior.

4. Problems with intimacy may develop, leading to difficulties in spending time alone; self-medication with food, alcohol, or drugs; or engaging in compulsive behaviors (shopping, exercise, sex). These problems can also lead to isolation from others and withdrawal from relationships (family, friends, and professional colleagues).
5. The more control the caregiver feels has been lost, the more control he or she tries to exert over self and others. Efforts may also be made to narrow or restrict the scope of one's world in the hope of avoiding anything that may be experienced as being outside of one's control.

• Positive as well as negative impacts are noted. Choices must be made to support positive rather than negative transformational changes.

Who Is Affected?

• Vicarious traumatization has occurred in emergency workers, physicians, nurses, police officers, firemen, journalists, clergy, social service workers, colleagues, family members, and other witnesses and bystanders to disasters and other trauma.

• The rate of vicarious traumatization appears to be related to years of experience or exposure to trauma.

• Risk factors:

1. Having a past history of traumatic experience
2. Overwork
3. Ignoring health boundaries

4. Taking on too much
5. Lack of experience as a therapist
6. Too much experience as a therapist
7. Dealing with large numbers of traumatized children, especially sexually abused children
8. Working with large numbers of patients who suffer from dissociative disorders
9. Having too many negative clinical outcomes

- Protective factors:

1. Good social support
2. Strong ethical principles of practice
3. Knowledge of theory
4. Ongoing training
5. Development of competence in practice strategies and techniques
6. Awareness of the potential of vicarious traumatization and the need to take deliberate steps to minimize the impact

Causes

- Vicarious traumatization can be viewed as a normal reaction to abnormal stress or a picture of adaptive coping skills gone wrong.
- Biologic, psychologic, social, and moral, spiritual, and philosophical components of the individual interact with the professional and sociopolitical context of the individual's life space to produce the final outcome.

Biologic Causality: Emotional Contagion

- Listening to victims of trauma can produce a noxious physiologic and psychologic state in the listener that is strongly defended against.

- Victims' social groups take measures to prevent the victims from sharing their experience and thereby spreading the contagion.

- Stress, in activating the complex human stress response, produces many kinds of powerful neurochemicals, including cortisol, an immune system suppressor.

- Chronic inhibition of negative emotions produces increasing work for the autonomic nervous system; this increased load functions as a chronic stressor with the result that biologic survival systems that should be "on" only under emergency conditions are reset to be "on" all the time.

- People who are traumatized are often overwhelmed by their emotions, particularly in the acutely traumatized state. Suppressing emotional states is bad for their health.

- Caregiving relationships help surface those emotions, often long buried, and the helper is the one who is most likely to be exposed to the overwhelming nature of the victim's emotional state. Good caregiving requires that the caregiver respond to this state in certain limited and prescribed ways and respond by containing rather than expressing the caregiver's own physiologic states of hyperarousal, fear, anger, and grief.

Psychologic Causality: Loss of Positive Illusions

- As we let the reality of "it really happened" in, we recognize that "it could happen to me" and feel all of the vulnerability that goes along with that recognition.

- The recurring sense of helplessness that victims feel may also affect the helpers, bringing with it a sense of hopelessness, expressed as "there's nothing I can do."

• Positive illusions about oneself, other people, and the world are destroyed by the constant exposure to traumatized people.

• The greatest conflict, the one most likely to produce symptoms, occurs in cases of family violence, including child abuse, spousal abuse, rape, and child sexual abuse because it threatens one of our most cherished cultural notions—the family as a safe place.

Social Causality: Inability to Use Normal Social Obstacles

• Traumatic experiences shatter basic personal and cultural assumptions about the primary way we order reality. There is no safety, the world no longer makes sense, other people cannot be trusted, the future is no longer predictable, and the past is no longer known because of dissociation. After trauma, one of the most perplexing experiences for the individual victim is that the world goes on as before.

• The need to talk, confess, and release stored tension is powerful and important for health, but the culture actively inhibits the individual's response.

• Listeners avoid having their own cognitive schemas disrupted, and they avoid the hyperarousal that is frequently an accompaniment of emotional contagion.

• Good caregivers are carefully trained to avoid using the kinds of social defenses that other people use against the impact of this recognition of the effects of violence on individuals. Clinicians and other caregivers are taught to screen for violence, listen carefully, avoid giving in to their own inclinations to distance themselves, and empathize with the experience and emotions of others. The inability

to use the social barriers available to other people makes helping professionals more likely to experience vicarious traumatization.

Organization Causality: Sick Systems

• Organizational settings that refuse to accept the severity and pervasiveness of traumatic experience in the population they serve thereby refuse to provide the social support caregivers require to do adequate work.

• Dysfunctional systems resemble dysfunctional families, having some or all of the following 9 characteristics:

1. An ongoing culture of crisis where long-term and preventive solutions are not formulated because all time and resources are spent "putting out fires"
2. The replacement of democratic processes with authoritarian decision making and rigid hierarchies
3. A culture of shaming, blaming, and judgmentalism
4. Maintenance of order through isolation, splitting, overcontrol, manipulation, and deceitful practices, leading to mistrust and avoidance
5. Little humor, with positive emotions discouraged and negative emotions tolerated or encouraged
6. Eventual development of a culture of toughness and meanness or actual violence
7. Denial that any real problems exist
8. A high degree of hypocrisy in daily functioning
9. Active discouragement of confronting reality

Moral, Spiritual, and Philosophical Causality: Theoretical Conflicts

• Most of these conflicts are not direct but instead comprise a background of disorder and include the following:

1. Desacralization of healing
2. Commodification of healthcare
3. Shortcomings of the medical model
4. A bias toward individualism
5. The issue of individual violence embedded within a context of cultural violence

• The resulting environment has been described as a "pressure cooker" where no one is served well except, perhaps, profiteers.

• It becomes increasingly difficult for caregivers to find the time or psychic energy to provide the compassion that victims of violence require if they are to take the first steps in recovery.

• Healthcare professionals may succumb to physical fatigue and compassion fatigue.

• In the traditional medical model, the patient is largely passive, waiting for cure or at least alleviation of symptoms to be delivered by a medical practitioner.

• The trauma therapist knows that one of the keys to recovery for the victim is empowerment, not passivity, and that further experiences of helplessness are often damaging.

• The role of the caregiver is different in sickness versus injury, so that the caregiver must face various role strains and stresses, as follows:

1. How do I keep my patient safe when only my patient has the power to keep herself safe?

2. What is the best way to empower people?
3. What is my responsibility and what is not my responsibility?
4. When do my interventions promote recovery and when do they inhibit or discourage recovery?
5. If this person is suffering from an injury as the result of a social, fixable problem, what is my role in preventing further injury to this person and to others?

- If caregivers attempt to stay politically disengaged, or "scientifically neutral," they may find themselves medicalizing or pathologizing disorders that are actually not a result of a medical problem but of a social, political, or economic problem. They may find themselves part of an oppressive system rather than countering that system.
- In contrast, if caregivers stand up and powerfully bear witness to the violence that they have observed, they are likely to be labeled as outcasts, troublemakers, lacking in scientific rigor, and subverters of the system.

Solutions

Caregivers must develop their own personal and professional strategies for bringing about change in key areas that will help reduce or prevent the further evolution of a process that could lead to burnout. **Table 15-1** offers some suggestions.

SANE-SART History and Role Development

The development of sexual assault nurse examiner (SANE) programs began in the early 1970s although different terminology was used to describe the role during the early years. Their development

Table 15-1. Prevention Stategies for Caregivers

PERSONAL-PHYSICAL

— Engage in self-care behaviors, including proper diet and sleep
— Undertake physical activity, such as exercise and yoga

PERSONAL-PSYCHOLOGIC

— Identify triggers that may cause you to experience vicarious traumatization
— Obtain therapy if personal issues and past traumas get in the way
— Know your own limitations
— Keep the boundaries set for yourself and others
— Know your own level of tolerance
— Engage in recreational activities, eg, listening to music, reading, spending time in nature
— Modify your work schedule to fit your personal life

PERSONAL-SOCIAL

— Engage in social activities outside of work
— Garner emotional support from colleagues
— Garner emotional support from family and friends

PERSONAL-MORAL

— Adopt a philosophical or religious outlook and be reminded that you cannot take responsibility for the client's healing but rather must act as a midwife, guide, coach, or mentor
— Clarify your own sense of meaning and purpose in life
— Connect with the larger sociopolitical framework and develop social activism skills

(continued)

Table 15-1. *(continued)*

PROFESSIONAL

- — Become knowledgeable about the effects of trauma on self and others
- — Attempt to monitor or diversify case load
- — Seek consultation on difficult cases
- — Get supervision from someone who understands the dynamics and treatment of PTSD
- — Take breaks during workday
- — Recognize that you are not alone in facing the stress of working with traumatized clients—normalize your reactions
- — Use a team for support
- — Maintain collegial on-the-job support, thus limiting the sense of isolation
- — Understand dynamics of traumatic reenactment

ORGANIZATIONAL/WORK SETTING

- — Accept stressors as real and legitimate, impacting individuals and the group as a whole
- — Work in a team
- — Create a culture to counteract the effects of trauma
- — Establish a clear value system within your organization
- — Develop clarity about job tasks and personnel guidelines
- — Obtain supervisory/management support
- — Maximize collegiality
- — Encourage democratic processes in decision making and conflict resolution
- — Emphasize a leveled hierarchy
- — View problem as affecting the entire group, not just an individual
- — Remember the general approach to the problem is to seek solutions, not assign blame
- — Expect a high level of tolerance for individual disturbance
- — Communicate openly and effectively
- — Expect a high degree of cohesion

(continued)

Table 15-1. *(continued)*

— Expect considerable flexibility of roles
— Join with others to deal with organizational bullies
— Eliminate any subculture of violence and abuse

SOCIETAL

— General public and professional education
— Community involvement
— Coalition building
— Legislative reform
— Social action

was facilitated by the landmark Violence Against Women Act (VAWA) of 1994.

NEED FOR SANE PROGRAMS

• Because women are so often the victims of violence, women who come to emergency departments (EDs) for even minor trauma must be thoroughly evaluated. ED staff must be aware of the types of injuries most likely to result from violence, and the potential victim must be asked about the cause of the trauma.

• In 1992, the guidelines of the Joint Commission on the Accreditation of Health Care Organizations (JCAHO) first required emergency and ambulatory care facilities to have protocols on rape, sexual molestation, and domestic abuse. By 1997, these guidelines also required healthcare facilities to develop and train their staffs to use criteria to identify possible victims of physical assault, rape or other sexual molestation, domestic abuse, and abuse or neglect of older adults and children.

- The SANE role continues to develop as an important component of the emergency medical response to survivors of sexual assault.
- The impetus began with nurses, other medical professionals, counselors, and advocates working with rape victims in hospitals, clinics, and other settings and was based on the fact that services to victims of sexual assault were inadequate and not equal to the same high standard of care as those provided to other ED clients.

History of SANE Program Development

- The first SANE programs were established in Memphis, Tennessee, in 1976; in Minneapolis, Minnesota, in 1977; and in Amarillo, Texas, in 1979. Unfortunately, these nurses worked in isolation until the late 1980s.
- In 1991, Gail Lenehan recognized the importance of this new role and published the first list of 20 SANE programs to facilitate communication and sharing of information among programs.
- In 1995, the American Nurses Association officially recognized forensic nursing as a new specialty of nursing.
- By October 2001, over 600 SANE programs were registered.

Definitions

- SANE: sexual assault nurse examiner; a registered nurse who has advanced education in the forensic examination of sexual assault victims
- SAFE or FE: sexual assault forensic examiner or forensic examiner; physician who conducts the evidentiary examination

SANE Scope of Practice

• Examine the sexual assault survivor to assess, document, and collect forensic evidence.

• Offer prophylactic treatment of sexually transmitted diseases (STDs) and prevention of pregnancy under a preestablished medical protocol or as approved by a consulting physician or advanced practice nurse.

• Treat minor injuries and refer care of major physical trauma to the ED or a designated medical facility.

• Explain to the client that the SANE only does a limited medical examination.

• Provide the rape survivor with information to ensure that the survivor can anticipate what may happen next, make choices about reporting and deciding whom to tell, and obtain the support that will be needed when he or she leaves the SANE facility.

• Provide emotional support and crisis intervention, working with the rape crisis center advocate when one is available.

• Train other healthcare and community agency professionals to provide services to sexual assault victims.

Operation of a SANE Program

Entry Into Hospital-Based Programs

• The victim calls local law enforcement, who will provide transportation to the hospital ED or SANE examination clinic.

• The victim goes directly to the hospital ED or hospital clinic.

• The victim calls the designated crisis line for assistance.

Entry Into Community-Based Programs

- The victim calls local law enforcement agencies, where he or she will be checked for injuries and, if only minor or no injuries are present, will be transported to the community-based SANE facility.
- The victim goes to the ED of a local hospital, where staff will check for injuries and, if only minor or no injuries are present, will arrange transportation to the community-based SANE facility.
- The victim goes directly to the community-based SANE program facility during office hours.
- The victim calls the designated crisis line for assistance and receives a referral to the community-based SANE facility.

SANE Responsibilities

- When the victim is uncertain about reporting, the SANE should discuss any fears and concerns and provide information as needed to make an informed decision. The SANE explains available options and the limitations of making a delayed report and offers to complete an evidentiary examination kit that can be held in a locked refrigerator for a specified time in case the victim chooses to report later.
- The SANE follows mandatory reporting laws for felony crimes or child abuse.
- When the victim does not want to report, the SANE should still offer medications to prevent STDs; evaluate the risk of pregnancy and offer pregnancy prevention; make referrals for follow-up medical care and counseling; and provide the victim with written follow-up information.

- When a report is made, the following occurs:

1. A complete evidentiary examination is conducted following the SANE agency protocol, generally within 72 hours of the assault.
2. The SANE obtains written consent, then performs a complete examination, including the collection of evidence in a rape kit.
3. The SANE assesses and documents injuries, provides prophylactic care for STDs, evaluates pregnancy risk and offers preventive care, initiates crisis intervention, and provides referrals for follow-up medical and psychologic care.

- When the victim is alone, the SANE discusses who should be called and where to go from the hospital on discharge, making every effort to find a place for the victim to go where he or she will feel safe and will not be alone, perhaps making arrangements for shelter placement or providing a place to sleep in a specified area of the hospital.

SANE Training

- Certification is being considered at the state and national levels.
- The International Association of Forensic Nurses (IAFN) adopted recommendations for SANE training curriculum, consisting of 40 or more hours of didactic instruction. Some programs also designate a number of clinical hours after completing the classroom training, generally ranging from an additional 40 to as many as 96 hours.
- Most SANE programs require specific criteria for maintaining certification.

Sexual Assault Response Team

• To be optimally effective and provide the best possible service, the SANE must function as part of a team, which may be organized formally as a SART or informally.

• SARTs vary from a team of individuals who respond together and jointly interview the victim at the time of the sexual assault examination to individuals who work independently on a day-to-day basis but who communicate regularly, possibly daily, and meet weekly or monthly to discuss mutual cases and solve mutual problems to make the system work more smoothly.

• Team members typically include the following:

1. SANE
2. Law enforcement officer
3. Detective
4. Prosecutor
5. Rape crisis center advocate or counselor
6. ED medical personnel
7. School counselors, battered women advocates, counselors who work with prostitutes, and any combination of representatives of programs in the community who address the problems of sexual assault

• Membership changes with changes in needs and goals.

Two SART Models

• Joint interview SART model

1. Multiple members of the SART respond to the ED together to conduct the sexual assault

examination interview. Members usually include law enforcement, the SANE, and a rape crisis center advocate. They are all present so that the victim only has to make a statement once.

2. Limitations: additional pressure may exist to report the assault; calls to law enforcement may be needed to authorize payment for services; and there is limited access to healthcare for STDs or pregnancy risk or prevention.

- Cooperative SART model

1. Team members meet regularly and communicate routinely about cases, but they do not actually respond at the same time. When law enforcement personnel are called to the scene of the assault, they protect the client from further harm, protect the crime scene evidence, and take a limited statement from the victim. They may call the hospital or rape center responsible for paging the SANE and rape crisis advocate.
2. Limitations: the memory and completeness of the various accounts required may vary somewhat; separate interviews require more effort on the part of all team members to be sure that they meet or communicate all that is required; all agencies must work together.

Advantages of SANE Programs

Communities that have SANE programs can experience the following benefits:

- Better collaboration with law enforcement
- Higher reporting rates
- Shorter examination times

- Better forensic evidence collection
- Improved prosecution

Role of Emergency Medical Service Prehospital Care Providers

Not only do prehospital providers need to assess injuries and provide appropriate treatment, but they are responsible for protecting potential evidence during medical evaluations and interventions and for working closely with law enforcement personnel.

Psychology of Victims

- Prehospital providers should help victims maintain a sense of control and safety after an assault.
- One of the most important steps in the emotional support and healing process is to return control to the victim.
- Victims must not be judged, regardless of their circumstances, appearance, lifestyle, race, or class.
- A victim is never responsible for a sexual assault.
- Compassionate care begins with verbal and nonverbal communication.

1. Use the victim's name and introduce yourself and your role.
2. Sit at eye level if possible and speak with a low voice, using a calm, soothing tone.
3. Express admiration for the victim's courage in reaching out for help.
4. Remember that victims have suffered a life-threatening experience and reassure them they are safe.

5. Ask permission to touch rape victims, even to take their blood pressure or assess injuries.
6. Make efforts to ensure privacy and maintain confidentiality regarding the victim's identity, history, and examination findings.
7. Explain various options and respect victims' decisions.
8. Provide information and resources as required.

Forensic Evidence

• Remember that the victims are a major part of the "crime scene."

• Preserve possible evidence found on victims' skin, clothing, wounds; preserve bodily fluids, such as urine or blood.

• Focus your physical assessment on complaints or injuries. Gather only the information needed to provide appropriate medical care and ensure the victim's safety.

• Begin with an objective assessment and documentation of behavior. Document victims' actions and behaviors with words that would permit a viewer of the document to be able to visualize the victims' demeanor.

• Document what is visible on arrival beginning with victim location, especially if that location is different from the location of the event.

• Preserve crime scene evidence found on clothing, documenting any modifications to clothing that were made after the assault, such as clothing put on backward, grooming, or debris removal.

1. Ensure that victims wear or bring to the hospital the clothing worn during the assault.

2. Instruct them to bring a change of clothing, including underwear to wear after the medical evaluation and forensic examination.

- Preserve crime scene evidence regarding wounds.

1. Focus the prehospital assessment on areas of discomfort, tenderness, or pain, without disturbing or removing clothing when possible.
2. According to Locard's exchange principle, when any 2 objects come into contact, there is a transfer from one object to the other, so evidence may be located within wound areas.
3. Describe the wounds objectively in terms of anatomical location and note the approximate size, amount of bleeding, deformity, swelling, and tissue color surrounding the area.
4. Limit first aid to these wounds to preserving life and limb because anything biological has potential DNA evidence. Do not clean wounds, but instead wrap any that are bleeding and splint deformities. Postpone application of cold compresses to tissue swelling so that skin changes or soft tissue swelling is not affected by vasoconstriction until the medical facility has an opportunity to see and photodocument the wounds.

- Preserve crime scene evidence regarding bodily fluids.

1. If sexual assault victims need to empty their bladders before transport, instruct them not to wipe their genitals and to collect urine samples in jars or leak-proof containers. These are handled as follows:

   Label the containers with the victim's name, date, and time collected.

Place containers in biohazard bags.

Turn the bags over to the hospital staff.

2. Instruct victims not to change any sanitary device after an assault until forensic evidence collection at the medical facility can be accomplished. Discarded sanitary devices should be collected if possible.
3. Document a "chain of custody" for each item of clothing, body fluid, or debris collected (see Chapters 4 and 10).

- Document everything legibly, clearly, and objectively.

1. Objective documentation comprises those things that one can visualize, hear, feel, or sense in terms of observation.
2. Subjective documentation comprises information related by the victim regarding history, degree of pain, or level of discomfort.
3. Use quotation marks to document chief complaints from the victim when possible. If these data come from other persons, document those sources.
4. Information about perpetrators or assailants may be documented but should not be solicited or questioned because it is not pertinent to prehospital medical assessment, treatment, or stabilization.

Transporting Victims to Hospitals

- Do not delay transport to a medical facility.
- Inform victims that they will have choices related to examinations, permission to photograph, collection of evidence for DNA screening, and medical treatment prophylaxis options.

- Allow victims to have control over which facility is sought for care.
- Advise victims of their options based on the following:

1. Forensic examiners (SANE programs)
2. Forensic equipment capabilities
3. SART support services (rape crisis counselor, social worker, and/or law enforcement)
4. Support of close friend or significant other

- Make victims aware of the forensic tools that may be employed, as follows:

1. Standardized sexual assault evidence collection kit
2. Colposcope, a binocular microscope able to magnify minor tissue trauma
3. Photographic capability to document tissue trauma
4. Rulers
5. Ultraviolet light sources (Wood's lamp)
6. Chemical markers (toluidine blue dye)
7. Body diagrams

References

Antognoli-Toland P. Comprehensive program for examination of sexual assault victims by nurses: a hospital-based project in Texas. *J Emerg Nurs.* 1985;11:132-136.

Baden M, Roach M. *Dead Reckoning: The New Science of Catching Killers.* New York, NY: Simon & Schuster; 2001.

Bloom SL. *Creating Sanctuary: Toward the Evolution of Sane Societies.* New York, NY: Routledge; 1997.

Bloom SL, Reichert M. *Bearing Witness: Violence and Collective Responsibility*. Binghampton, NY: Haworth Press; 1998.

Bullock K. Domestic violence and EMS personnel. *Ann Emerg Med*. 1998;31:286.

Burgess AW. *Violence Through a Forensic Lens*. Prussia, Pa: Nursing Spectrum Publishing; 2000.

Burgess AW, Holmstrom LL. Rape trauma syndrome. *Am J Psychiatry*. 1974;131:981-986.

Catherall DR. Coping with secondary traumatic stress: the importance of the therapist's professional peer group. In: Stamm BH, ed. *Secondary Traumatic Stress: Self-Care Issues for Clinicians, Researchers, & Educators*. Lutherville, Md: Sidran Press; 1995:80-92.

Ciancone AC. Sexual assault nurse examiner programs in the United States. *Ann Emerg Med*. 2000;35:353-357.

Coates D, Wortman CB, Abben A. Reactions to victims. In: Frieze IH, Bar-Tal D, Carroll JS, eds. *New Approaches to Social Problems*. San Francisco, Calif: Jossey-Bass; 1979:21-52.

Crowley SR. *Sexual Assault, the Medical-Legal Examination*. Stamford, Conn: Appleton & Lange; 1999.

Cunningham M. The impact of sexual abuse treatment on the social work clinician. *Child Adolesc Social Work J*. 1999;16:277-290.

DiNitto D, Martin PY, Norton DB, Maxwell SM. After rape: who should examine rape survivors. *Am J Nurs*. 1986;86:538-540.

Ehrman WG. Approach to assessing adolescents on serious or sensitive issues. *Pediatr Clin North Am*. 1998;45:189-204.

Figley CR. Compassion fatigue: toward a new understanding of the costs of caring. In: Stamm BH, ed. *Secondary Traumatic Stress: Self-Care Issues for Clinicians, Researchers, & Educators*. Lutherville, Md: Sidran Press; 1995:3-28.

Fox EB, Davidson J, Frances A, Culpepper L, Ross R, Ross D. The expert consensus guideline series. Treatment of Posttraumatic Stress Disorder. The Expert Consensus Panels for PTSD. *J Clin Psychiatry*. 1999;60(suppl):4-76.

Gabriel MA. Group therapists and AIDS groups: an exploration of traumatic stress reactions. *Group*. 1994;18:167-176.

Garrett C. *Stress, Coping, Empathy, Secondary Traumatic Stress and Burnout in Healthcare Providers Working With HIV-Infected Individuals* [dissertation]. New York: New York University; 1999.

Hallett SJ. *Trauma and Coping in Homicide and Child Sexual Abuse Detectives* [dissertation]. San Diego: California School of Professional Psychology; 1996.

Harber KD, Pennebaker JW. Overcoming traumatic memories. In: Christianson SA, ed. *The Handbook of Emotion and Memory: Research and Theory*. Hillsdale, NJ: Lawrence Erlbaum Associates; 1992:359-387.

Holloway M, Swan A. A&E management of sexual assault. *Nurs Stand*. 1993;7(45):31-35.

International Association of Forensic Nurses (IAFN). *SANE Standards of Practice*. Thorofare, NJ: IAFN; 1996.

Janoff-Bulman R. *Shattered Assumptions: Towards a New Psychology of Trauma*. New York, NY: The Free Press; 1992.

Joint Commission on Accreditation of Health Care Organizations (JCAHO). *Comprehensive Accreditation Manual for Hospitals: The Official Handbook.* Oakbrook Terrace, Ill: JCAHO; 1997.

Kiffe B. *Perceptions: Responsibility Attributions of Rape Victims* [master's thesis]. Minneapolis, Minn: Augsburg College; 1996.

Kostouros PA. *Vicarious Traumatization Among Sex Offenders* [master's thesis]. Victoria, British Columbia: University of Victoria; 1998.

Landis JM. Victims of violence: the role and training of EMS personnel. *Ann Emerg Med.* 1997;30:204-206.

Ledray LE. Sexual assault nurse clinician: an emerging area of nursing expertise. In: Andrist LC, ed. *Clinical Issues in Perinatal and Women's Health Nursing.* Vol. 4, No. 2. Philadelphia, Pa: JB Lippincott Co; 1993.

Ledray LE. *Sexual Assault Nurse Examiner (SANE) Development and Operation Guide.* Washington, DC: Office for Victims of Crime, US Dept of Justice; 1999.

Ledray LE, Chaignot MJ. Services to sexual assault victims in Hennepin County. *Evaluation and Change.* 1980;(special issue):131-134.

Lemmey D. Violence against women. In: Bobak IM, Jensen MD, Lowdermilk DL, eds. *Maternity and Gynecologic Care.* St. Louis, Mo: Mosby; 1992: 1336-1361.

Lenehan GP. A SANE way to care for rape victims. *J Emerg Nurs.* 1991;17:1-2.

Li J. Gamma-hydroxybutyrate intoxication and overdose. *Ann Emerg Med.* 1999;33:476.

Linden JA. Sexual assault. *Emerg Med Clin North Am.* 1999;17:685-695.

Lynch VA. President's report: goals of the IAFN. Paper presented at: Fourth Annual Scientific Assembly of Forensic Nurses; November 1-5, 1996; Kansas City, Mo.

Lynch VA. *Clinical Forensic Nursing: A New Perspective in Trauma.* Divide, Colo: Bearhawk Consulting Group, Co. & Publishing; 1997.

McCann IL, Pearlman LA. Vicarious traumatization: a framework for understanding the psychological effects of working with victims. *J Trauma Stress.* 1990;3:131-147.

Meyers TW. *The Relationship Between Family of Origin Functioning, Trauma History, Exposure to Children's Traumata and Secondary Traumatic Stress Symptoms in Child Protective Service Workers* [dissertation]. Tallahassee: Florida State University; 1996.

O'Brien C. Sexual assault nurse examiner (SANE) program coordinator. *J Emerg Nurs.* 1996; 22(6):532-533.

Pennebaker JW. *Opening Up: The Healing Power of Expressing Emotions.* New York, NY: Guilford; 1997.

Riggs N. Analysis of 1,076 cases of sexual assault. *Ann Emerg Med.* 2000;35:358-362.

Rosenbloom DJ, Pratt AC, Pearlman LA. Helpers' responses to trauma work: understanding and intervening in an organization. In: Stamm BH, ed. *Secondary Traumatic Stress: Self-Care Issues for Clinicians, Researchers, & Educators.* Lutherville, Md: Sidran Press; 1995:65-79.

Saakvtne W, Gamble S, Pearlman LA, Lev BT. *Risking Connection: A Training Curriculum for Working With Survivors of Childhood Abuse*. Lutherville, Md: Sidran Press; 2000:168.

Sandrick KM. Medicine and law. Tightening the chain of evidence. *Hosp Health Netw*. 1996; 70(11):64, 66.

Schauben LM, Frazier PA. Vicarious trauma: the effects on female counselors of working with sexual violence survivors. *Psychol Women Q*. 1995;19:49-64.

Simonds SL. *Vicarious Traumatization in Therapists Treating Adult Survivors of Childhood Sexual Abuse* [dissertation]. Santa Barbara, Calif: The Fielding Institute; 1996.

Speck P, Aiken M. 20 years of community nursing service. Memphis Sexual Assault Resource Center. *Tenn Nurse*. 1995;58(2):15-18.

Stamm BH. Work-related secondary traumatic stress. *PTSD Res Q*. 1997;3:1-3.

Thomas M, Zachritz H. Tulsa sexual assault nurse examiners (SANE) program. *J Okla State Med Assoc*. 1993;86(6):284-286.

Tjaden P. *Prevalence, Incidence, and Consequence of Violence Against Women: Findings From the National Violence Against Women Survey*. Washington, DC: National Institute of Justice; 1998:1-16. NCJ172837.

Tobias G. Rape examinations by GPs. *Practitioner*. 1990;234:874, 877.

Yorker BC. Nurses in Georgia care for survivors of sexual assault. *Ga Nurs*. 1996;147:335-341.

Chapter 16

Legal Issues, Investigation, and Prosecution

Patsy Rauton Lightle
Maureen S. Rush, MS
Jeanne L. Stanley, PhD
Mimi Rose, JD
Tracy Bahm, JD
Duncan T. Brown, JD
Mary-Ann Burkhart, JD
Caren Harp, JD
Susan Bieber Kennedy, RN, JD
Lisa Kreeger, JD
Susan Kreston, JD
Millicent Shaw Phipps, JD
Laura L. Rogers, JD
Christina Shaw, JD
Cari Michele Steele, JD
Victor I. Vieth, JD
Dawn Doran Wilsey, JD

Law Enforcement Issues

Law enforcement personnel must be cognizant of the indications of sexual abuse and understand that some techniques have proved useful in these investigations. The investigator assigned to the case must be thorough and methodical, have a basic understanding of sexual offenses, and be comfortable seeking other experts' advice when needed.

Processing the Scene and Collecting Evidence

- The steps for a sexual assault investigation are often the same as would be taken in any criminal assault.

• Record exact time and location of the assault, employing 9-1-1 tapes and law enforcement dispatch tapes as needed for court purposes.

• While traveling to the scene, carefully note fleeing persons, vehicles, witnesses, etc.

• If the first notification of the assault is received in person, detain this person for investigation and written statement.

1. If unable to detain this person, obtain enough information to locate him or her at a later time.
2. If a third party reports the assault, document identification information for follow-up interview(s).

• Record exact time of the arrival and notify communications that you are on the scene. Do not use a telephone at the crime scene to report your arrival. Use your mobile radio, hand-held radio, or agency-issued cell phone, but never a telephone at the scene because it may have the suspect's fingerprints on it.

• If the victim is injured, request emergency medical services (EMS) and provide first aid.

1. Do not move seriously injured persons unless it is to protect them from additional harm.
2. Be sure to document if the emergency medical technician (EMT) moves or touches anything within the crime scene. Document what, when, and why the alterations were made and if any medications were given to the victim.
3. The emergency medical staff or a law enforcement officer will take the victim to a licensed healthcare facility where a sexual assault evidence collection protocol can be performed.

This protocol provides a standardized and coordinated approach to the collection of information and forensic evidence, treatment of injuries, and prevention of sexually transmitted diseases (STDs) or pregnancy.

4. Remind the victim to take an additional set of clothing because the clothing he or she is wearing will be collected for forensic evidence processing.

• An initial incident report detailing information to support a crime should be taken.

1. Record the names and addresses of all persons present when you arrive.
2. Record the names of all officers present with you at the time of arrival and any officers who come later to assist.

• Only one officer should enter the scene.

• Isolate a large area around the assault scene to prevent loss of evidence. Establish a perimeter and secure it using crime scene tape, ropes, cones, barricades, etc., and at least one officer to provide security until evidence collection and documentation by the forensic crime scene unit and lead investigator are completed.

• Consider the weather conditions for crimes occurring outside and protect the scene.

1. Document weather conditions, persons present, and any nearby vehicle information, including license number, make, model, and color.
2. Avoid discussion of the crime; the suspect may appear as a neighbor or an onlooker.

• Once the scene is secured and the victim is safe and located away from the scene, conduct a complete, thorough background investigation.

1. Keep a crime scene log-in or sign-in sheet at all crime scenes. The officer in charge of security for the crime scene can also be in charge of the sign-in sheet. It includes the name, agency, and telephone number of all individuals who enter and depart from the scene.
2. The security officer ensures that only authorized individuals enter through one designated entrance to the scene. Cross-contamination occurs when individuals are allowed to use more than one entrance into the building. In addition, it is extremely difficult to account for everyone who enters and departs from the scene when more than one entrance is used.

• Isolate and separate witnesses or suspect(s). Do not permit any conversation among them, and detain witnesses and suspects for investigators.

• Do not allow anyone to smoke, chew gum, or use the toilet or the sink in the crime scene area. Remember that the cigarette butt or gum they throw down or put in an ashtray will contaminate the scene, or their hands may distort fingerprints on the toilet handle or evidence on a hand towel. It will be tested for saliva, secretor status, and DNA and will add "evidence" that is not involved with the crime.

• Observe, photograph, and sketch the scene before conducting any search and before evidence is seized. The photographer should also document the date, time, weather and light conditions, and type of film and camera, and must initial each roll of film.

- Note the surrounding area of the house and identify the point of entry of the suspect.
- Make a sketch using measurements from fixed points such as doors, walls, stairs, etc., not necessarily drawn to scale.
- Photograph all physical evidence and place it in a separate paper bag sealed with evidence tape, labeled, and initialed.
- Process the crime scene for fingerprints.

1. Latent, or hidden, fingerprints should be photographed with an identifying marker and documented as to location, date, and time.
2. Patent prints are visible and usually made by the fingertips, which are impregnated with body oil, blood, or dirt, or when the surface is soft and pliable such as putty or wax. These fingerprints are simply photographed and need nothing more to enhance their ridge detail.
3. An etched print occurs when a person handles an object, usually metal, and a chemical reaction from that person's body fluid on the fingers etches a print on the object. These prints look just like those lifted with powder and are easily identifiable by a fingerprint expert. These prints can then be compared with known fingerprint standards of the suspect(s).

- If applicable, a blood spatter expert must photograph and measure bloodstain patterns to reconstruct the scene before blood samples are collected.
- A good rule of thumb to remember is that, with every crime, the suspect leaves identifiable evidence behind at the scene or takes something of the

victim with him. This theory justifies the need to thoroughly and methodically conduct the crime scene search.

• If the assault occurred outdoors, choose the search method.

1. The grid method and strip method are the best for outdoor searches that encompass a large area.
2. An alternate light source is used to process evidence for body fluids, hairs, fibers, and fingerprints.
3. If the assault occurred in a wooded area, the alternate light source, using a battery pack or generator, can be mobilized to locate seminal stains on objects such as leaves and grass.

• If the assault occurred in a vehicle, document the make, model, year, license number, vehicle identification number (VIN), and color.

1. If possible, move the vehicle to a forensic or law enforcement garage for processing.
2. If a vehicle is involved in another way, such as transporting the suspect and/or victim, check the engine to see if it is cold, warm, or hot to the touch to corroborate the victim's statement and help in setting the timeframe.

• Submit a copy of the photographs, crime scene sketch, inventory of evidence seized, and the logbook to the investigator for court purposes.

• The inventory of evidence seized includes a description of the evidence, the name of the officer who collected it, the location, date, and time collected, and a checkmark indicating that the evidence was photographed in its original position and location before collection.

• A good investigator collects evidence, uses forensic evidence from the medical examination, interviews all parties involved, canvasses the neighborhood, conducts background checks, locates the suspect, conducts interviews or interrogations of the suspect, makes the arrest, and is successful in bringing the suspect to court for a conviction.

The Interview Process

• The goal of the interview is to obtain information that will lead to an arrest and conviction of the assailant.

• Although it is uncommon, the suspect may be at the scene when the first officer arrives. If this occurs, the officer should take accurate notes, arrest the suspect if evidence is present to indicate guilt, and determine if the suspect is armed.

1. Search for and seize any weapon and record the number, description, and location of the weapon seized.
2. Secure any evidence found on the suspect and document any spontaneous statements.
3. Tell the suspect that he or she is under arrest, use the Miranda warning as appropriate, and do not allow any conversation between suspect and other parties.
4. Do not interview or interrogate the suspect.
5. Isolate the suspect from other witnesses.
6. If he or she is arrested inside the crime scene, remove him or her as quickly as possible.
7. Do not allow the suspect to return to the crime scene if he or she is arrested outside of that area.

8. Do not allow the suspect to wash his or her hands, change clothes, or use the toilet because evidence will be lost.
9. Do not leave the suspect alone; observe and document his or her behavior.
10. Note the suspect's mental and physical condition, especially such signs as nervousness; potential influence of drugs; torn and/or stained clothing; glass, leaves, or fibers in his or her hair; and injuries to his or her skin.
11. Transport the suspect to a secure facility as soon as possible, where a Suspect Evidence Collection Kit and Protocol will be performed.

• The suspect will then be interviewed by an investigator skilled in interviewing techniques, ensuring that the interview is conducted in a way that maximizes the potential for discovering the truth.

• Obtain a criminal history or background check on the suspect.

• Build a rapport when interviewing as detailed in Chapters 4, 8, and 10.

• Make inquiry into the suspect's employment history, education, means of transportation, past prison time, relatives, leisure activities, and relatives with whom he or she associates.

• Obtain basic information, including full name, nickname(s), alias, gender, race, date of birth, Social Security Number (SSN), height, weight, build (eg, small, medium, thin, average, stocky, obese), hair color, hair length, facial hair, eye color, glasses, contacts, scars, tattoos, teeth, unusual physical features, detection of body odor, speech

impediment, language/accent, mental or physical impairments, emotional condition, address that includes the name and number of people living there, and marital status.

- The suspect's body is inspected during the collection of the Suspect Evidence Collection Kit and Protocal for injuries, bruises, wounds, scars, and bite marks. The officer will ask the suspect how he or she obtained the injuries and document and photograph all injuries and marks.
- Differentiating an interview from an interrogation:

1. Interview: a structured conversation presented in a nonaccusatory manner referencing the interviewee's involvement in the crime.
2. Interrogation: a conversation in which the person being interviewed is accused of being involved in the crime and is closely regulated legally.

- Interview strategy

1. Acknowledge that the offender has a problem and that you are concerned with helping him or her.
2. Deemphasize the criminal nature of the perpetrator, avoiding threatening words, tone, or actions.
3. Interpret the suspect's body language, listen sympathetically, and ask open-ended questions.
4. Allow the suspect to make a full statement, then follow up with more probing questions.
5. Reduce the statement to writing and ask the suspect to sign it.
6. Document all alibi statements and changes in the statement.

7. When handwritten notes are involved, as in stalking cases, request a handwriting exemplar from the suspect.
8. Strategies to expect of the suspect include denial, minimization of his or her behavior, justification for his or her actions including suggestions that the actions were beneficial for the victim or that he or she was under undue stress, and fabrication of events to explain his or her behavior.

- Determining who interviews the victim:

1. The victim's age, his or her mental and/or physical impairments, and the availability of a forensic interviewer versus a specially trained investigator with good interview skills will play an important part in selecting the interviewer.
2. Sensitivity and experience on the part of the interviewer may determine the successful apprehension and conviction of the assailant.

- Ask the victim basic questions, such as the following:

1. Did you know the suspect? (If not, describe his or her race, height, weight, color of hair, hair length, facial hair, glasses, body odor, scars, tattoo or other physical markings, and clothing.)
2. Do you know the suspect's name, address, family, friends, daily routine, hobbies, work history, or present occupation?
3. What do you remember of the assault?

- Thank the victim for doing his or her best to help you gather information to identify the assailant.

• Remember that you are interested in the victim's recall of the type of restraint (if any) that was used, conversation that the assailant had with the victim, instruments used to draw or write on the victim's body, any physical or mental torture, photographs or videos taken of the victim, and sexual preference or dysfunction exhibited by the assailant.

• Follow up with the victim on a regular basis in the event that additional details of the assault are remembered and to assure the victim that law enforcement is continuing its investigation and has not forgotten about the victim or the case. Never promise the victim that you will apprehend the assailant, but provide assurance that everything will be done to obtain this end.

• Interview the victim's family and friends.

• Perform a neighborhood canvass. Most law enforcement agencies have a standard neighborhood canvass questionnaire to serve as a guide.

1. Basic questions include the neighbor's name, address, date of birth, employment, work address, and telephone number.
2. Ask whether they were aware of the crime, when they first learned of the crime, and whether they know the victim.
3. If they know the victim, ask for the date, time, and location they last saw or talked to the victim, whether they were present at the crime scene, and what they have heard about the crime.
4. Take a statement if the neighbor has any knowledge of the crime.

Search Warrants

• Search warrants are a significantly underutilized investigative tool.

• Developing probable cause begins at the investigation's onset.

• Officers should keep a log of information obtained daily that helps to validate the charges to be filed. These should be as detailed as possible when describing a person, place, or object.

1. Person: record all the basic personal traits such as race, gender, height, weight, eye color, hair color, hair length, build, and physical marks such as tattoos and scars.
2. Place: note whether it is a residence or a place of business, the address, description of the building, landmarks, neighboring houses or buildings, outbuildings on the property; maps and/or aerial photographs may be useful. The description should be detailed enough so that the officer who has never been to the particular location can locate it by following the portrait set forth in the search warrant.
3. Search: after obtaining probable cause, a search is made of the suspect's house, car, office, storage shed, garage, lockers, etc.

• A legal search can provide material regarding additional suspects and/or victims and corroborate the victim's statements.

• Remember that physical evidence goes beyond blood, hair, semen, and saliva and can include colors, wallpaper, photos, books, television shows, or a certain song.

Corroborating Evidence

• Corroborating evidence supports the victim's statement, strengthens the prosecutor's case, reduces the victim's stress by supporting testimony, and makes it difficult for the defense attorney to attack the victim's credibility.

• To aid officers in searching for corroborating evidence, a multidisciplinary team should go over the victim's statement sentence by sentence and word for word. After each sentence, ask yourself: Can anything be corroborated?

• The suspect's statement is treated the same way.

Bite Marks

• Bite marks are valuable evidence and have been overlooked and missed for years as an essential part of a criminal investigation. Bite marks are latent or patent images left on a victim or subject.

• Photograph all bite marks. It is possible to match the bite mark to a dental impression and matching or not matching could prove the suspect did or did not create the bite mark.

• Bite marks can be used much like fingerprints, with their individual morphologic characteristics and relationship with each other in the dental arch leaving a distinct mark on the victim.

• Additional bite marks may be seen elsewhere on the body, particularly a child's, in various stages of healing, indicating chronic abuse.

• Bite marks are most often found on the chest, face, abdomen, and extremities. They may be covered with blood but will almost always be covered with saliva, which contains nucleated squamous epithelial cells, valuable in DNA analysis. Be sure to swab the bite mark to collect the saliva before photographs are taken.

• The odontologist or forensic dentist relies on bite mark evidence photography to serve as a permanent record of the mark. The photography should be performed as soon as possible after the assault and follow-up photos should be taken in 3 days and again at 10 days. Reflective ultraviolet photography of the bite mark may be performed at later dates to show any latent images. By using ultraviolet lighting with photography, bite marks have shown up as long as 4 months after the assault because of the collection of blood under the skin as a result of bruising.

• All photographs should be taken by a forensic odontologist or a dentist trained by a forensic odontologist. When photographing the bite mark, it is advisable to indicate size by using a ruler certified and approved by the American Board of Forensic Odontology (ABFO).

• Photographs and impressions should be taken from the suspect as well as the victim.

Computer-Assisted Sexual Exploitation of Adult Victims

• Computer-facilitated sexual assault and cyberstalking have become high-profile crimes.

• The new issues relevant to gathering computer evidence must be incorporated into the interview to give law enforcement the best chance of amassing the optimal amount of digital evidence from the suspect and consequently from the computer(s).

Preparing for the Interview

• During the interview phase, investigators are pitting their knowledge of computers and the Internet against that of the offenders.

• Investigators should consider the following when determining the approach to use in interviewing a suspect in a computer-facilitated sexual exploitation case:

1. Assess their own computer knowledge to avoid trying to bluff a suspect who knows more than they do.
2. Assess the computer knowledge of the suspect from all other evidence to determine who you are up against.
3. Obtain as much information as possible concerning the hardware and software used by the subject, for example, the suspect's username or user ID; suspect's online profile; suspect's Internet service provider (ISP); suspect's account information; and the time of day or night the suspect is usually online.

• It is best to conduct the suspect interview in a private room away from the location when a search warrant is being carried out. Audio and videotaping should be carried out to protect the detective and the department and to provide important evidence for later presentation at trial.

• Any telephone call the suspect is allowed to make may result in the removal or destruction of digital or other evidence. Many computers can be accessed remotely. Alternatively, the suspect may request that the person called destroy the contents of the computer(s) either by physically removing the computer(s) involved or by accessing the suspect's computer(s) and destroying the evidence at the source.

- Search and seizure information

1. Obtain basic information from the suspect on the computer(s) used by him or her and how they may be protected from external scrutiny.
2. Determine hardware, software, number of computers the suspect had access to, and location.

- Password and encryption issues

1. The password helps ensure that unauthorized users do not access a computer, program, or file. The investigator should ask if there is password protection, what the passwords are, and who else has knowledge or access to those passwords.
2. Encryption is the most effective way to achieve data security. The investigator should ask if any of the computer files have been encrypted and if so what the names of the files are, what encryption software was used, and what the keys or passwords are to decrypt the files. If the encrypted files contain incriminating evidence, this will show knowledge and intent on the suspect's part to hide or conceal that information.

- Defeating the "Some Other Dude Did It" defense

1. Investigators should ask who else uses the computer, who else goes on the Internet from this computer, and who else goes on the Internet using the suspect's username.
2. By getting the suspect to admit exclusive dominion over the computer(s) and his username, later claims that another person was the wrongdoer may be avoided.

- Amassing character evidence

1. Information should be elicited regarding the suspect's Internet usage and habits.
2. Later defenses that focus on the concept of victim bashing may be precluded by the suspect's own statements in these areas.

- Storage location

1. Not all images are necessarily stored on-site in the suspect's computer(s). Off-site storage is entirely possible.
2. Investigators should ask where the images are stored on the computer (files, folders, and directories) and where else the suspect stores correspondence, including floppy disks, CD-ROMs, and tapes.

Forensic Evaluation

- Investigators armed with the answers to the questions from the interview can begin the forensic analysis of the computer. A single stand-alone computer will take an average of 40 hours to analyze.

- Although the crime of sexual assault does not directly involve the use of a computer, the information found on the computer can greatly aid in the prosecution of the crime.

- The search begins with remembering that a computer is like any other crime scene and should be treated as such.

- Accessing the computer's hard drive should be done only after a number of typical and procedural steps are taken.

1. First, if the computer is off, leave it off and if it is on, leave it on and photograph the screen.

2. Photograph the back of the computer hard drive to show where all the plugs were plugged in and what ports were empty at the beginning of the investigation.
3. When the computer must be turned off, do not follow the normal shutdown procedures but simply disconnect the power cord from the back of the computer. Properly shutting down a computer creates the possibility that some information, especially in temporary memory, might be lost. Some computers start the normal shutdown process if the power from the wall is interrupted. By pulling the plug from the computer, the computer does not take these steps.

• Once the decision to seize the computer is made, remove the computer so that reconstructing it will be simple and exact.

1. Photograph the computer as it was found if this has not already been done.
2. Isolate the computer from any telephone or cable connections.
3. Clearly mark all plugs and ports so that they can be replaced once the machine is in custody.

• When transporting seized items, use great caution.

1. Pack and cushion the items well and treat each piece of hardware as extremely fragile.
2. Keep all items away from magnetic devices, microwaves, radio transmitters, and other sources of energy that might delete information.
3. Transport items on the floor of the back seat of a car if possible.

• During the search, be aware that several different types of files and documents can yield a great deal of useful evidence.

1. Files, images, and saved e-mails: look at the file names under which the suspect may have the account divided. A scan of the sent item folder is also recommended. A check of the delete file is needed because most programs require users to delete twice; a file is not deleted merely because it has been sent to the delete file. E-mail headers also provide a wealth of information if read properly (**Table 16-1**).
2. Web sites: when a person logs onto the Internet, the computer begins a series of electronic transfers of information with the ISP server. The transfers are the equivalent of the 2 machines talking with each other and are the source of the annoying screeching noise heard from modems. These transfers include information about the suspect's computer as well as information sent by the ISP about the Web sites. The Web site's computer is also accessing information about the suspect's computer, specifically the type, speed, and size of the computer, and organizing that information in a file on the suspect's hard drive, commonly called a cookie. When the suspect's computer logs back onto the Web site, the Web site's computer simply goes to the cookie file on the computer, finds the appropriate cookie, and identifies the computer as a past user. Cookies can be opened up and the investigator can obtain the Web address of the site and possibly even what pop-up ads were displayed on the screen.

Table 16-1. How to Read an E-mail Header

MESSAGE HEADER AND TRANSLATIONS

Return-path: jqpublic@email.com
Translation: Informs receiving computer who sent the message and where to send error messages if the message does not go through.

Received: from ruguilty@netmail.com (4.1/SMI-4.1) id BB11011; Mon, 1 Mar 99 12:34 EST
Translation: Shows the route the message took from sending to reception. Every time a computer receives a message, it adds a "Received:" field with address and time stamp.

Received: from localhost byjqpublic.email.com (4.1/SMI-4.1) id BB10011; Mon, 1 Mar 99 12:33 EST
Translation: Same as example 2.

Message-ID: <1234567890.BB1011@ruguilty.netmail.com>
Translation: Message ID line is the only line that cannot be altered. The ID is logged by the computer and may be traced through the computers it has been sent from if needed.

Date: Mon, 1 Mar 1999 12:35 -0800 (EST)
Translation: Shows date, time, and time zone when the message was sent.

From: "JQ Public" <jqpublic.email.com>
Translation: Gives e-mail address of sender.

To: Joey Bagadonuts bagadonuts@internet.org
Translation: Shows e-mail name and address of the recipient. In this case ".org" denotes an organization, ".com" a commercial vendor, and ".edu" an educational institution.

CC: Reggie Osborn reggoz@law.fgu.edu
Translation: Shows names and addresses of any "CC's." This can also be a "BCC," or blind CC, in which case the name and address would be hidden.

3. History directory: computers keep a list of recently visited Web sites in a directory called history.
4. Temporary Internet files: these contain bits and pieces of downloads and Web site information from Web sites that were visited by the suspect's computer. Cookies are also deposited in these files.

- Created/Modified/Access Dates

1. The "created date" is the date that the file was created, first saved, or downloaded onto the suspect's hard drive. This date is important because it records the date when the file first appeared on the suspect's computer.
2. The "modified date" shows whether and when the suspect altered or changed the file. Modification can imply knowledge of the file as well as use and possession of it.
3. The "access date" is useful because it shows how recently the suspect opened the file. However, the access date only records the most recent action taken. If a forensic examiner is too hasty and opens a file before properly creating a duplicate copy of the hard drive, all the access dates will reflect the dates law enforcement accessed them, not the suspect.

- Instant messaging

1. Instant messaging is a useful tool for investigators who are conducting online stings.
2. The difficulty with the software is that there is no automatic logging of conversations, nor are the chats saved.

- Looking for files on a hard drive or disk

1. Check the allocated space, which is space that has data written to it.
2. Check the unallocated space, the space that is available for writing.
3. Check the slack space, which is space left over from allocated space.
4. Remember that information contained in RAM space can be lost if the investigator opens large files on the hard drive or reboots the computer or if programs that depend on RAM space are run before the proper software is engaged to search it. Therefore, first check all temporary files and run a thorough search of the RAM space to preserve any potentially useful information contained therein.
5. Contact the American Prosecutors Research Institute's (APRI) National Center for Prosecution of Child Abuse for technical assistance (703-549-4253).

Other Considerations

- Investigators must be familiar with their state laws regarding issues such as criminal sexual conduct, privacy and wiretapping, emergency protective custody, termination of parental rights, obscenity, sexual exploitation with a minor or elder, mandated reporting statutes, and penalties for failure to report.

- Case management is vital. Investigation of criminal sexual assault generates a tremendous amount of paperwork, and the ability of the investigator to collect, document, organize, and process the information is critical. The ultimate goal of any criminal investigation is to identify the

assailant, prevent him from harming any more citizens, and successfully provide information to the prosecution for conviction.

• When an investigator is preparing a case file for court, the following information must be included:

1. Cover sheet
2. Brief synopsis that includes a chronology of events
3. Offense report with all supplemental reports
4. Arrest reports
5. Follow-up reports, statements, arrest and/or search warrants
6. Forensic laboratory reports as applicable, including DNA, trace or latent prints, question documents, polygraph results, toxicology findings, evidence, evidence forms, and chain of custody
7. Background sheets
8. Criminal histories
9. Medical information
10. Victim and Suspect Sexual Assault Evidence Collection Protocols
11. Photographs
12. Sketches
13. Videotapes, audio tapes
14. List of witnesses with their addresses and telephone numbers and their involvement in the case

• Law enforcement personnel depend on the medical professional who collects the evidence and interprets it. Thus, the medical and law enforcement professionals must work together to build a case.

• Once the case file is complete, the investigator should set up a meeting with the appointed prosecutor to provide this information in an orderly fashion.

• The investigator is also responsible for being well prepared for giving testimony in court. Suggestions are as follows:

1. Know your case, your victim, the circumstances, and the connection of the evidence between the suspect and the victim.
2. Look professional, be courteous, and speak distinctly.
3. Respond to questions with brief answers, and address your answers to the jury and judge.
4. If you do not understand a question, be comfortable enough to ask the individual politely to repeat the question. Asking the defense or prosecution to repeat the question also allows you a bit more time to think about the question and formulate an answer.
5. Describe in detail the steps taken in the investigation.

The Role of Police as First Responders

The role of police personnel as first responders focuses on providing empathetic care and services to victims of sexual assault and ensuring the proper performance of investigative work to support the criminal prosecutions of such cases.

Preparation for First Responders

• First responders must have access to initial and continuing education designed to address sexual assault issues, including the following:

1. The broad range of victim reactions to sexual assaults
2. The various methods of empathetic questioning
3. The most up-to-date forensic procedures
4. The many myths, stereotypes, and assumptions about victims of sexual assault
5. The various ways victims present themselves after a sexual assault
6. The importance of avoiding value judgments regarding the impact of sexual assaults on victims
7. Changes and modifications of laws
8. The roles of race, ethnic background, age, gender, religion, economic status, disabilities, and sexual identity in sexual assault cases

• First responders must understand that from a legal standpoint, stranger rape and acquaintance rape are equally important and they are given equal weight throughout the investigation and prosecution.

• First responders must also establish relationships with available community resources and social services for sexual assault victims, which will allow the first responder to make appropriate and useful recommendations focusing on the specific needs of each victim.

• It is useful to establish relationships with service providers to address the unique issues facing male victims as well as lesbian, gay, bisexual, and transgender victims.

• Knowing which referral sites have multilingual counselors or interpreters is also helpful.

Victim Contact

• Victims' initial contact with first responders often creates an indelible perception about the entire justice system.

• Police must begin by learning what is beneficial in interactions with victims.

• Police dispatchers

1. Begin by assessing the safety of victims, investigating whether the victim is still in immediate danger and whether immediate medical attention is required.
2. Provide important information regarding victim care to responding police personnel.
3. Collect information used in criminal prosecutions, including basic data (name, age, current location) and time-sensitive or "flash" information that relates to the time and location of the assault, descriptions of the assailant(s), vehicles, other physical identifiers, and direction of the assailant's flight.
4. Immediately broadcast this information to all available patrol and detective units in the field so that officers can survey their patrol areas for such perpetrators.
5. May ask the victim for specific locations where the assailant may be found if the victim knew the perpetrator.
6. Give specific directions to victims to preserve important prosecution evidence and assist the forensic components of investigations.
7. Instruct victims to remain at their current location until police arrive (if safe).

8. Remain on the phone with victims until police arrive to ensure victims' safety and provide psychologic support.

- Police officers

1. Provide the initial on-scene contact.
2. Maintain confidentiality by using unmarked police cars and plainclothes officers, as well as a low-profile approach.
3. Make efforts to be aware of other situational factors that are important to victims, such as arranging support services for children or childcare while victims are engaged in medical examinations and police interviews; determine if the presence of family members or friends is helpful or harmful; enlist family or friends to assist in gathering needed information; and determine whether trained interpreters would be more helpful.
4. Take victims to the apprehension location to identify assailants, remaining mindful of victims' vulnerabilities and informing the victim in advance of what will take place and what is expected of the victim.
5. Be mindful of factors that affect their ability to fulfill these roles, including the psychologic and physical status of victims that hinder officers' ability to gather detailed and accurate information.
6. Respect victims' request to speak with a same-gender officer.
7. Interview EMS personnel who arrived before police to obtain information they may have gathered from the victim and include it in final police reports.

8. Understand the need for accuracy because such records will eventually affect the criminal prosecution.
9. Take copious notes about the scene, the condition of the victim, and any statements given by the victim, detailing all irregularities at the scene.
10. Maintain written resources and referral information to give to victims who do not want the services of police or who do not want to follow through with the prosecution of the case; these should include a basic description of the medical and legal issues and procedures after a sexual assault, the location and description of sexual assault and rape crisis agencies, and lists of programs that provide services for the prevention and treatment of STDs, HIV infection, and pregnancy.

Medical Examinations

• Medical evaluations may take place in designated hospital emergency centers, requiring transport of the victim to the facility. Unless victims are medically impaired, police rather than EMS transport victims to hospitals.

• Offer a brief explanation of the medical examination process (Chapters 9 and 10).

Investigative Interviews

• Investigating officers conduct a detailed interview with the victim after the medical evaluation and treatment.

• Victims may choose to postpone giving their statement so that they have some time to rest, but most researchers find that victims are more at ease discussing the details of the assault within the first

24 hours and statements should be taken as soon as possible to avoid losing memories.

- Allow victims to give their statements at their own pace and without interruption before asking additional clarification questions.
- Interview locations are important and should usually be statement rooms that are comfortable and out of the bustle of main squad rooms; sometimes it will be necessary to give victims a choice. If interviews must be taken at the medical facility, interviewers may find it helpful to use private spaces or private patient rooms instead of sterile examination rooms.
- Interviewers must be flexible, open, and aware of the victim's needs, as well as avoid subtle insinuations about the victim's veracity.
- Focused questions assist in gathering specific information.
- Open-ended questions may be used to expand victims' responses.
- Other fundamental interviewing skills include active listening and attending skills.
- Even if the victim chooses not to prosecute the assailant(s), police should follow normal procedures.

Criminal Prosecution

- First responders must be aware that every element may become part of the "discovery," or the evidence used to prosecute criminal cases.
- Defense attorneys may be entitled to review all statements, including flash information, given by victims to police and dispatchers; 9-1-1 radio tapes, which may have victims or friends providing

descriptive information regarding attacks and perpetrators; first responders' initial reports; investigators' interviews and final investigative reports; and forensic evidence gathered at the scene and by examining medical personnel at the hospital.

• The same criminal investigative procedures must be used whether or not the perpetrator is known to the victim, even in cases of spousal assault.

Victim Reactions

• First responders require a significant level of insight into the emotional state of victims.

• Look for general overarching themes in the victim to better understand a victim's reaction to an assault.

• Be aware that reactions differ from person to person in the degree, length, and sequence of emotional, behavioral, and analytical responses shown.

1. Varying reactions may also affect the length of time taken by victims to contact police; minutes, hours, days, months, and years may pass before victims are able or willing to approach police.
2. Length of time is not an indicator of severity or realness; rather it reflects different reactions of the survivor to the incident.

• Other factors that influence the range of reactions include victims' situational and psychologic circumstances before, during, and after the assault.

• Rape trauma syndrome

1. First responders are likely to experience victims in the acute phase of the syndrome, a period marked by disorganization and a broad range of emotions, from strongly expressive to subdued affect, calmness, or composure.

2. Emotional reactions are often related to the fear, anxiety, humiliation, self-blame, shame, and anger experienced by victims.
3. Physical outcomes include bruising, contusions, breaks, and bleeding as well as genital disturbances such as discharge, bleeding, cuts, and pain.
4. Immediate behavioral reactions include disturbances in the ability to concentrate, form cohesive sentences, and focus on questions and statements.
5. The long-term reorganization process occurs and survivors experience feelings of depression, restlessness, and exhaustion (similar to what is seen in posttraumatic stress disorder [PTSD]); nightmares, flashbacks, disturbed eating and sleeping patterns, sexual dysfunction, and difficulty in social adjustments; and finally, with time, a reorganization of the victim's understanding of the world before and after trauma, potentially leading to a degree of resolution and integration of the event into life.

Ongoing Contact and Victim Support

• Maintain ongoing contact with victims to keep victims informed and updated throughout the legal process.

• Remain in contact to ensure a successful conclusion for victims, which may or may not mean a conviction.

• Support victims as they gain the ability to move on with their lives, reassuring them that their assault was indeed significant and it is recognized by the police as such.

Legal Issues From a Prosecutor's Perspective

Personal injury is a criminal and a civil matter. Thus, the victim of a sexual assault may be involved in both the criminal and the civil legal systems.

Crimes of Sexual Assault

- Criminal law is always changing to reflect shifting community values.

- Criminal laws and penalties are created by each state and reflect unique variations peculiar to that state. Therefore, it is necessary to study specific crimes, laws, and penalties for the state in which you are practicing.

- Generally, sexual offenses involve 4 types of conduct, as follows:

1. Sexual intercourse
2. Deviate sexual intercourse (oral or anal sex)
3. Digital penetration or penetration of the genitals with an object
4. Indecent contact, which involves touching the genitals or other body parts for sexual gratification without penetration

- If such conduct occurs under any of the following conditions, it is a crime:

1. The act occurs without the complainant's consent.
2. Force or threat of force is used; this is not limited to physical force but also includes psychologic, moral, or intellectual pressure of sufficient magnitude.
3. The victim is unconscious or involuntarily

intoxicated by drugs or alcohol, and the assailant knows this.

4. The complainant suffers from a mental disability rendering him or her incapable of giving consent.
5. The complainant is less than age 13 years.
6. The complainant is less than age 16 years and the assailant is 4 or more years older.

Statute of Limitations

• All crimes (except murder) have a statute of limitations that puts a limit on how much time a person has to report a crime to the police for purposes of arrest and prosecution.

• Generally, felonies are more serious offenses and carry a longer possible sentence than misdemeanors.

• The different time requirements for children that allow a minor to reach adulthood before disclosing abuse to authorities is a recent change in the law.

The Criminal Justice Process

• Sexual assault may be reported through the 9-1-1 system, as a result of hospital protocol, or through reports received by county child welfare agencies, among other ways.

• Police usually take the victim for a medical examination for health reasons and for possible forensic evidence collection.

• Investigators interview the victim and any eyewitnesses, go where the assault occurred, take photographs, and collect evidence from the crime scene.

• Evidence collection often requires a search warrant if evidence is believed to be within the perpetrator's control.

• If the suspect is known to police, he or she is informed of the investigation and given the opportunity to make a statement.

• Suspects in police custody cannot be questioned without being advised of their right to refuse to give a statement, their right to have a lawyer present during police questioning, and a warning that any statement could be used against them. The recitation of these rights is commonly known as Miranda warnings.

• If the assailant is a stranger to the victim but he or she had the opportunity to observe the assailant during the attack, the victim may be shown a series of photographs or a line-up of several individuals similar to the description of the assailant and be asked to identify the perpetrator.

• If the victim is unable to identify his or her assailant, circumstantial evidence or DNA obtained from forensic examination of the victim may be sufficient to prosecute.

• At the conclusion of evidence gathering and after all statements are taken, the police submit their investigation to the district attorney (also known as the prosecutor or state's attorney).

1. The district attorney or assistant district attorney determines if there is enough evidence to arrest the suspect and with what crimes the suspect is to be charged based on the evidence.
2. Some jurisdictions convene a grand jury comprising community members who make the determination if there is sufficient evidence to bring the accused to trial.
3. The standard used by police and prosecutors to decide whether or not a suspect should be

arrested for a crime is the finding of probable cause. Probable cause is found when a law enforcement officer believes that a crime probably has been committed and that the suspect is probably the perpetrator.

Preliminary Arraignment

- After arrest, the preliminary arraignment begins the judicial process.
- The defendant (the term used after arrest) is fingerprinted, photographed, and computer-checked to determine if he or she has ever been arrested for other crimes.
- Bail

1. The purpose of bail and pretrial detention is not to punish the offender; all arrested persons are presumed innocent until proven guilty.
2. The monetary amount is set based on the nature of the offense, the defendant's prior criminal history, any ties to the geographic area, and any prior willful failure to appear at court hearings.
3. Bail is collateral to compel the defendant to appear at court dates.
4. If the defendant fails to appear, bail is forfeited.
5. The higher the risk of flight from trial, the higher the bail imposed.
6. Community safety and victim safety are also factored into determining bail amount.

- At the preliminary arraignment, the person is given formal notice of the charges and notice of the next court hearing.

• Conditions such as prohibiting contact with the victim, abstention from drugs or alcohol, house confinement, or electronic monitoring of the defendant may also be imposed.

Appointment of Counsel

• At the preliminary arraignment, the defendant is entitled to a lawyer.

• Depending on income, a person must either hire an attorney or, if income-eligible, the public defenders office is appointed to represent the accused.

The Preliminary Hearing

• The next court proceeding in a sexual assault case in many states is the preliminary hearing.

• It is usually held within a few weeks after an arrest and is designed as one of the safeguards to ensure the accused's right to fairness.

• A judge reviews the charges and hears brief testimony, usually from the victim, to determine if the legal requirements of the crime are met so that the case may ultimately go to trial.

• The judge reviews the police and the prosecution's decision to arrest a suspect on the charges. The credibility of the witness is not decided nor is any corroborating evidence required. The victim simply needs to give a brief account of the essential facts to determine if there is legally sufficient evidence to have the case go to trial.

• The sexual assault victim's first encounter with the judicial system is during the preliminary hearing. It is the victim's first time to speak of the assault before a judge, a defense attorney, and the defendant in a courtroom open to the public by law.

1. This difficult experience can be empowering or retraumatizing, depending on the sensitivity of the judge, prosecutor, and court staff.
2. Some sexual assault preliminary hearings are held in a designated courtroom with prosecutors who are victim-sensitive and competently trained in the law and the dynamics of sexual assault to handle these cases.
3. Often, when the victim must appear, advocates are present in the courtroom to offer support and social service referrals.

• The time between the preliminary hearing and the trial varies, taking weeks or months.

• Once the preliminary hearing has ended, the case is assigned to the prosecutor who will take the case to trial.

1. The prosecutor is the director of the case; the police reports, witness interviews, hospital records, etc., that tell of the events leading up to the assault and its aftermath are the script.
2. The incident is recreated for the jury by testimony from the witnesses and the production of physical and/or scientific evidence.
3. Meeting with witnesses, finding additional witnesses or evidence not initially uncovered by the police, researching the law, and thinking about trial strategy occupy the defense attorney and the prosecutor in anticipation of a trial.

• When an alleged sexual assault is committed by an unknown assailant, lack of consent by the victim is presumed, and the central issue is the identity of the assailant.

• Generally, the alleged perpetrator is known to the victim, so consent is frequently raised by the defense.

• What constitutes legal consent changes with changing community attitudes about sexuality and gender-based violence.

Corroboration

• The law does not require corroboration to arrest or convict a person of sexual assault; the testimony of the victim, if believed, is sufficient. At the close of a case, the judge will instruct the jury that they may convict on the victim's word alone.

• The victim's account may be the only testimonial evidence available, so physical evidence collection is critical.

• It is important to document and photograph bruising and injury, torn clothing, or a room in disarray after a struggle and to collect physical evidence such as bed sheets, towels, and clothing for forensic testing to determine the presence of sexual fluids, hairs, or blood. DNA testing is conducted by obtaining blood samples from the accused.

• A sexual assault trial often occurs several months after the incident, and it may be difficult for a complainant to convey to the court the emotional state and demeanor during a traumatic assault. Medical personnel must, therefore, accurately document observable emotional states. Accurate, timely documentation of statements from a victim or witness is also important.

• Witnesses are not permitted to give opinions or impressions about what they have observed; it is the

jury's function to draw opinions and conclusions about the credibility and weight of the evidence. The exception to this rule would be the expert witness.

• Physicians, nurses, or social workers can be subpoenaed by either the prosecution or the defense to testify as a fact witness or an expert witness **(Table 16-2)**.

1. Fact witness: a person who has seen or heard something that the prosecution or the defense believes supports their theory of the case. Fact witnesses are asked to testify about their observations. Because the accuracy of memory can diminish over time, these observations should be documented close in time to their occurrence. If required to testify, the healthcare provider is usually allowed to bring any records to court and to refer to them during testimony.
2. Expert witness: if the subject matter is ruled by the judge to be beyond what a jury member would be expected to understand and if it is determined to be generally accepted in the scientific, medical, or other professional community to which the witness belongs that the witness has the requisite education and experience concerning the subject matter at issue, then that witness may be qualified as an expert in a given field and permitted to give an opinion about the evidence. Expert testimony in sexual assault cases is often given by physicians or sexual assault nurse examiners (SANEs) concerning the significance of physical findings or lack of physical findings from a forensic examination performed on an alleged sexual assault victim. The physician's or nurse's ability to educate the jury may make all the difference between a just and an unjust verdict.

Table 16-2. The Direct Examination

PROSECUTOR QUESTIONS AND
EXPERT WITNESS RESPONSE SUGGESTIONS

— Full name and spelling

— Current occupation
State full title
Duties and responsibilities in current position

— Prior occupation (if experience enhances credibility with the jury, such as rape crisis counselor, police officer, evidence technician, etc.)
State full title
Duties and responsibilities in past position
Describe relevance of past position to current testimony

— Educational background
Associate degree: date, institution, and discipline
Undergraduate degree: date, institution, and discipline
Graduate degree: date, institution, and discipline

— Medical training and experience
Residency: date, institution, and specialty
Internship: date, institution, and specialty
Fellowship: date, institution, and specialty

— Specific sexual assault training
Child sexual abuse training (be specific in amount and practicality of training)
Physical abuse training (be specific in amount and practicality of training)
Sexual assault training (be specific in amount and practicality of training)

— Peer review participation
  — What is peer review?
  — How often does peer review occur?

(continued)

Table 16-2. *(continued)*

- — How is peer review conducted?
- — What is/are the benefit(s) of peer review?
- — How often do you participate in peer review?
- — Describe your participation in peer review.

— Teaching
- — Do you train other professionals in the area of sexual assault examination?
- — What percentage of your current position involves training others in this expertise?
- — Does your teaching include lecturing or hands-on training?
- — How long have you been responsible for training others in the area of sexual assault examinations?
- — Approximately how many other professionals have you trained?

— Continuing education
- — Do you participate in continuing education?
- — Define for the jury what constitutes continuing education.
- — How much continuing education do you receive on an annual basis?
- — How is the continuing education applicable to your expertise as a sexual assault examiner?

— Publications
- — Have you published any scholarly articles, studies, etc., in the area of sexual assault or abuse?
- — Have you published any scholarly articles, studies, etc., in any other areas of medical research?

— Is there anything else that you should tell the jury about your training, experience, or background that would assist the jury in making a decision?

(continued)

Table 16-2. *(continued)*

— In the course of your professional duties, have you ever performed a sexual assault examination to determine if a person was sexually assaulted?
  - — How many sexual assault examinations have you personally performed?
  - — How many sexual assault examinations have you observed being performed?

Have you ever supervised the performance of a sexual assault examination?

— You stated earlier that you are involved in training other professionals in the performance of sexual assault examinations.
  - — Who do you train to perform sexual assault examinations?
  - — How do you perform this training?

— Have you previously qualified as an expert in the area of sexual assault forensic examination?
  - — Which courts?
  - — How many times have you qualified?
  - — In what areas of expertise have you qualified as an expert?

— Is the manner in which a sexual assault examination is conducted regulated by a protocol?
  - — What is a protocol for purposes of a sexual assault examination?

— Is there a protocol in place in your jurisdiction for sexual assault examination?
  - — When was the protocol for sexual assault examination established?
  - — Is the protocol ever evaluated and revised?

    History of protocol being reevaluated and revised.

(continued)

Table 16-2. *(continued)*

— Please explain the procedure required in the protocol for sexual assault examination.
This should include a short generalized answer, including information such as:
Obtain a verbal history of the sexual assault.
Conduct an external physical examination.
Conduct a genital examination.

— What is a history?
- — Why do you obtain a history?
- — From whom do you obtain the history?
- — Why is a history obtained at the beginning of the examination?
- — Does a history assist you in forming your ultimate medical opinion or diagnosis?
- — How does the history assist you in forming a medical opinion?

— Do you document the history that you receive?
- — On what form do you document your findings?

— Does the protocol require this form to be completed?
- — Have you received training on how to correctly complete the form?
- — Approximately how many times have you completed this form?

— When do you document the information that you receive while obtaining the history?
- — Why do you document the information at this time?

— After obtaining and documenting the history received, what do you do next?

(continued)

Table 16-2. *(continued)*

— What is involved in performing the external examination?
This should outline the items to note during the examination, such as:
  Temperature, blood pressure, weight, age, etc.
  Demeanor and attitude of patient
  Bruising, scratches, etc.

— Do you document the information and findings that you obtained during the external examination?
  — How?
  — When?
  — Where?

— After completing the external examination, what do you do next?

— Please explain how the genital examination is conducted.
Examination of external genitalia:
  Labia majora
  — Where is this?
  — What is the purpose of the labia majora?
  Labia minora
  — Where is this?
  — What is the purpose of the labia minora?

— Continue through all parts of external genitalia.
— I would assume that your next step is to conduct an examination of the internal genital area.
— Are there various positions used when conducting this part of the examination?
  — What are the different position(s) used to complete the examination?
  — Please describe the various positions used.
— Why are multiple positions used to complete the examination?

(continued)

Table 16-2. *(continued)*

- What are the names of the body parts that are examined?
  Vagina
  Hymen
- What do you look for when examining the hymen?
  - Are all hymens shaped the same?
  - What are the different shapes possible?
  - What is the significance of the shape of a hymen?
  - Does the shape of the hymen affect your examination?
  - Does the shape of the hymen affect whether it can be injured?
  - Is the hymen located on the interior or exterior of the female body?
  - How far inside the female body is the hymen located?
- Continue with other significant body parts.
- Does the protocol require that you document these findings in a certain manner?
  - How?
  - When?
  - Where?
- How long does a typical sexual assault examination last?
  Waiting time
  History
  Physical examination
- On ________, did you conduct a sexual assault examination on ________?
- In conducting this examination, was the protocol followed?

(continued)

Table 16-2. *(continued)*

— In following the protocol, you obtained a history from the victim prior to conducting the examination. What is the history that you received?
— Did you receive additional historic information from any other source(s)?
Family members
Detectives, beat officers, social workers, etc.
Hearsay problems

— In accordance with the protocol, did you record the information that you received?

— While you were taking the history, did you have an opportunity to observe the victim's demeanor and attitude?

— What was her demeanor and attitude?
  — Based on your training and experience, was her demeanor and attitude consistent with a person who has suffered a traumatic event?
  — Why?

— Did you record her demeanor on the required form?
  — When did you do this?

— Does the victim's demeanor affect your ultimate medical opinion?
  — How?
  — Why?

— After obtaining the history, your protocol requires an external examination to be conducted. Did you do this?

—Describe the examination that you conducted.

— What were your findings?
  — Were your findings consistent with a person who has suffered a traumatic event?
  — Why?
  — How so?

(continued)

Table 16-2. *(continued)*

— Did you document your findings from the external examination as required by protocol?
  — When?
  — How?

— What specifically did you document on the form?

— Did you do anything to document your findings visually from the external examination?
  Hand-drawing on the required form
  Photographs:
    Make sure photographs have perspective.
    Use a ruler.
    Use a color scale.
  — How do you identify the photographs as being of this victim if no face can be seen?
  — Did you do this in this case?

— Is there anything else regarding the external examination that we have not discussed?

— According to protocol, did you next conduct the genital examination?
— Did you follow the procedures as required by the protocol?
— How did you perform the examination?
— Please describe how the examination began.
  External genitalia
  Internal genital area
  Position(s) used to complete examination
    Use diagram/board to demonstrate to jury.
    Define the different parts of genital area.
    Explain in plain English.
— What were your findings with respect to the examination of the external genitalia?
  Labia majora
  Labia minora

(continued)

Table 16-2. *(continued)*

— Did you document your findings in accordance with protocol?
— Did you next conduct an examination of the internal genital area?
— Did you examine the part(s) of the body that you earlier described to us:
  — Vagina?
  — Hymen?
  — Etc.

— What tools did you use to complete the examination?
  Swabs (size?)
  Speculum
  Colposcope
  — What is a speculum?
  — What is the purpose of a speculum?

— What did you discover during the internal genital examination?
  Vagina
  Hymen
  Injuries found:
    Type of injury
    Location of injury

— I am showing you what has been marked as _____. What is it?
— Please explain this diagram to the jury.
— Please explain the significance of the numbers.
— Please mark on the diagram the injuries that you found.
— You've placed a mark on the _____. What does that mark represent?

— Is the placement of an injury significant?
  — Why?
    Explain in detail.
— Were your findings different depending on the position of the victim?
  — Why is this significant?

(continued)

Table 16-2. *(continued)*

— You stated earlier that you also used a colposcope during the examination. What is a colposcope?
  — Please explain what the function of a colposcope camera is during a sexual assault examination.
  — How is it used?
  — Does it actually touch the victim?
  — What is the benefit of using a colposcope rather than a traditional camera?
  The subject matter is magnified by the colposcope.
  — Why are colposcopic photographs taken during the sexual assault examination?

— I am showing you what has been marked as _____. What is it?
— How do you recognize this as being a photograph of _____?
— Please identify the injuries that you have described finding on the victim.
— You earlier stated that the placement of the injury is significant. Using the photograph, demonstrate and explain why placement is significant.

— Were you able to determine the age of the injuries?
  — How is it possible to determine the age of an injury?
  — Do you have an opinion regarding the age of the injury?
  — What is your opinion?
  — What do you base your opinion on?

— Did you form an expert opinion regarding the cause of the genital injury?

— What is your expert opinion?

— What did you base your opinion on?
Examination, history by victim and others, experience, continuing education, etc.
— Based on your examination, do you have an opinion as to whether your findings are consistent with the victim's history of sexual assault?
— What is your opinion?
— What do you base your opinion on?

• To be a successful expert witness, the following 10 factors are extremely helpful:

1. Make careful pretrial preparation: the medical witness must read and digest the entire medical record, including the laboratory reports on all of the samples taken and have an overview of all of the information pertinent to the patient. Medical witnesses must prepare a curriculum vitae or resume before testifying, including education, training, and experience.
2. Attend a pretrial meeting with the prosecutor: the prosecutor will outline the topics that will be discussed at trial and the medical witness should educate the prosecutor regarding significant medical facts that will be of assistance. The medical expert may be able to direct the prosecutor in forming questions that will provide the expert with the right opportunity to testify regarding pertinent information. Possible topics of cross-examination should also be discussed, and the witness should ask if any information or report is available regarding the case to help him or her better prepare for giving testimony.
3. Practice professionalism and promptness: develop a good working relationship with the prosecutor and call the day before the date of the subpoenaed appearance to determine if attendance is required. Prosecutors should inform witnesses if they are not needed. If they are needed, medical professionals should be on time to avoid problems with the judge. Plan for problems with traffic, parking, and getting lost when going to court. Dress appropriately

because jurors often make preliminary decisions on credibility based on the witness' appearance. Scrubs or traditional medical attire is not appropriate for the courtroom environment.

4. Make it simple: because the average educational level of a jury panel is eighth grade, remember to structure answers in a simple and nontechnical manner. Before testifying, take a moment and consider all the words used in daily conversation that can be considered technical language and avoid them.
5. Incorporate demonstrative aids: because we are a visual society, some jurors may lose interest if no photographs or other physical evidence is presented. In addition, jurors are more likely to remember evidence if it is communicated 3 times; demonstrative aids will allow for a repeated presentation of important facts. If you are using demonstrative aids, practice and consider how to incorporate the exhibit into the testimony. If you must leave the witness chair and approach an exhibit, ask the questioning attorney or judge if this is possible; permission will always be granted. Face the jury or have your side toward the jury; remember that your audience is the jury, not the judge or the prosecutor. Do not stand where you obscure the exhibit from the jury's sight. If you are using a felt-tipped marker, bring one to court with you and ensure that it works. Consider what color will be most visible. Be aware that it may be difficult to talk, mark, stand correctly, and make sure that every member of the jury can see the exhibit during the testimony and practice.

6. Be polite to the defense attorney: it is important to remain calm and polite even if the cross-examination is being conducted in a rude, condescending, or arrogant manner. Trust the jury to acknowledge the attitude of the defense attorney.
7. Be aware of your body language: recognize the existence of bad habits and nervous reactions and suppress them so they are not a distraction to the jurors, perhaps undercutting the impact of your testimony.
8. Be assertive on cross-examination: questions are often couched to allow for a "yes" or "no" response, yet you may have a great deal of information to provide that would be helpful to the jury. It is extremely helpful to the prosecutor if the medical witness simply states, "I would like to explain, but my answer will be (yes or no)." This statement notifies the prosecutor that a follow-up question should be asked on redirect examination and notifies the jury that there is additional relevant information that needs to be elicited.
9. Do not become a target: do not testify to expert information for which you are not qualified. During the pretrial meeting, you should explore all of the areas of information so that you know if you are qualified to render testimony. Extending beyond your expertise allows questions that can destroy your credibility in the present case as well as in future cases.
10. Debrief with the prosecutor: a follow-up meeting with the prosecutor is beneficial to both parties and should focus on each party providing constructive criticism or feedback to the other.

DNA Evidence

• Forensic DNA typing has become an integral part of the criminal justice system used by prosecutors to prove identity.

• DNA is used in many applications other than forensics, such as paternity determinations; identification of remains in mass tragedies and war; determination of plant, animal, and microorganism origins; and in pharmaceutical, wildlife, and diagnostic laboratories. The use of DNA in other fields assists the prosecutor's use of such evidence by demonstrating acceptance and reliance on DNA in scientific areas.

• The biologic materials collected by police officers and analyzed by forensic laboratories most commonly are blood and seminal fluid. These materials are the most likely to be left at the scene of a murder or sexual assault and are also replete with genetic material.

• Defense attorneys faced with DNA evidence linking their clients to the crimes charged may attack the validity of the evidence in an effort to prevent the jurors from ever seeing it. The appropriate time for such an attack is pretrial in an admissibility hearing.

• The Supreme Court provided a nonexclusive and nonexhaustive list of factors that judges should consider when determining reliability, as follows:

1. The testability of the theory or technique
2. Publication and peer review
3. Known or potential error rate
4. The existence of standards or protocols
5. General acceptance

• The prosecutor should avoid giving the fact finder a molecular biology lesson, offering detailed explanations of testing techniques, using technical and confusing demonstrative exhibits, and expecting the judge or jury to be fluent in the many scientific terms and acronyms associated with DNA (see Chapter 10).

• When presenting any DNA evidence, a qualified and competent expert is the witness who will be called to offer a brief, basic explanation of DNA. This person may be the scientist who performed laboratory testing of samples with DNA evidence or the director or supervisor of the laboratory.

• This witness will define essential terms and present the test results. Visual displays may be helpful in demonstrating the profile rarity to the fact finder. How the statistical analysis was undertaken should be discussed.

• The witness' education and training, forensic experience, nonforensic experience, publications, familiarity with professional literature, memberships and associations, and previous qualification as an expert are all elucidated for the jury or judge.

• The prosecutor can build trust in the witness' laboratory by questioning the expert about issues such as the laboratory following national forensic standards, quality assurance and control, internal validation of testing procedures, proficiency testing, laboratory and personnel accreditation, and peer review of the laboratory's work.

• The prosecutor can support the technology used and the results obtained by the testing laboratory by using the expert presented by the defense. The prosecutor must be prepared to question that

expert on issues of bias, lack of forensic DNA typing experience, and amount of income derived from expert testimony.

• DNA database

1. Rather than linking only a known suspect to a known crime scene sample, databases facilitate breakthroughs without traditional investigation, called "cold hits." Crime scene samples can immediately match suspects to cases, revealing serial crimes and prompting coordinated investigations.
2. While the statutes that create these databases vary widely, most detail the convictions that require sample submission and the procedure employed to limit access and ensure privacy.

• DNA has taken a prominent role in postconviction proceedings such as habeas corpus and new trial petitions; pardons and clemency hearings; and parole and probation hearings.

The Trial

• A criminal trial puts the burden on the state (or the commonwealth) to prove the legal elements of a crime beyond a reasonable doubt. There is no burden on the accused to prove anything.

• The accused need not testify or offer any witnesses, although he may elect to offer defense witnesses. From the time of the arrest, the accused is cloaked with the presumption of innocence that is removed only if there is a conviction.

• The role of the defense is to attack the state's evidence. This may be accomplished by offering evidence, defense witnesses, or the defendant's testimony.

Jury Selection

• Sexual assault trials may be decided by a jury or a judge.

1. In some states, only the defense may choose between having a case heard before a judge or jury.
2. In other states, the prosecution may demand a jury trial even if the defense wants to waive the right to trial by jury and have a judge determine the verdict.

• The jury selection process is designed to create a forum of 12 persons who can listen to a case in a fair, impartial, and unbiased manner.

• The 12 jury members must agree to apply the judge's instructions about the law to the evidence as it is presented.

• Because sexual attitudes, including gender, sexual orientation, and morality, are usually deeply ingrained opinions determined by personal experience, education, and social class, jury selection is critically important.

Admissibility of Evidence

• For evidence to be considered admissible in a criminal trial, it must be relevant, reliable, and material to the issues at hand.

• The probative value must outweigh the prejudicial impact of the evidence.

• Preparation is key in establishing relevance and admissibility of evidence. The 5 general guidelines to preparation are as follows:

1. Know everything about the rule of evidence to be argued.

2. Know every detail about the testimony or physical evidence to be offered under the proposed rule and the purpose for its introduction.
3. Know how the evidence and current facts relate to existing case law.
4. Lay a solid foundation for the evidence at the pretrial hearing.
5. File all motions and briefs of record.

• Legislatures have passed rape shield laws to prevent the introduction of a victim's sexual life if it has no relevancy but to put the victim on trial.

• Evidence of other crimes is only admissible in narrowly drawn exceptions to the general rule of inadmissibility for evidence of previous bad acts.

• The jury must decide that the defendant committed the crime based on proof, not prejudice created by prior criminal convictions.

• However, prior convictions for crimes that support the defendant's commission of the crime on trial may be admissible if there is a common pattern that serves to prove intent or identity.

Defenses

• The most common defenses in adult sexual assault cases are the following:

1. Consent, if the parties know each other and if there is corroboration of sexual contact
2. Misidentification, if the assailant is a stranger
3. Fabrication, if there is no corroboration of sexual contact

• The most common defenses with very young, preschool-age child victims are the following:

1. Suggestibility of the child to adult questioning
2. Allegations that the child is fantasizing
3. Developmental immaturity leading to unreliable testimony

• The most common defenses in latency-age children and adolescents are the following:

1. The child's retaliation for strict parenting and discipline.
2. If the alleged offender is a stepparent or the companion of a parent, the child is accused of falsely disclosing abuse to get the defendant out of the house.
3. Consent is not usually raised with young victims because it is generally not a legal defense to child sexual abuse.

Outcomes

• In our criminal justice system, the law enforcement officers and prosecutors must investigate sexual assault cases with great sensitivity and skill before arrest or trial. The prosecutor's job is not to seek convictions but to obtain justice.

• At the conclusion of a trial, the fact finder (whether a jury or a judge) reviews the evidence and arrives at a verdict. Usually, the fact finder must consider more than one criminal charge.

• The defendant may be acquitted or convicted of all charges, or convicted of some and acquitted of others.

• If a jury cannot reach a unanimous verdict after a long period of deliberation, the jury is declared deadlocked and a mistrial (often referred to as a hung jury) is declared by the judge. A mistrial necessitates the case being tried again before another fact finder.

• If the defendant is convicted of a sex crime, the penalty is determined by state law. Most states have sentencing guidelines that give a suggested sentence for the crime in mitigated, standard, and aggravated ranges.

1. The mitigating or aggravating factors are decided by the sentencing judge.
2. Although a judge may deviate from the guideline recommendations, the reasons must be substantial.
3. In some states, certain sex crimes carry mandatory lengthy prison sentences. While treatment for sex offenders is available in prison facilities and outpatient clinics, the outcome of any treatment depends on many factors. Compulsive sexual behavior carries a great risk of recidivism.

References

Avner JI (Chairperson). New York State Governor's Task Force on Rape and Sexual Assault. *Rape, Sexual Assault and Child Sexual Abuse: Working Towards a More Responsive Society*. Albany: New York State Division for Women; 1990.

Best Practices for Seizing Electronic Evidence. Washington, DC: US Secret Service, International Association of Chiefs of Police, National Institute of Justice; 2002.

Brown ML. Dilemmas facing nurses who care for MSBP patients. *Pediatr Nurs.* 1997;23:416-418.

Bulkley JA, Feller JN, Stern P, Roe R. Child abuse and neglect laws and legal proceedings. In: Briere J, Berliner L, Bulkley JA, Jenny C, Reid T, eds. *The APSAC Handbook on Child Maltreatment.* Thousand Oaks, Calif: Sage Publications; 1996:271-296.

Burgess A, Holmstrom L. Rape trauma syndrome. *Am J Psychiatry.* 1974;131:981-986.

Ells M. Forming a multidisciplinary team to investigate child abuse. *Portable Guide to Investigating Child Abuse*. Washington, DC: US Dept of Justice; 1998.

Fisher AJ, Svensson A, Wendel O. *Techniques of Crime Scene Investigation*. New York, NY: Elsevier Science Publishing Co, Inc; 1987.

Goldner JA, Dolgin CK, Manske SH. Legal issues. In: Monteleone J, ed. *Recognition of Child Abuse for the Mandated Reporter*. St. Louis, Mo: GW Medical Publishing; 1995:171-210.

Hazelwood RR, Lanning KV. Collateral materials in sexual crimes. In: Hazelwood RR, Burgess AW, eds. *Practical Aspects of Rape Investigation: A Multidisciplinary Approach*. 3rd ed. Boca Raton, Fla: CRC Press; 2001:221-232.

Heiman W, Ponterio A, Fairman G. Prosecuting rape cases: trial preparation and trial tactic issues. In: Hazelwood RR, Burgess AW, eds. *Practical Aspects of Rape Investigation: A Multidisciplinary Approach*. 3rd ed. Boca Raton, Fla: CRC Press; 2001:347-364.

Henry JB. *Clinical Diagnosis and Management*. Philadelphia, Pa: WB Saunders Co; 1979.

Holmes WC, Slap GB. Sexual abuse of boys: definition, prevalence, correlates, sequelae, and management. *JAMA*. 1998;280:1855-1862.

Kinnee KR. *Practical Investigation Techniques*. Boca Raton, Fla: CRC Press; 1995.

Kirkpatrick DG, Edmunds CN, Seymour AK. *Rape in America: A Report to the Nation.* Arlington, Va: National Victim Center; 1992.

Leo R. Interrogations and false confessions in rape cases. In: Hazelwood RR, Burgess AW, eds. *Practical Aspects of Rape Investigation: A Multidisciplinary Approach.* 3rd ed. Boca Raton, Fla: CRC Press; 2001:234-242.

MacDonald JM. *Police Response to Rape.* Springfield, Ill: Charles C. Thomas; 1995:140.

Myers JEB. *Legal Issues in Child Abuse and Neglect Practice.* 2nd ed. Thousand Oaks, Calif: Sage Publications; 1998a.

Myers JEB. Expert testimony. In: JEB Myers, ed. *Legal Issues in Child Abuse and Neglect Practice.* Thousand Oaks, Calif: Sage Publications; 1998b:221-281.

National Cybercrime Training Partnership. *Cyber Crime Fighting: The Law Enforcement Officer's Guide to Online Crime.* Washington, DC: Computer Crimes and Intellectual Property Section, US Dept of Justice; 1999.

National Institute of Justice. *Electronic Crime Scene Investigation: A Guide for First Responders.* Washington, DC: National Institute of Justice, US Dept of Justice; 2001.

Panichas GE. Rape, autonomy, and consent. *Law Soc Rev.* 2001;35(1):231-270.

Schulhofer SJ. *Unwanted Sex: The Culture of Intimidation and the Failure of Law.* Cambridge, Mass: Harvard University Press; 1998.

Spaulding RP, Bigbee PD. Physical evidence in sexual assault investigations. In: Hazelwood RR, Burgess AW, eds. *Practical Aspects of Rape Investigation: A Multidisciplinary Approach.* 3rd ed. Boca Raton, Fla: CRC Press; 2001:261-298.

State v. Love, 936 SW2d 236 (Mo Ct App 1997).

Wicklander DE, Zulawski DE. *Practical Aspects of Interview and Interrogation*. Boca Raton, Fla: CRC Press; 1993.

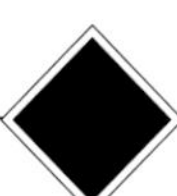

Photographic Appendix

Presented in order by age group of the victim, from young children to elderly persons, the photographs in this gallery are intended to supplement the information contained in the text—to reflect the findings most characteristic of the various age groups, whether normal or pathologic. While many findings are seen across the life span, generally only one example is offered, placed within the age group where it is most prevalent. For a comprehensive photographic representation of sexual assault, please consult *Sexual Assault Victimization Across the Life Span: A Color Atlas*, ISBN 1-878060-61-9.

Infant Sexual Abuse: 0-3 Years Old

History of Sexual Abuse

Normal and Nonspecific Findings

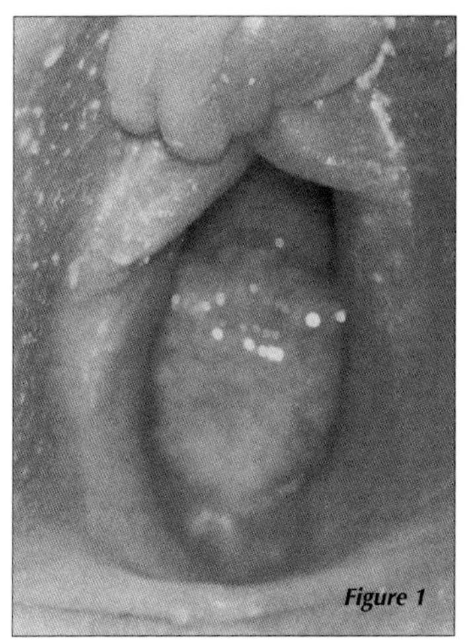

Figure 1

Case Study 1

This 2-year-old was brought by her mother because the mother suspected that the child's father had fondled her. Older siblings had reported this repeated occurrence over time. The most recent incident was over 72 hours before the time of the examination. Other female children in this family had also been "rubbed" by their natural father. Disclosure occurred because an older sibling saw a program at school.

Figure 1. *There is a normal color pattern throughout. The hymen is redundant. The continuity of the hymenal rim cannot be assessed in this view (supine position).*

The perpetrator pled guilty to child molestation of 2 children and was sentenced to 2 years in prison and registration as a child sex offender. The mother of the children divorced the father.

Special Cases

Males

Case Study 2

This 3-month-old circumcised male was brought for an examination while his parents were in a domestic violence conflict. The infant's toxicology screen was positive for amphetamines.

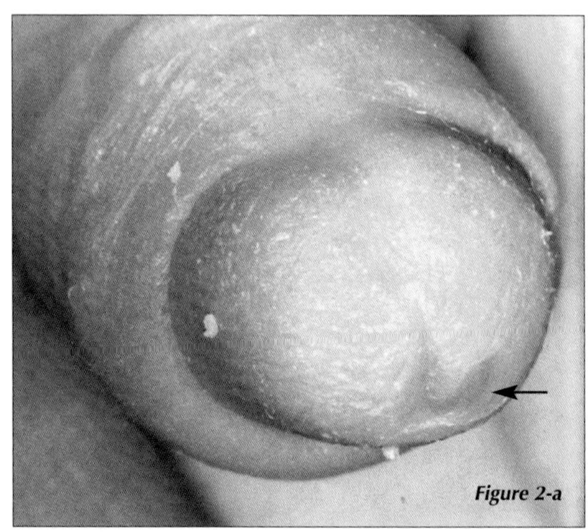

Figure 2-a. *Erythema at 5 o'clock on the glans penis.*

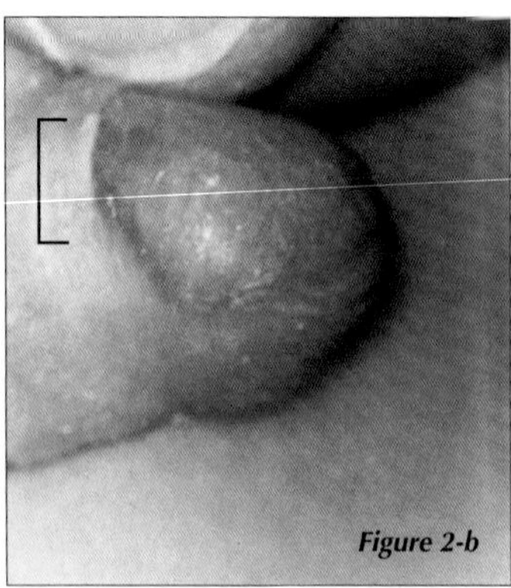

Figure 2-b. *Erythema at 8 o'clock on the undersurface of the glans penis.*

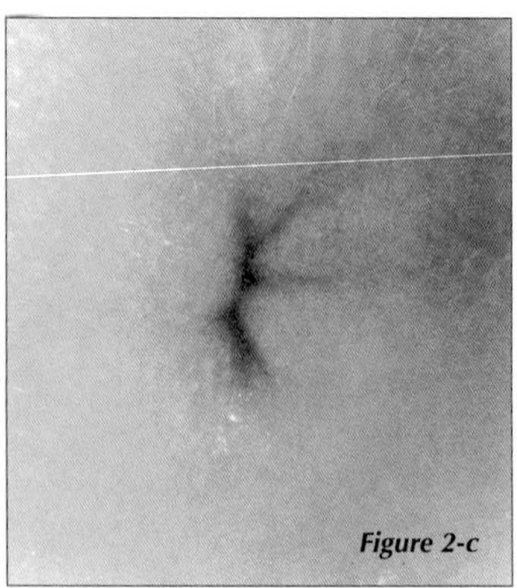

Figure 2-c. *Perianal erythema. There was no anal spasm or laxity. The perianal folds are flattened, consistent with his relaxed state.*

Disabled

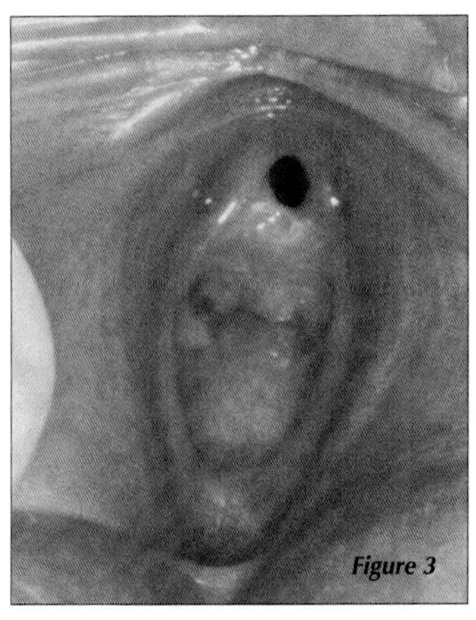
Figure 3

Case Study 3

This 3-year-old female has Prader-Willi syndrome. Her natural father penetrated her digitally and attempted penile-vaginal penetration multiple times. He did the same with her other 3 sisters and molested her brother. The last time she was penetrated was 2 weeks before the examination. She had a history of *Candida* infections.

Figure 3. *A crescentic hymen with a vaginal tag at 9 o'clock and a patulous urethra.* Candida albicans *was present on the culture from this examination.*

The father confessed to the abuse and is serving 18 years in prison with registration as a child sex offender.

Nonassault Variants

Labial Adhesions

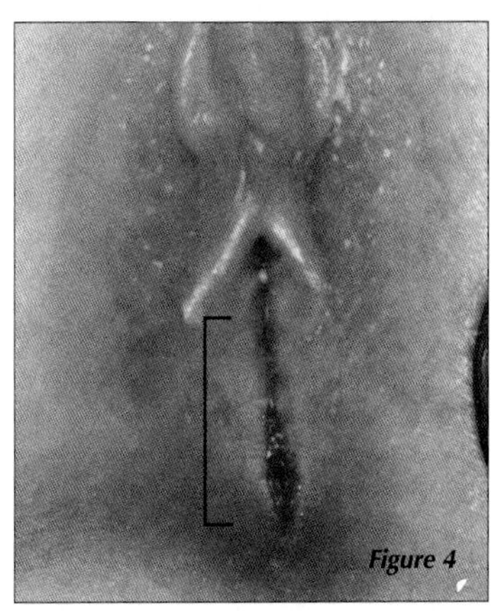
Figure 4

Case Study 4

This 2-year-old child had a history of blood in her diaper.

Figure 4. *Labial adhesions run from mid-labia posteriorly. The anterior opening is not evident in the photograph. The posterior aspect of the labial adhesion is beginning to separate, evident as the examiner gently separates.*

Infection

Bacterial

Case Study 5

One of 2 twin 3-year-old girls was examined because of a report that the father had been molesting the girls over the last 3 days. The father was the main care provider because the mother was in an inpatient drug recovery program.

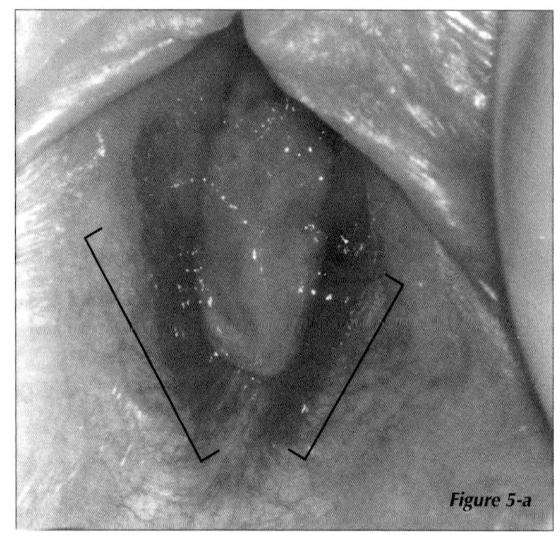

Figure 5-a. *A vivid erythema around the base of the hymen from 3 to 11 o'clock. Cultures of vaginal secretions revealed* Staphylococcus epidermidis.

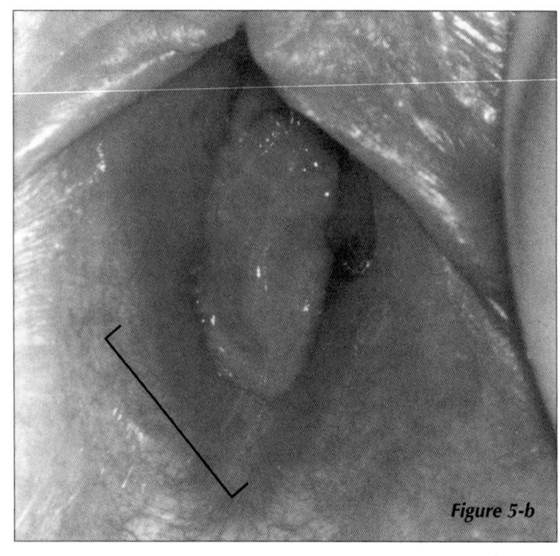

Figure 5-b. *Erythema is most distinct from 6 to 9 o'clock. The hymen is normal.*

Fungal

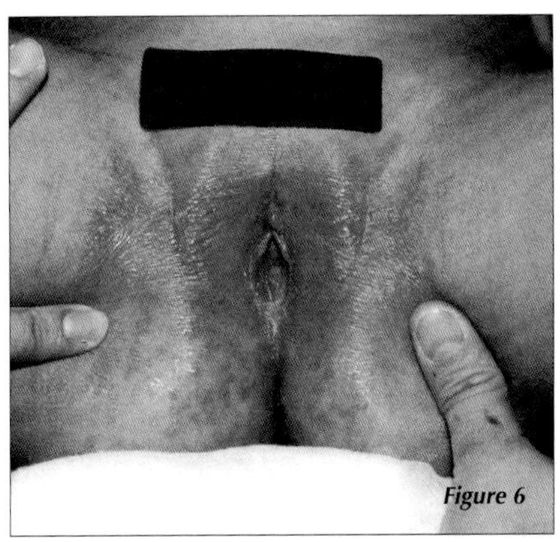

Figure 6

Case Study 6

This 3-year-old female has diaper dermatitis.

Figure 6. *Satellite lesions characteristic of diaper dermatitis associated with* Candida albicans. *Cultures revealed* Candida albicans. *Parents may assist in holding the child for examination (35 mm).*

Balanitis

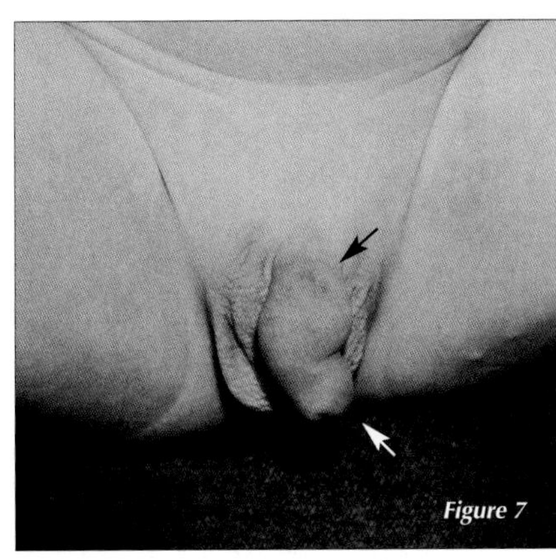

Figure 7

Case Study 7

This 2-year-old Native American Indian male arrived from a reservation with ecchymosis on the dorsal surface of the shaft of the edematous penis and on the side of the foreskin. The child has been in the care of his parents. Neither parent suspected abuse of the child. However, his hygiene is poor. The pediatrician referred the child for a medical-legal examination. It was determined that the child has balanitis.

Figure 7. *Ecchymosis on the dorsal surface of the shaft of the edematous penis and on the side of the foreskin (35 mm).*

Normal Findings

Annular Hymen

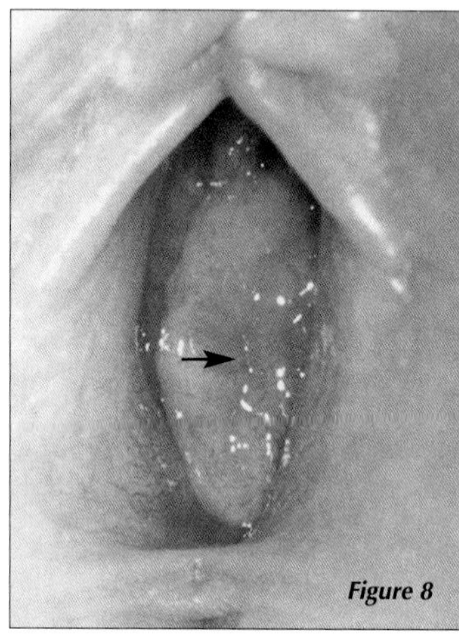

Figure 8

Case Study 8

This 2-year-old has a redundant, pink hymen.

Figure 8. *A redundant hymen. The vascular pattern is not prominent. Labial traction, knee-chest position, or probing the hymenal edge with a swab may help to evaluate for continuity of the hymen. The arrow points to the hymenal opening.*

Crescentic Hymen

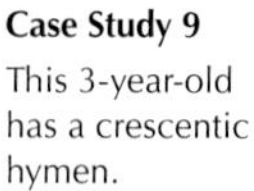

Case Study 9

This 3-year-old has a crescentic hymen.

Figure 9-a. *The crescentic hymen is open in the supine frog-leg position. The left and posterior rim edges are smooth and uninterrupted, but the right rim cannot be clearly visualized.*

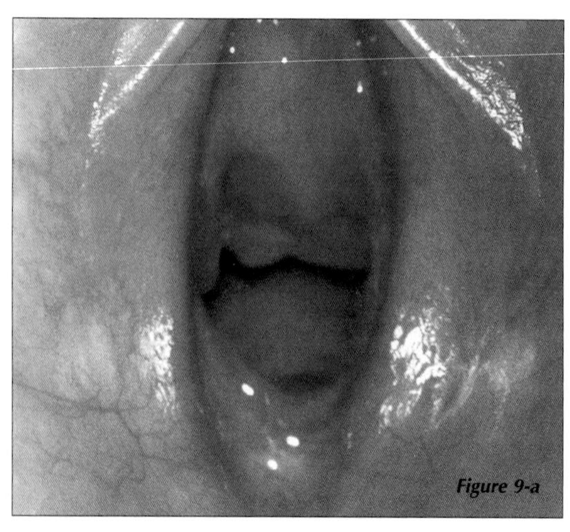

Figure 9-a

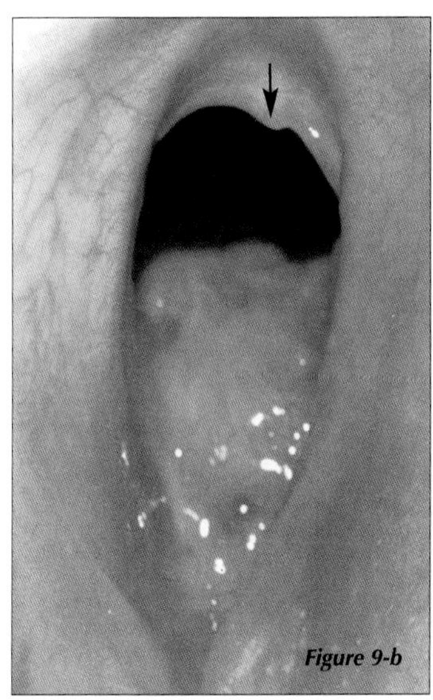

Figure 9-b. *In the knee-chest position, a mound is visible.*

Septate Hymen

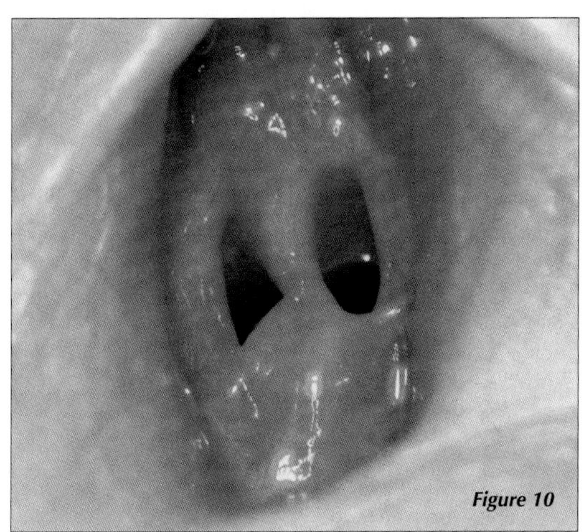

Case Study 10

This 3-year-old was referred for further gynecologic evaluation.

Figure 10. *Septate hymen. Even the vascularity of the septum can be seen with increasing magnification.*

Young Child Sexual Abuse: 4-8 Years Old

History of Sexual Abuse

Acute Findings

Digital Penetration of the Vagina

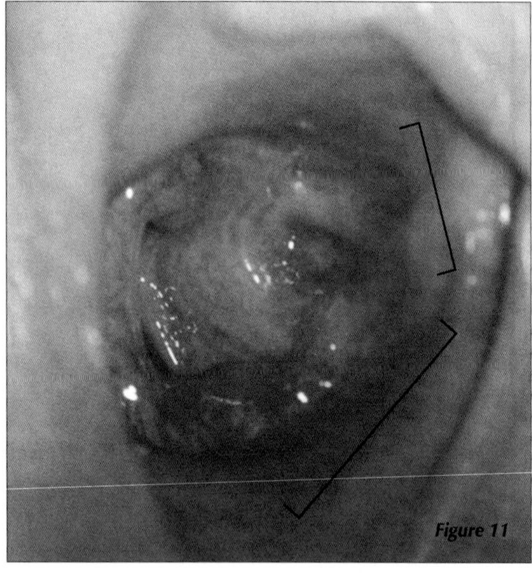

Figure 11

Case Study 11

This 5-year-old Caucasian was kidnapped from a playground near her apartment by a stranger who put his finger in her vagina one time. She was examined within 48 hours of her abduction.

Figure 11. *There is erythema and edema on the hymen from 1 to 7 o'clock.*

The perpetrator pled innocent to charges of abduction and child molestation but was convicted.

Normal and Nonspecific Findings

Penile Penetration of the Vagina

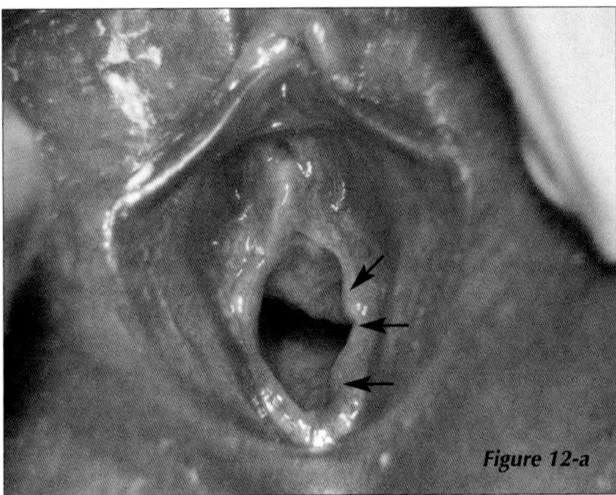

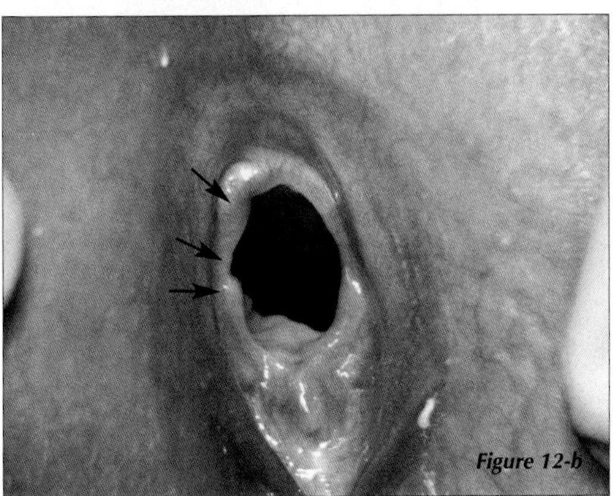

Figure 12-a. *Labial traction is used in this photo. There are mounds at 2 and 5 o'clock and a cleft at 3 o'clock.*

Figure 12-b. *This photo was taken with the child in knee-chest position. The mounds and cleft are still present in this thin, annular hymen.*

Case Study 12

This patient is 8 years old and African American. There is a history of beating with a belt and other physical abuse by her mother and stepfather. The stepfather's brother fondled the child over a period of 2 years and penetrated her vagina with his penis many times. The most recent is over 72 hours ago. She described bleeding during some of those times.

Special Cases
Males

Case Study 13

This 6-year-old male experienced penile-anal penetration by a 14-year-old male who lived in the same apartment building. The child stated "he used green lotion" as a lubricant. The 14-year-old called police to confess that he had forced anal penetration with several young male victims.

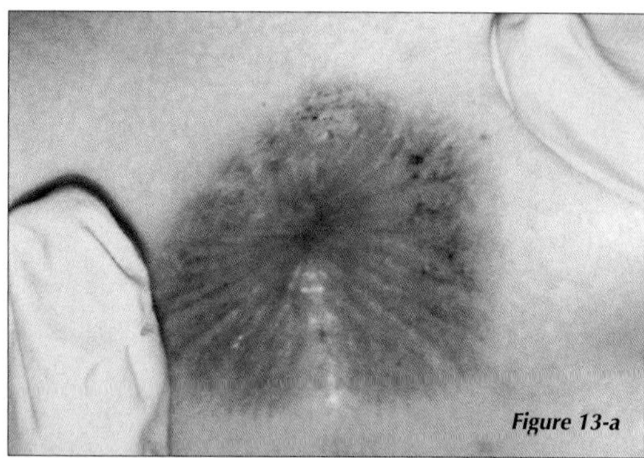

Figure 13-a

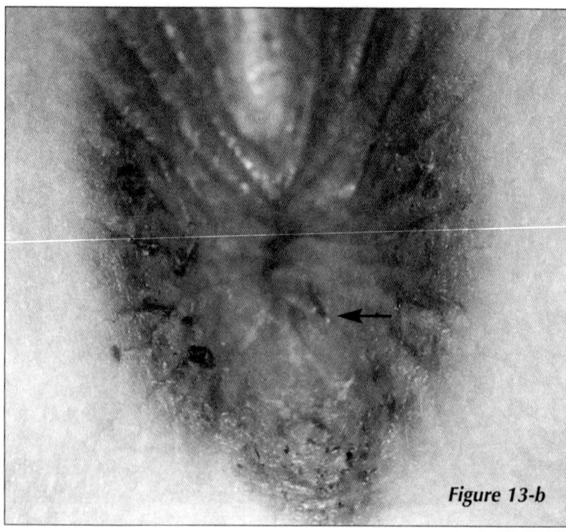

Figure 13-b

Figure 13-a. *There is perianal erythema with stool in the anal folds. There is another ring of erythema closer to the anal orifice from 11 to 5 o'clock. This child is in knee-chest position (35 mm).*

Figure 13-b. *There is a laceration at 5 o'clock in the perianal folds. Toluidine blue dye would have made this laceration more evident.*

Incest

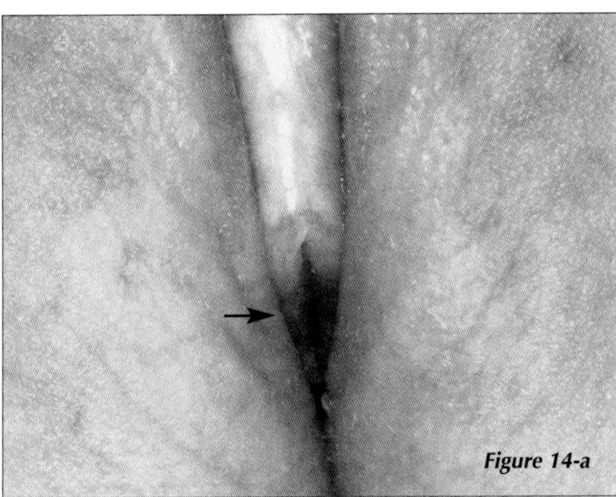

Case Study 14

This is an 8-year-old Caucasian female. She said, "My dad has bad touches." She would not reveal any details of the "bad touches." When she was being interviewed for potential abuse by her father, she explained that her "privates" were sore because she had recently fallen on the playground bars.

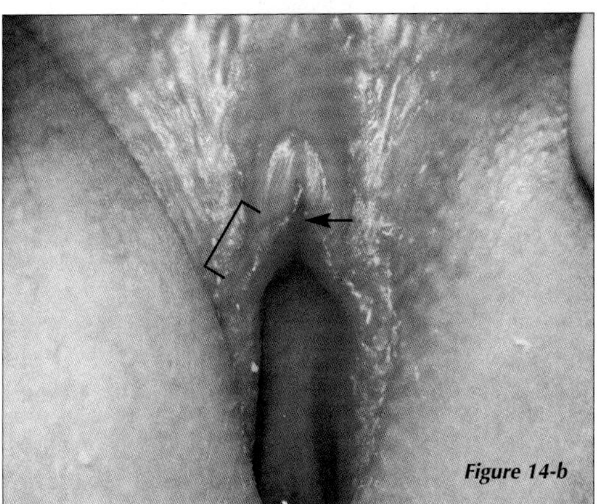

Figure 14-a. *There is a bruise on the clitoral hood.*

Figure 14-b. *There is erythema of the anterior commissure and periurethral area with punctate erythema at 10 and 11 o'clock.*

NONASSAULT VARIANTS
Infections
Viral

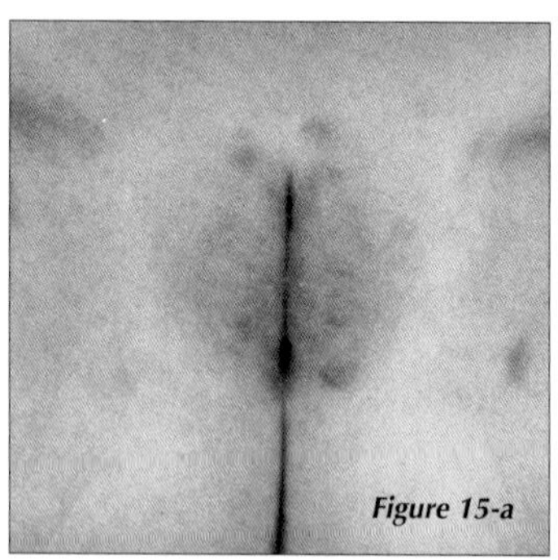
Figure 15-a

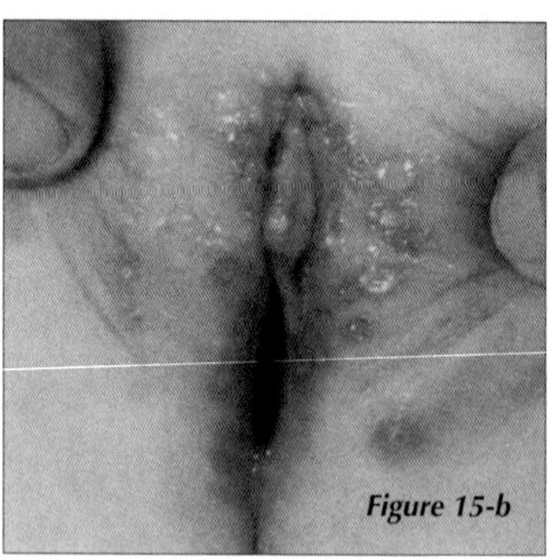
Figure 15-b

Case Study 15

This 6-year-old female was seen following a child protective services referral.

Figure 15-a. *Herpes simplex 2 vesicles on the labia majora (35 mm).*

Figure 15-b. *This photo shows vesicles on the medial aspect of the labia majora and around the introitus (35 mm).*

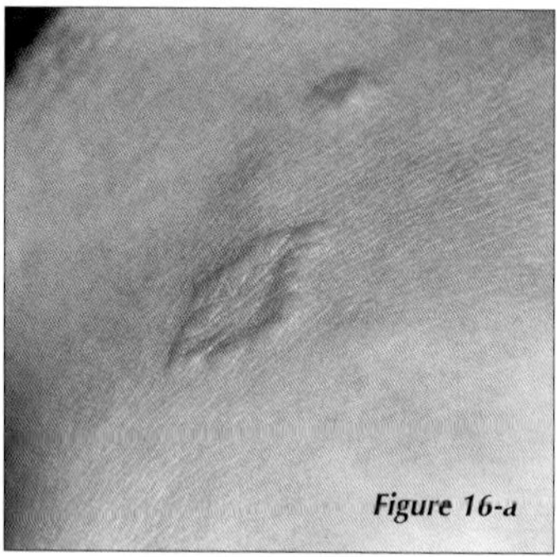
Figure 16-a

Figure 16-b

Case Study 16

This 4-year-old male presented for a physical exam. There was no history of molestation.

Figure 16-a. *Approximately 100 papular lesions were present in various places on this child, some in clusters. Some of the lesions were flat, others were raised.*

Figure 16-b. *There is perianal erythema with 3 papular lesions at 5 and 7 o'clock. There are brown stool particles around the anus.*

Parasitic

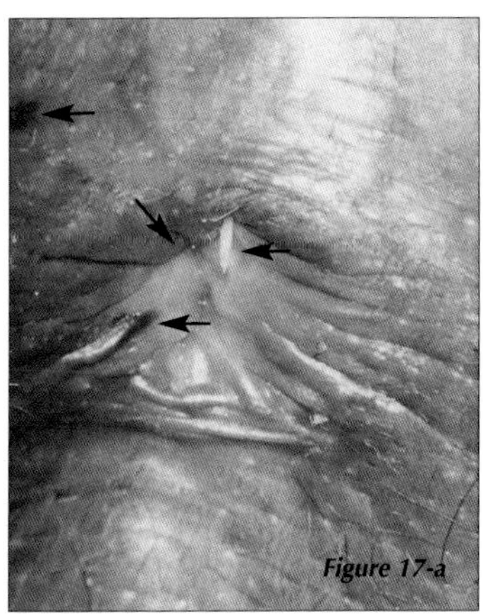

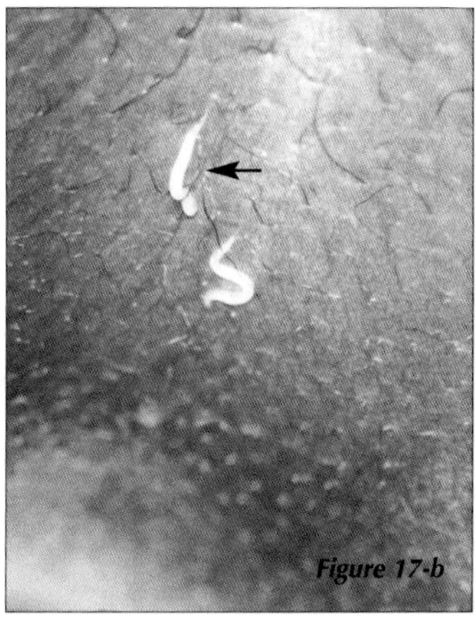

Case Study 17

This African American 7-year-old was referred for sexual abuse. She had pinworms.

Figure 17-a. *A pinworm going into the perianal tissue; there is a laceration adjacent to the pinworm. Two nevi are present at 8 and 10 o'clock around the perianal tissue.*

Figure 17-b. *Pinworms on the perianal area.*

Friable Fourchette

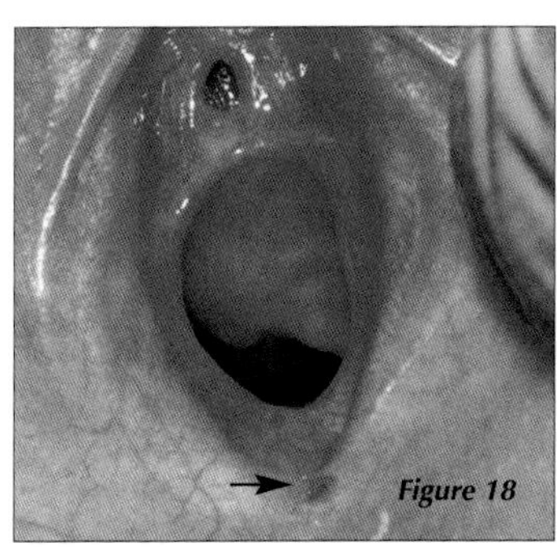

Case Study 18

This is a 9-year-old Caucasian with no history of abuse.

Figure 18. *An iatrogenic laceration of the posterior fourchette.*

Anal Findings

Case Study 19

This is a 6-year-old Hispanic with no history of molestation. She did have a history of hard stools.

Figure 19. *Fissures at 6 and 11 o'clock.*

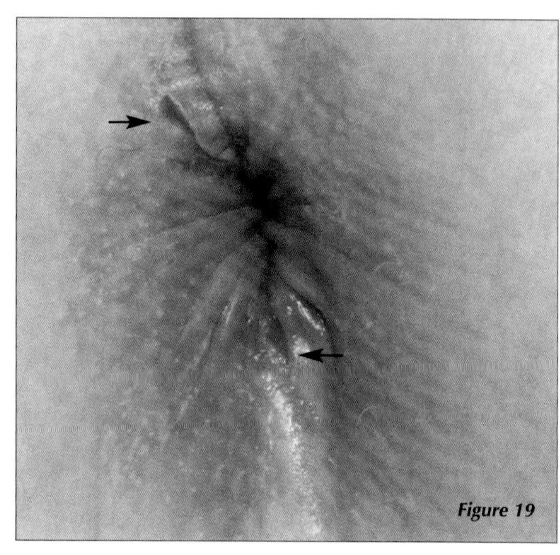

Figure 19

NORMAL FINDINGS

Annular Hymen

Case Study 20

This patient is 5 years old and Caucasian.

Figure 20. *This annular hymen has mounds at 1 and 2 o'clock. The periurethral bands are distinct especially on the right side. There is baby powder on the labia creating a border for the vestibule.*

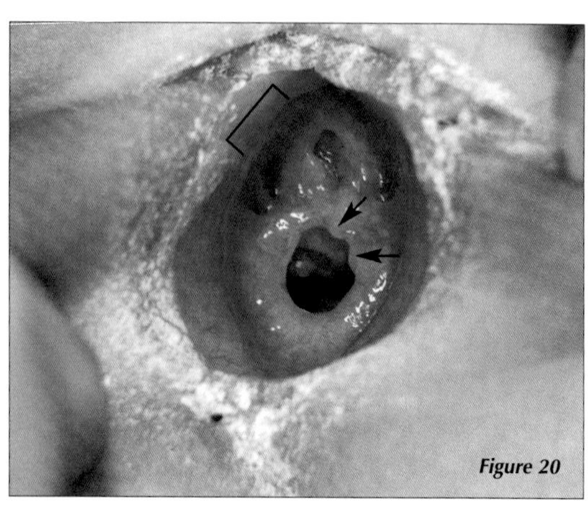

Figure 20

Preadolescent Sexual Abuse: 9-12 Years Old

History of Sexual Abuse

Friend of the Family Perpetrator

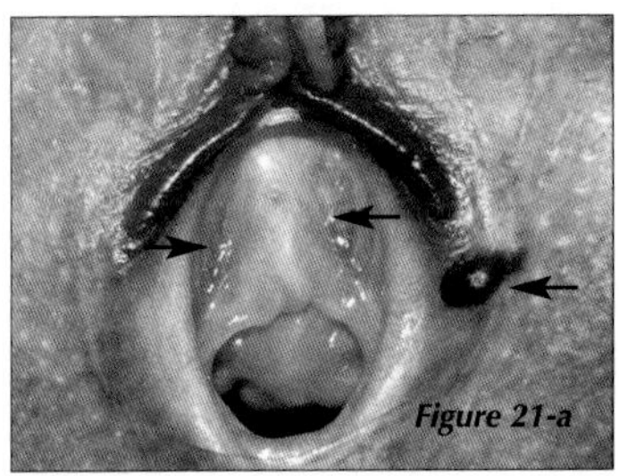

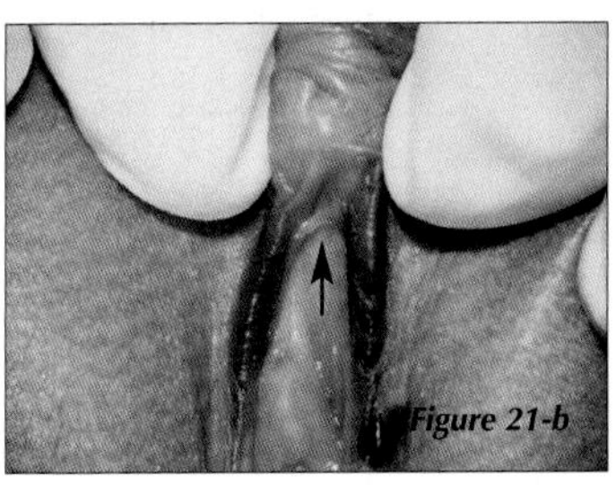

Case Study 21

This 7-year-old African American female and her sister were 2 of 5 frequent visitors to a 56-year-old male neighbor. He gave them money for ice cream, took pictures of them "humping" each other, and touched their privates, according to the child's history.

Figure 21-a. *This is a normal annular hymen with sharp edges. A nevus is noted at the left inferior labium minus. Periurethral bands are also visible.*

Figure 21-b. *Mild clitoral erythema is evident. There is a band inferior to the clitoris.*

The suspect pled guilty and was sentenced to 18 years in prison and must register as a sex offender.

Adolescent Perpetrator

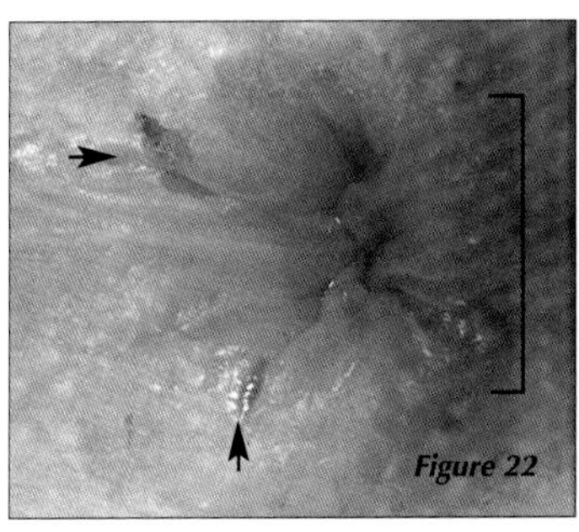

Case Study 22

This 9-year-old Hispanic male complained of anal pain and itching. He said a 16-year-old male forced penile-anal penetration many times. The examination was within 72 hours of the most recent incident.

Figure 22. *The child is in knee-chest position. There are 2 healing lacerations at 7 and 10 o'clock and venous congestion from 1 to 4 o'clock. Erythema is present from 8 to 11 o'clock.*

Nonassault Variants

Infection

Spirochetal

Case Study 23

This is a 12-year-old male.

Figure 23. *There is a syphilitic chancre visible on the upper lip (35 mm).*

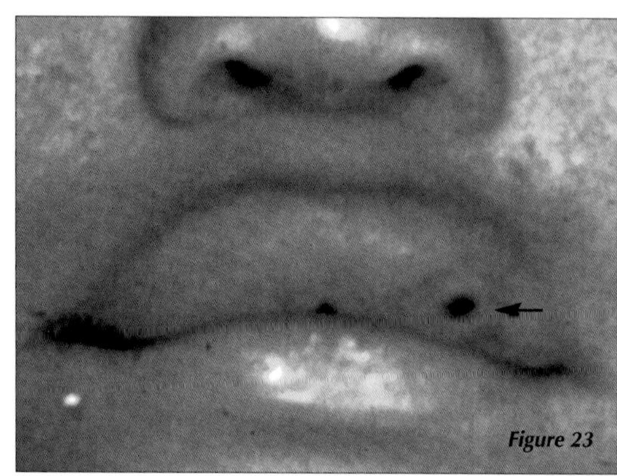

Normal Findings

Varied Examiner Technique

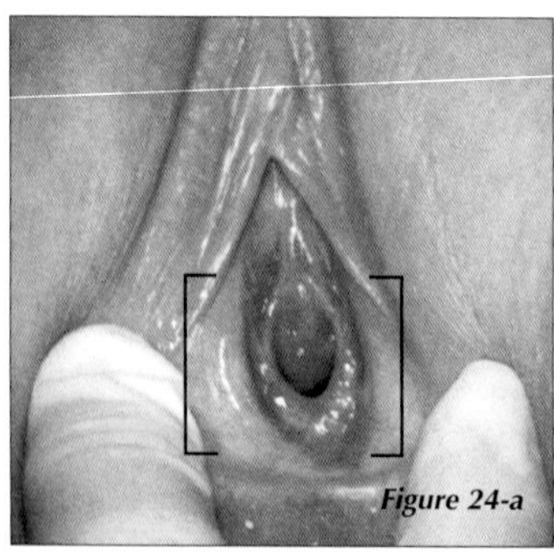

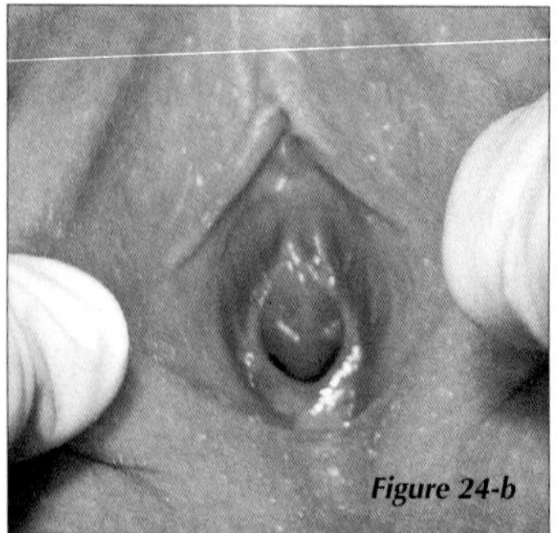

Case Study 24

This patient is an 11-year-old with no history of sexual abuse. This series of photographs shows the differences in visibility of anatomy with changes in examiner technique.

Figure 24-a. *A normal crescentic hymen is visualized using labial separation.*

Figure 24-b. *The hymenal rim comes into view more clearly with the labial traction technique.*

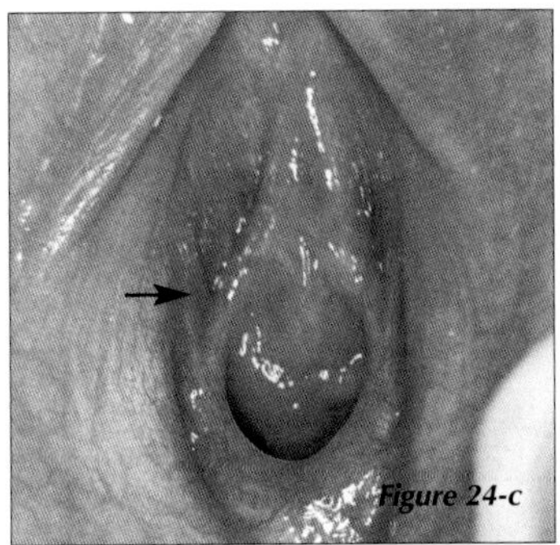

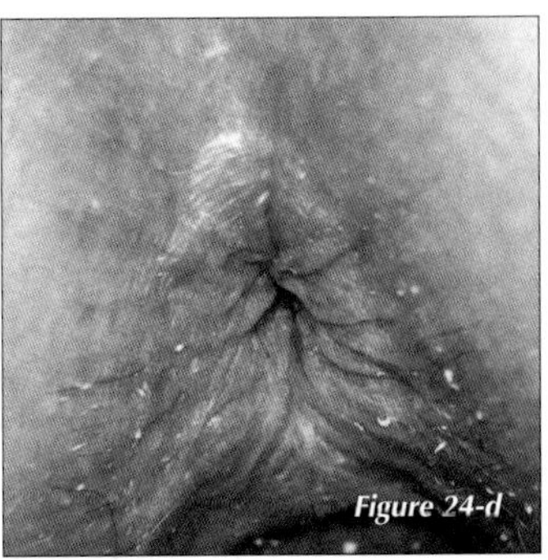

Case Study 24 *(continued)*

Figure 24-c. *With labial traction and greater magnification, the hymenal rim is more clearly visualized and perihymenal bands become evident.*

Figure 24-d. *A normal anus. Separation is used to visualize the perianal area.*

Hymen

Failure to Fuse

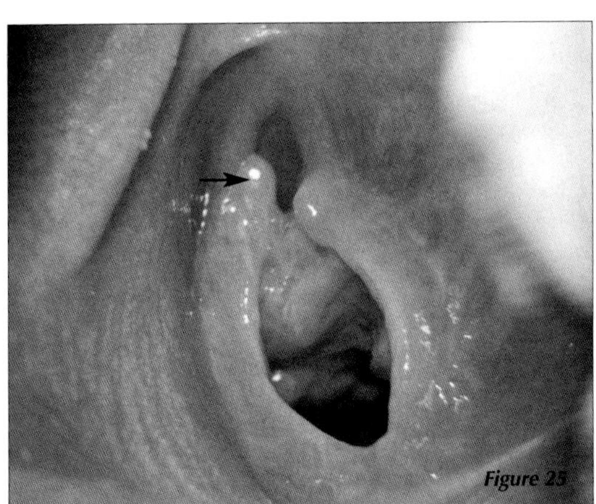

Case Study 25

This 12-year-old has a congenital anterior failure of the hymen to fuse.

Figure 25. *This hymen has failed to fuse. There is an intravaginal ridge at 3 o'clock.*

Adolescent Sexual Abuse and Assault: 13-17 Years Old*

History of Sexual Abuse or Assault

Penile-Vaginal Penetration

Characteristics of the Injury—Acute Findings

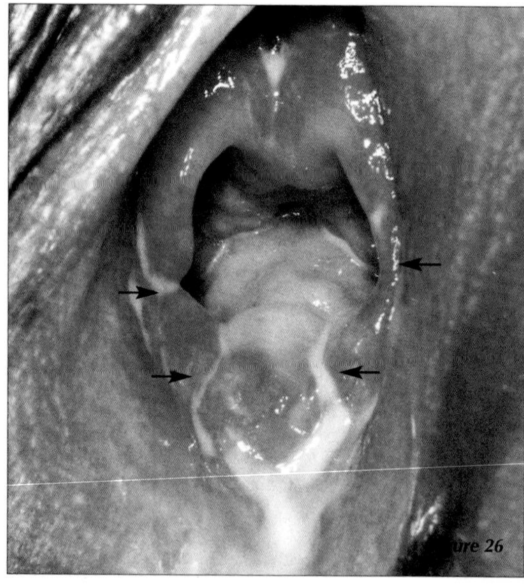

Case Study 26

This 12-year-old Hispanic female has a recent history of 2-time penile-vaginal penetration with ejaculation, fondling of buttocks, and kissing by her natural father. The child was examined within 72 hours of the assault. There is domestic violence in the home, and the child is distressed and depressed. She is not sexually active.

Figure 26. *The vaginal wall can be easily seen through the opened hymen. Further evaluation is needed to determine the continuity of the hymen, especially at 3, 5, 7, and 9 o'clock. There is a thick white discharge. Cultures were negative.*

*Some cases in the adolescent group are younger than 13 years but are Tanner stage 2 or greater.

Characteristics of the Injury—Healing Injury

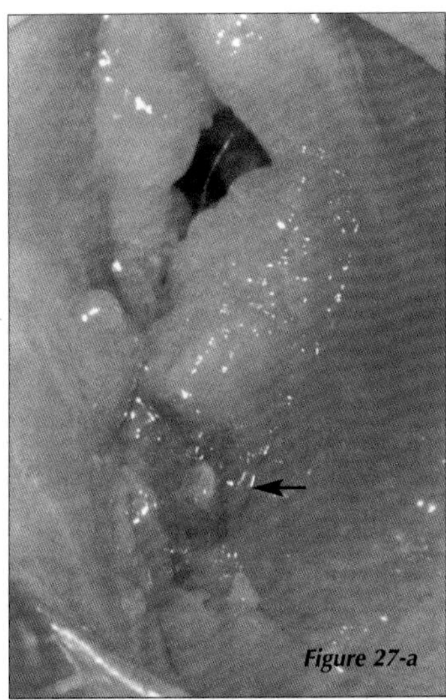
Figure 27-a

Case Study 27

This 12-year-old runaway was sexually assaulted by a 21-year-old male neighbor.

Figure 27-a. *There is acute bleeding from the laceration just below the hymen at 6 o'clock.*

Figure 27-b. *This photo shows more exposure of the same laceration. Exploring the hymen with a balloon-covered swab may have more clearly revealed the hymenal transection at 6 o'clock.*

Figure 27-c. *This photo was taken at a follow-up examination 2 weeks later and shows the healing laceration. Labial separation would help to better evaluate the hymen, fossa navicularis, and posterior fourchette.*

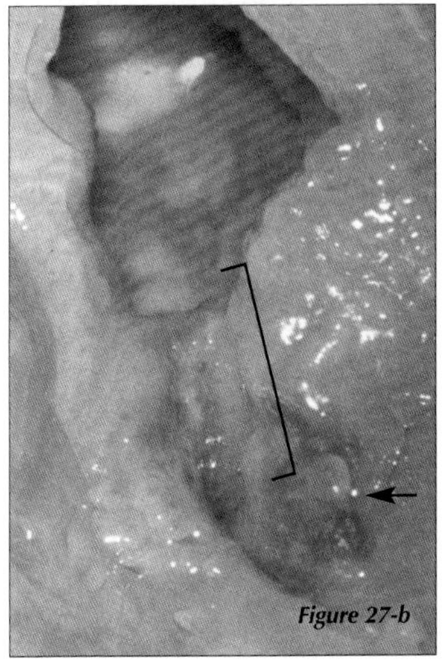
Figure 27-b

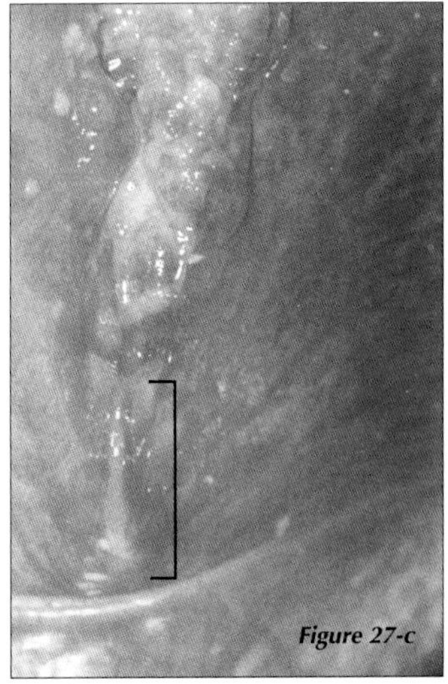
Figure 27-c

Characteristics of the Victim—Not Previously Sexually Active

Case Study 28

This 12-year-old Tanner stage 2 female has been postmenarchal for 1 year. She reported, "My parents beat and sexually abuse me." She reported forced fellatio, genital rubbing with penis, and penile-vaginal penetration with bleeding by her father. She was examined 2 weeks after the most recent episode of vaginal penetration.

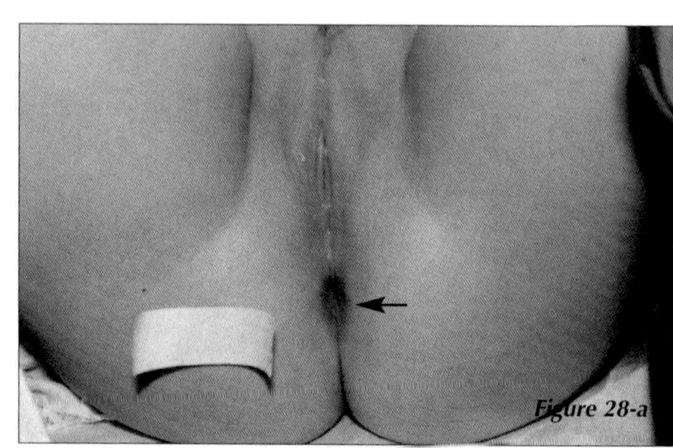

Figure 28-a. *There is anal hyperpigmentation visible (35 mm).*

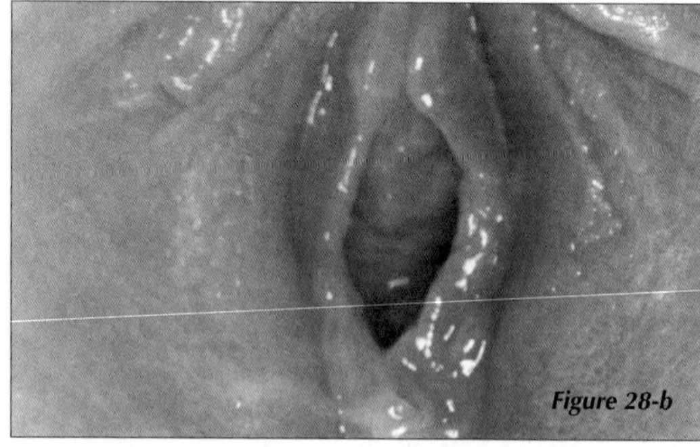

Figure 28-b. *The hymen has a normal color and contour.*

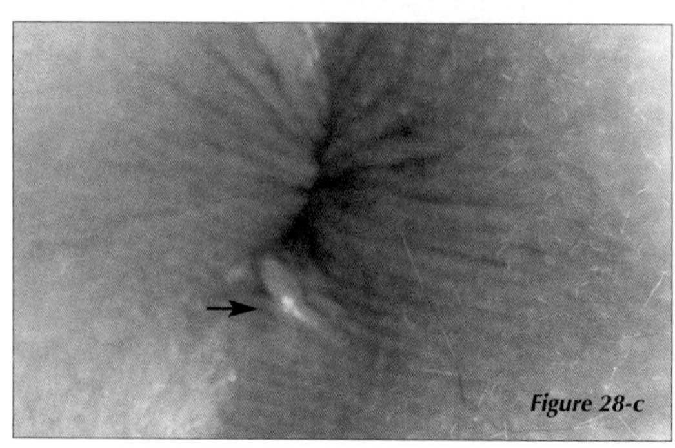

Figure 28-c. *There is an anal tag at 6 o'clock.*

Characteristics of the Victim—Pregnant

Case Study 29

This Tanner stage 2 12-year-old female and her 13-year-old sister gave a history of fondling by their 17-year-old brother for the past year. Her urine test for HCG was positive on 2 occasions, supporting her pregnancy. She was not aware of being pregnant, nor could she provide any history of how it occurred.

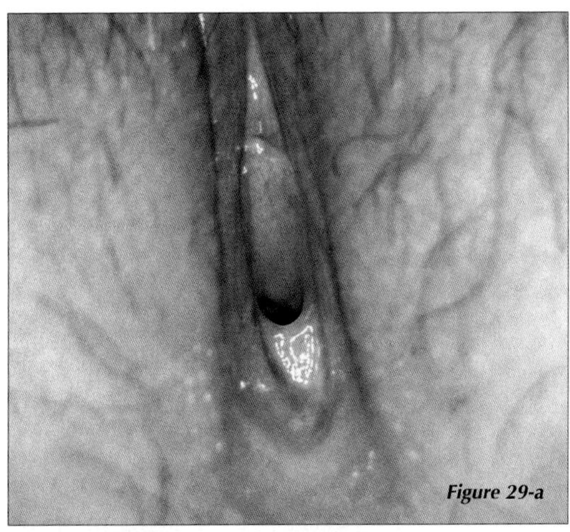

Figure 29-a

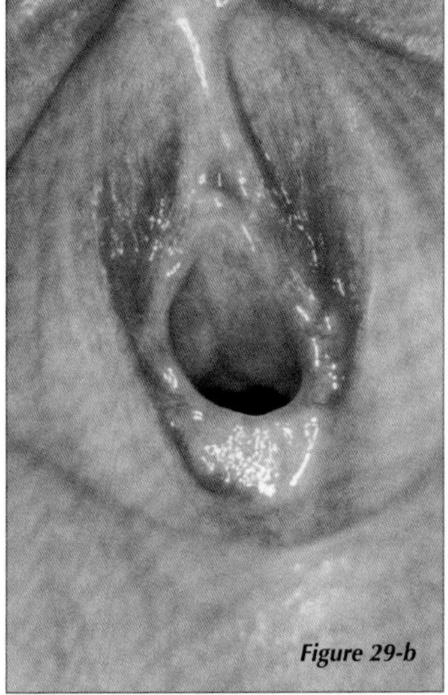

Figure 29-b

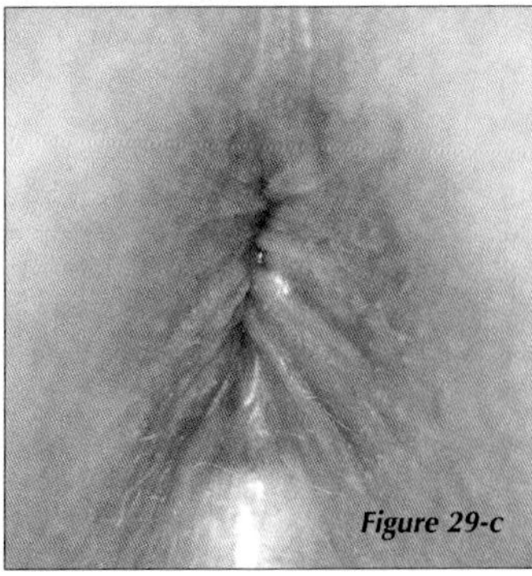

Figure 29-c

Figure 29-a. *The hymen is thin and has sharp edges. There is no separation being used here.*

Figure 29-b. *This is the same normal hymen, visualized with labial separation.*

Figure 29-c. *The perianal folds are asymmetrical in this normal anus.*

Digital-Vaginal Penetration

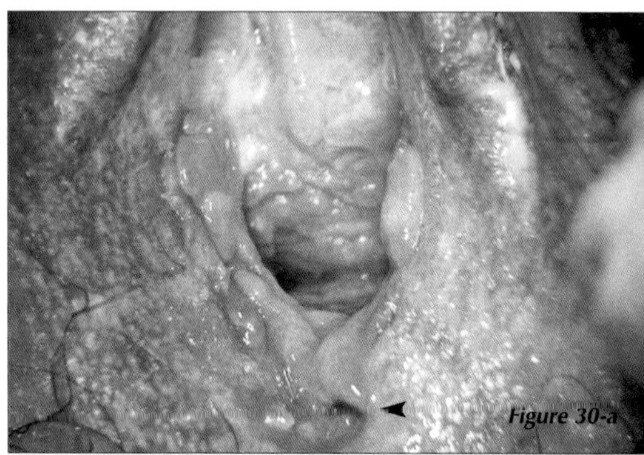

Figure 30-a

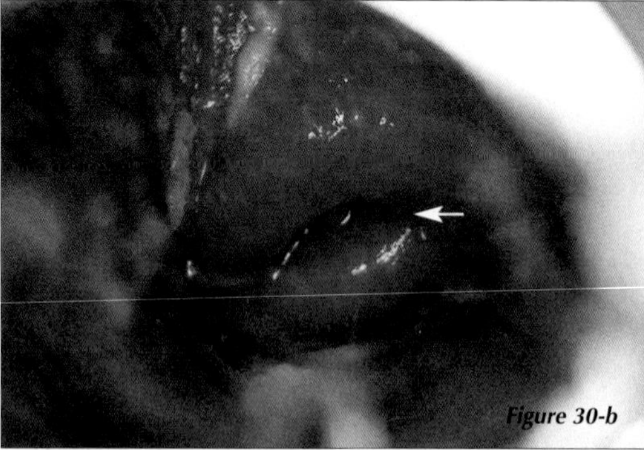

Figure 30-b

Case Study 30

This 15-year-old Tanner stage 3 female was molested by her 37-year-old stepfather but did not disclose the abuse to her mother because the mother was "fragile." The victim reported more than 75 incidents of fondling and digital penetration. The most recent incident took place 48 hours before the examination.

Figure 30-a. *The hymen is estrogenized and fimbriated. There is erythema at 6 o'clock in the fossa navicularis.*

Figure 30-b. *The pink cervix without injury. There is thick, white accumulation superior to the cervix, although the mucus in the cervical os is clear.*

The suspect pled guilty.

Sodomy

Case Study 31

This 15-year-old male was seen in the emergency department after having been brought in by ambulance. He explained that he was resting in his dorm room, and the next thing he remembers is the ambulance.

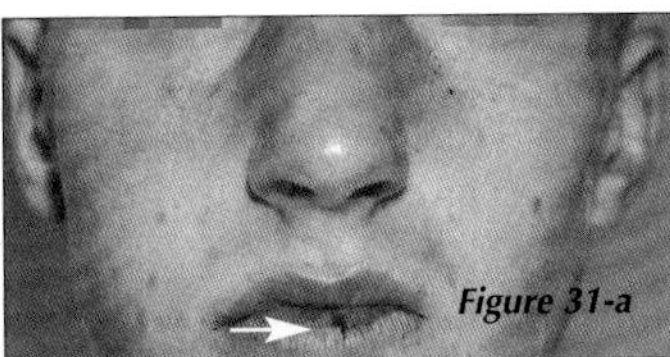
Figure 31-a

Figure 31-a. *There is ecchymosis below the right eye. The nose is swollen and a nasal fracture was confirmed by x-ray. There is also a laceration to the left of the midline on the lower, dry edematous lips (35 mm).*

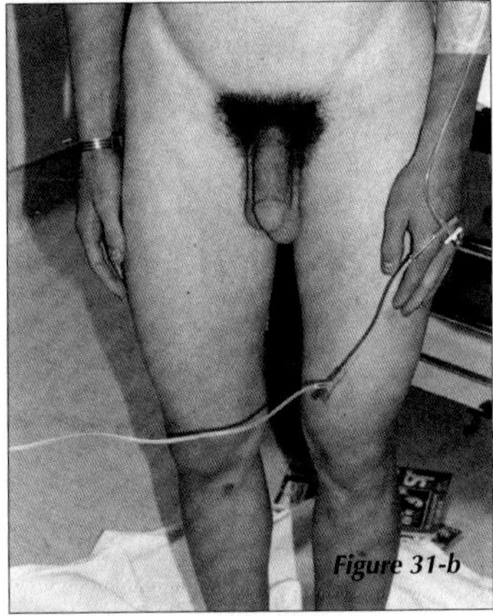
Figure 31-b

Figure 31-b. *Abrasions of the lower legs. The genitalia appear to be normal, Tanner stage 4 (35 mm).*

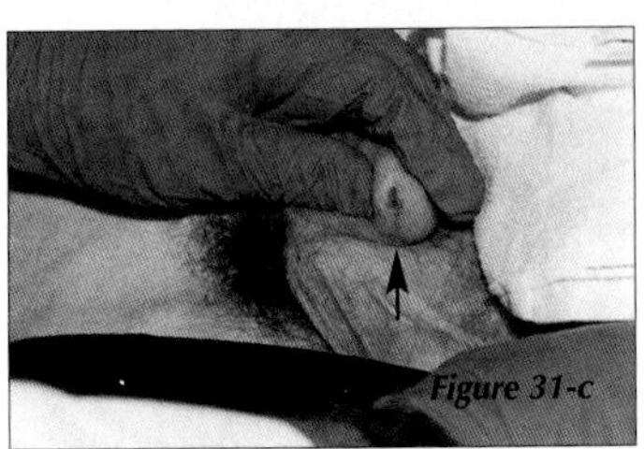
Figure 31-c

Figure 31-c. *There is an abrasion on the glans penis, starting near the urethra at 4 o'clock and extending downward. Note the erythema of the fingernails from biting them (35 mm).*

Figure 31-d. *Erythema and edema of the anus (35 mm).*

Figure 31-e. *This broken-off pencil was retrieved from his anus; the eraser end was in first. The victim was not aware that there was a pencil in his rectum. The point of the pencil was not identified by anoscopic examination. It may have been broken off in order to make removal painful (35 mm).*

The case was inactivated because there were no suspects and no leads.

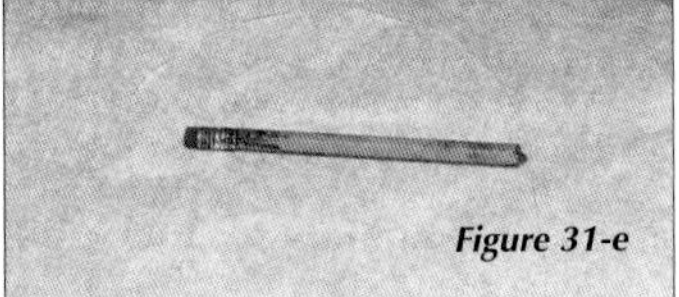
Figure 31-e

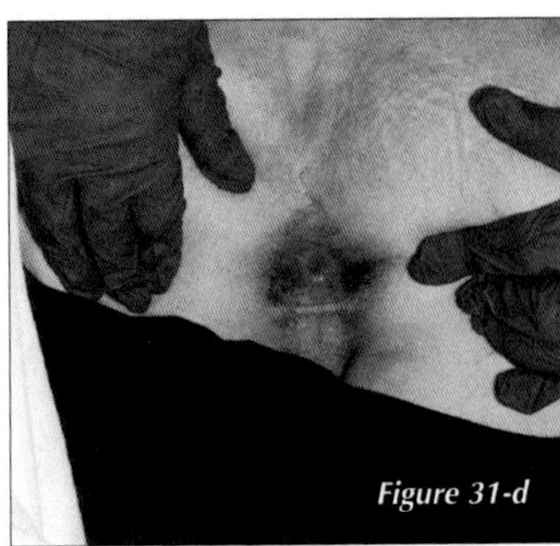
Figure 31-d

General Injuries

Case Study 32

This 14-year-old was beaten by her father because she was walking with a boy. She denied sexual assault by her father.

Figure 32-a. *This laceration to her upper lip was caused by a bracket of her braces when her father hit her mouth (35 mm).*

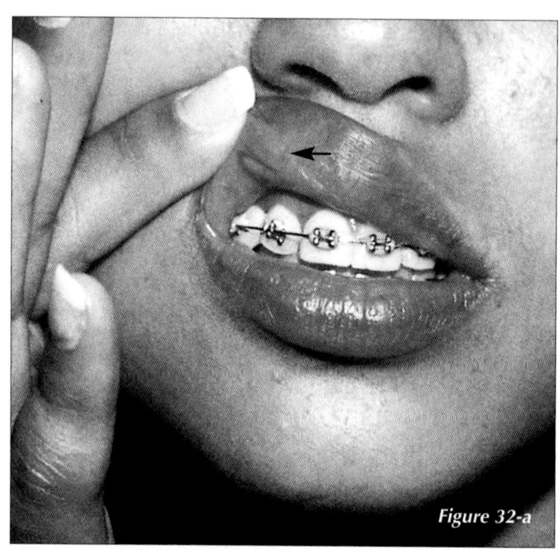

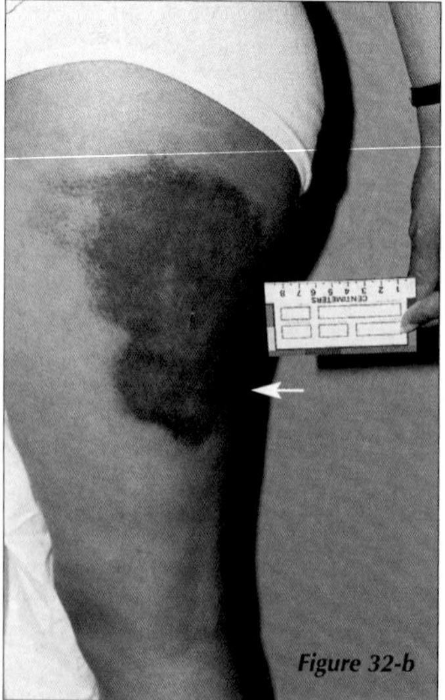

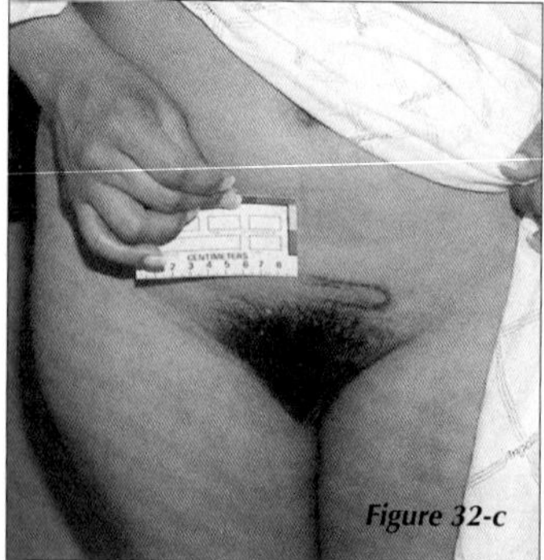

Figure 32-b. *An ecchymosis where her father kicked her (35 mm).*

Figure 32-c. *An ecchymosis from the end of a belt (35 mm).*

Her father pled guilty.

Nonassault Variants

Skin-Related

Lichen Sclerosis

Case Study 33

This 9-year-old Tanner stage 2 female was reported to child protection because she wore no underwear to school and repeatedly touched her genitalia. She lives with both of her natural parents, and there was no history of sexual abuse.

Figure 33-a. *A hypopigmented, thin friable area surrounding the genitalia. There is ecchymosis medial to the hypopigmentation, starting at the right labium minus and extending downward to the posterior fourchette. There is erythema lateral to the clitoral hood (35 mm).*

Figure 33-b. *A magnified view of the ecchymosis at the labium minus.*

Figure 33-c. *Ecchymosis at the posterior fourchette that ends in a hematoma. There are 2 lacerations evident. The hymen is pink, vascular, and has a continuous edge.*

It was determined that this was lichen sclerosis. She was successfully treated with steroid cream.

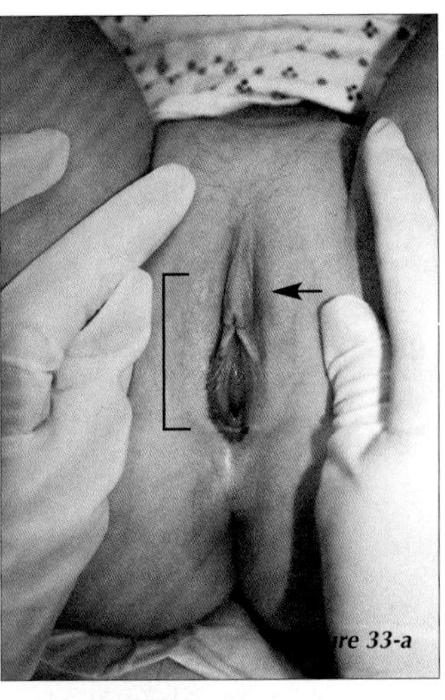

Figure 33-a

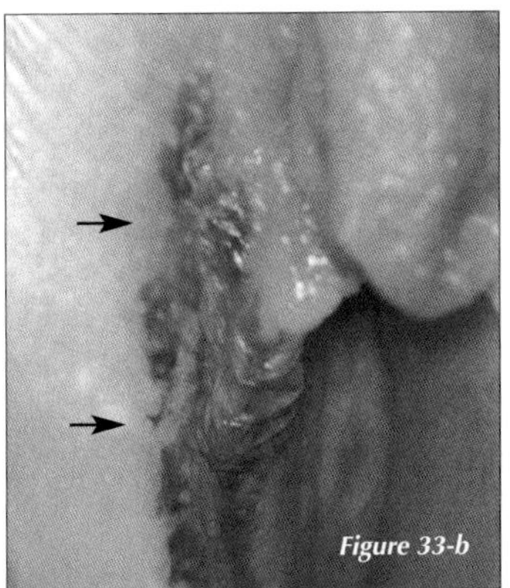

Figure 33-b

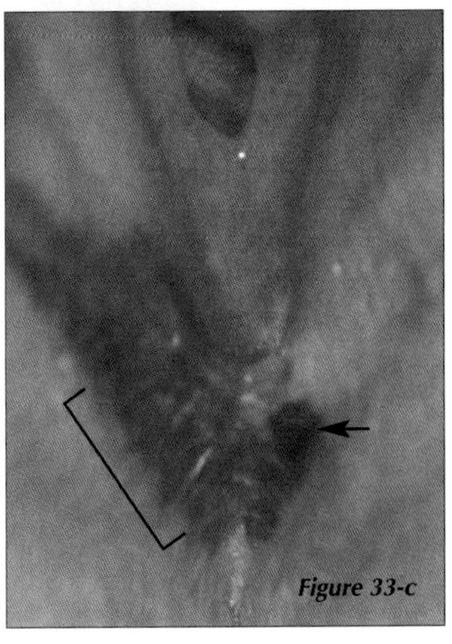

Figure 33-c

Normal Findings

Hymen

Never Sexually Active

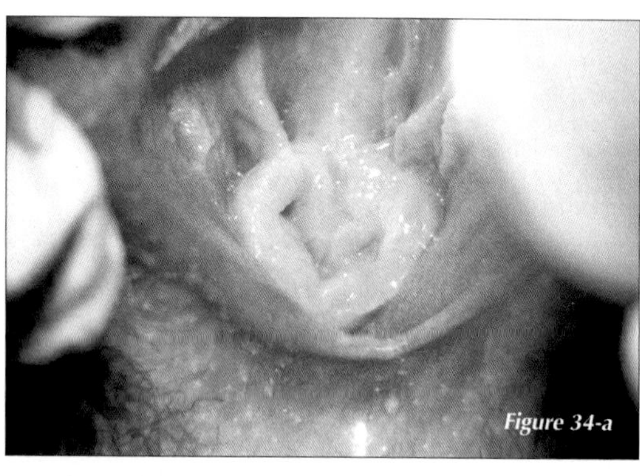

Figure 34-a

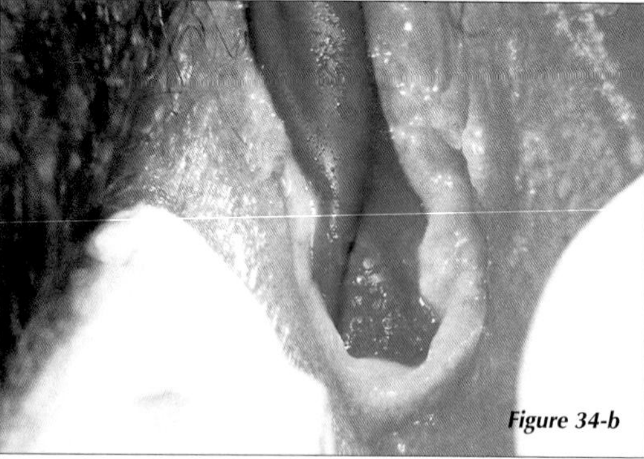

Figure 34-b

Case Study 34

This is a 14-year-old who has never been sexually active.

Figure 34-a. *The thick, pale hymen has an uninterrupted edge and thick, pale bands.*

Figure 34-b. *A balloon-covered swab is used to demonstrate the continuity of the lower border of the redundant hymenal edge.*

Asymmetrical Labia

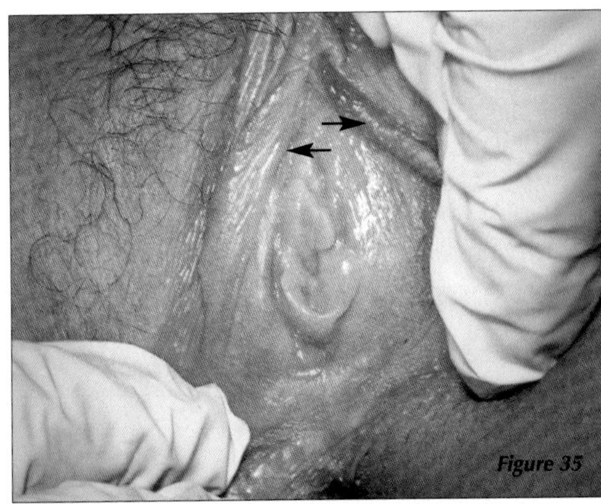

Case Study 35

This is a 12-year-old Hispanic female.

Figure 35. *Asymmetrical labia minora with the left labium minus larger and more pigmented than the right.*

Cervix

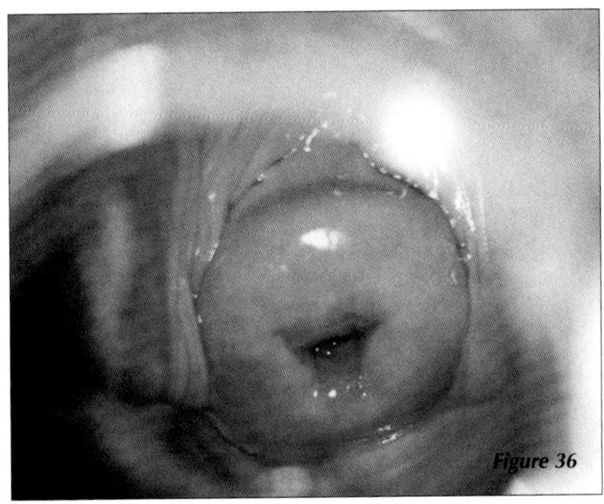

Case Study 36

This 18-year-old female is 7 weeks postpartum.

Figure 36. *The os is opened and normally irregular. Mucus is flowing from the os.*

Anal/Rectal

Case Study 37

These 3 photographs show a normal rectum at 3 positions of the anoscope.

Figure 37-a. *A view from 5 centimeters into the anus.*

Figure 37-b. *A view from half-way out of the anus. Yellow stool is present.*

Figure 37-c. *A view from just beyond the anal verge.*

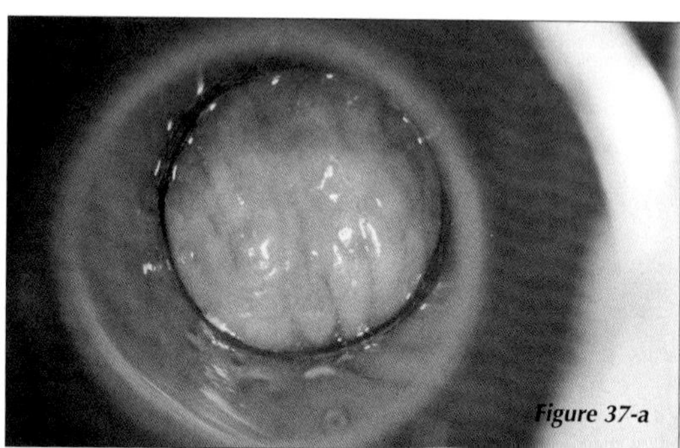

Figure 37-a

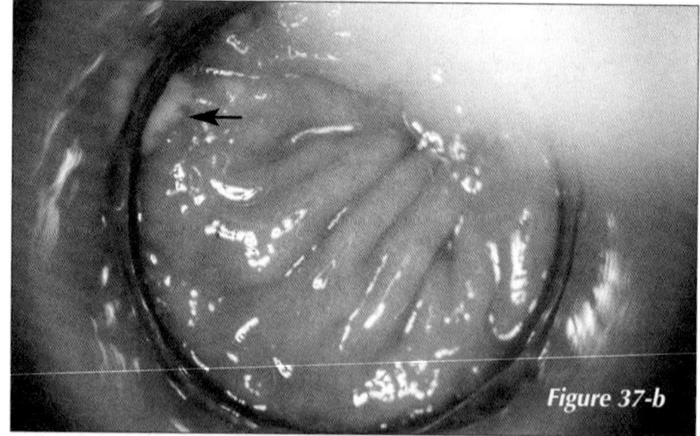

Figure 37-b

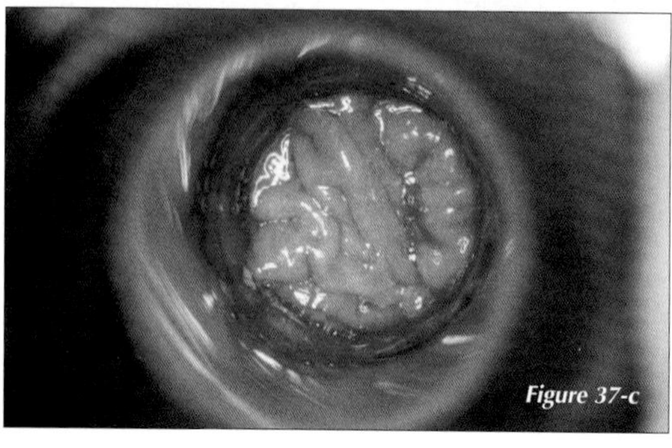

Figure 37-c

Adult Sexual Assault: 18-39 Years Old

History of Sexual Assault

Crime Scene

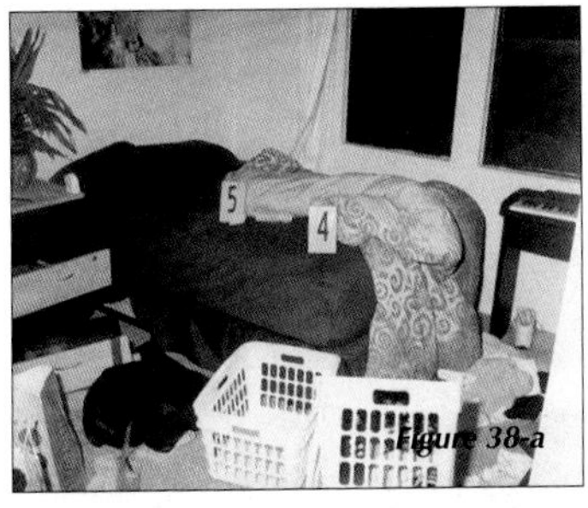

Figure 38-a

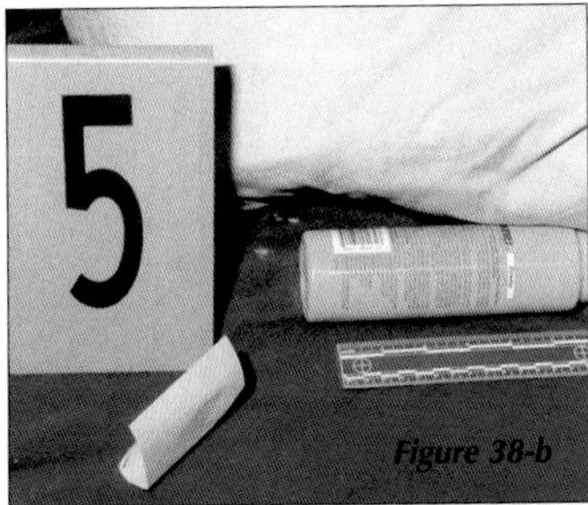

Figure 38-b

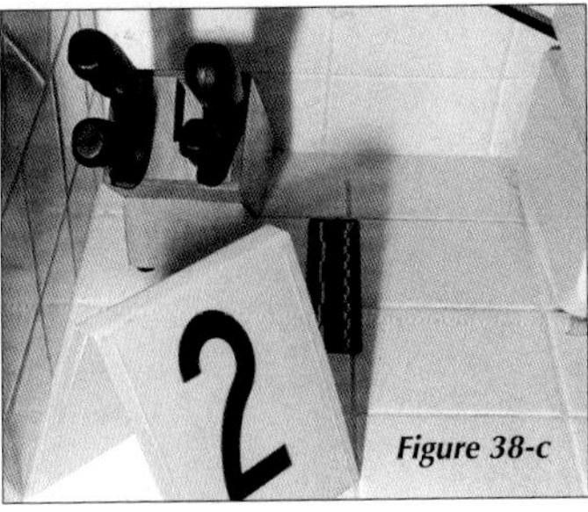

Figure 38-c

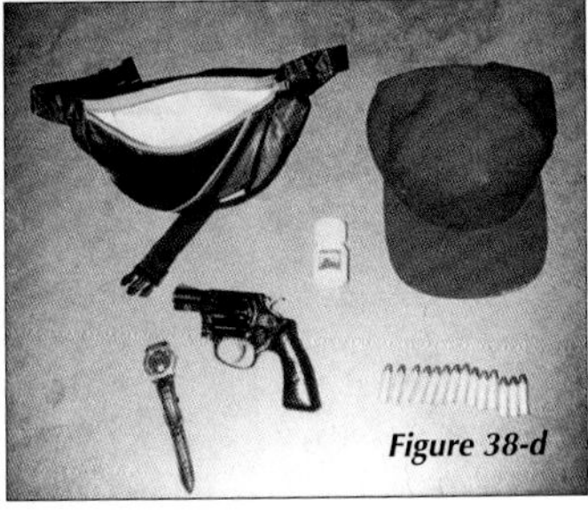
Figure 38-d

Case Study 38

This 35-year-old was in her apartment with her boyfriend when 2 African American males broke in, intending to rob her. The intruders forced the victim and her boyfriend into the bedroom. One of them threatened the victim with a kitchen knife. He held her prone and inserted a can of foot powder into her vagina 2 times. Then he pushed his penis into her vagina "for a couple of minutes." There was no ejaculation, but semen was found on the vaginal swabs. He attempted anal penetration.

Figures 38 a-d *are of the crime scene.*

Figure 38-a. *The victim's bedroom. The assault occurred on the bed (35 mm).*

Figure 38-b. *The foot powder can used in the assault (35 mm).*

Figure 38-c. *Knives, one of which was missing, were used to threaten the victim (35 mm).*

Figure 38-d. *These items were found in the perpetrators' possession. The watch belonged to the victim, as did some collectable coins which are not present in the photograph (35 mm).*

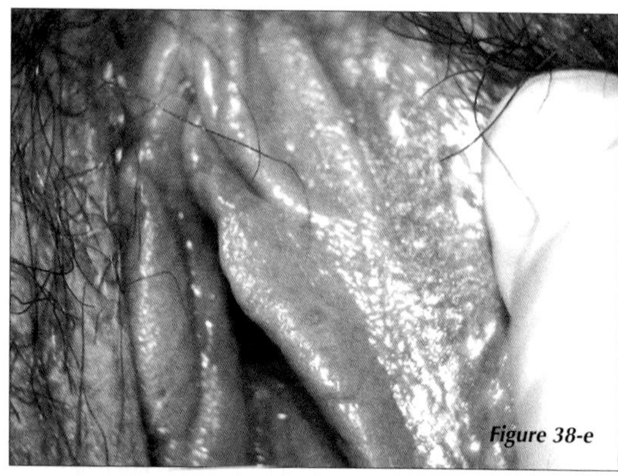

Figure 38-e

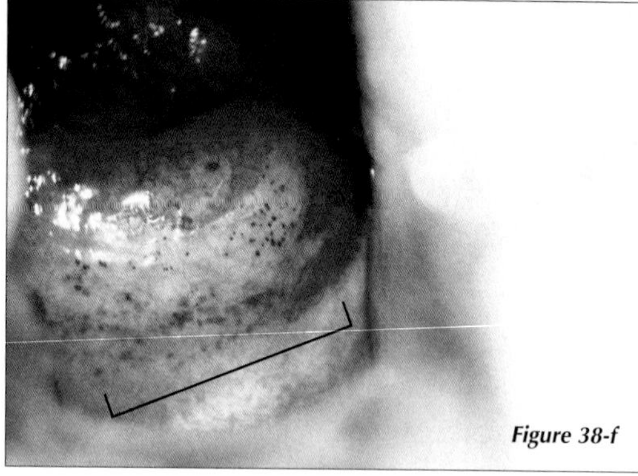

Figure 38-f

Case Study 38 *(continued)*

***Figures 38-e** and **38-f** are of the victim.*

***Figure 38-e.** There is ecchymosis of the labium minus at 9 to 11 o'clock.*

***Figure 38-f.** Petechiae are visible on the cervix.*

The victim called the police and was able to describe the perpetrator's car, which was quickly identified, and the perpetrators were apprehended. They were convicted of conspiring forcible rape in concert, forcible sodomy and sodomy in concert, robbery, and residential burglary. Male 1 was sentenced to 61 years to life and male 2, who had prior convictions, was sentenced to 80 years to life.

Disabled Victims

Case Study 39

This 19-year-old male is epileptic and autistic and lives at a residential facility. When he returned from a visit to his parents' house, he complained of anal pain to the care providers at the residential facility. He was examined 4 hours after his report of pain.

Figure 39-a. *This is the victim. Note his posture is consisent with his disability (35 mm).*

Figure 39-b. *There is a laceration of the anus, and dried blood is present in the perianal area.*

Figure 39-c. *There is visible erythema and edema of the anus and a laceration at 6 o'clock. An external hemorrhoid is present at 12 o'clock.*

Figure 39-d. *There is venous pooling around the anus with a large laceration at 6 o'clock.*

Investigation is being pursued.

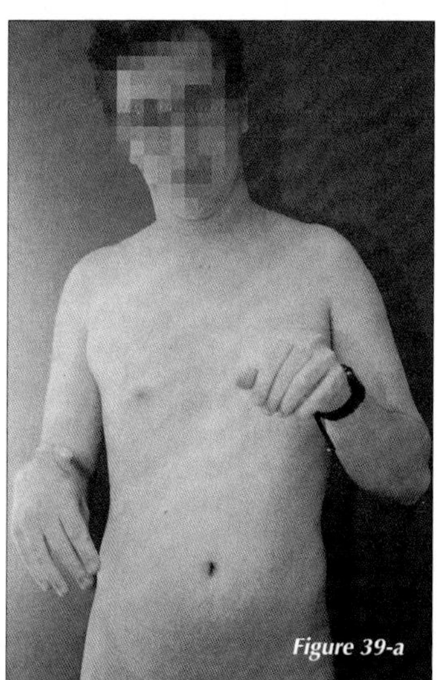

Figure 39-a

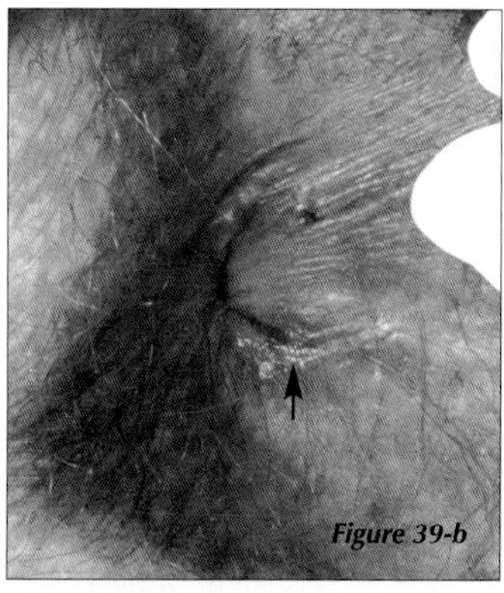

Figure 39-b

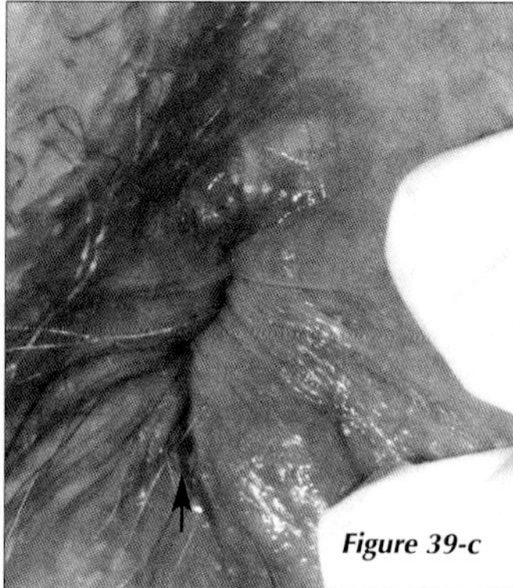

Figure 39-c

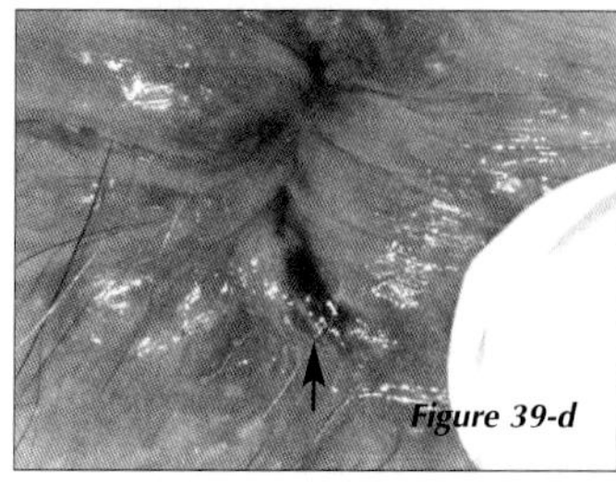

Figure 39-d

Oral Injury

Case Study 40

This 24-year-old female is a prostitute. Her pimp forced penile penetration of her mouth and then beat her because she wasn't making enough money. She was examined 17 hours after the assault.

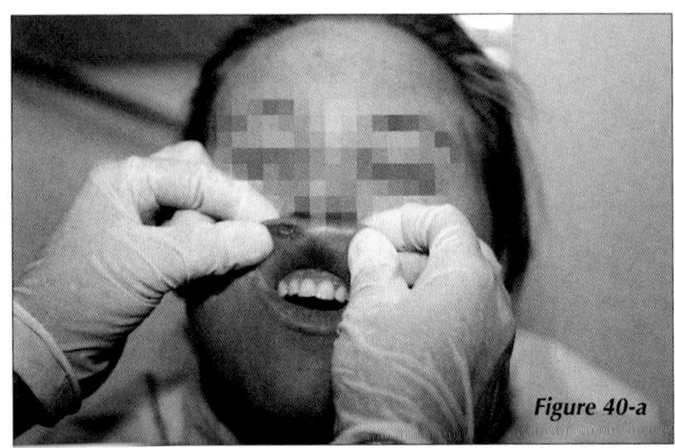

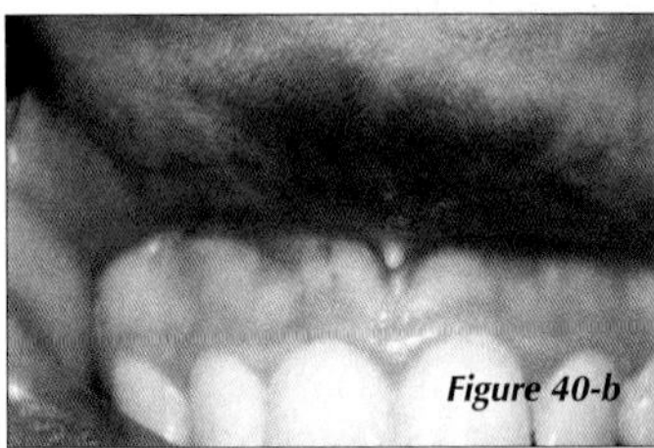

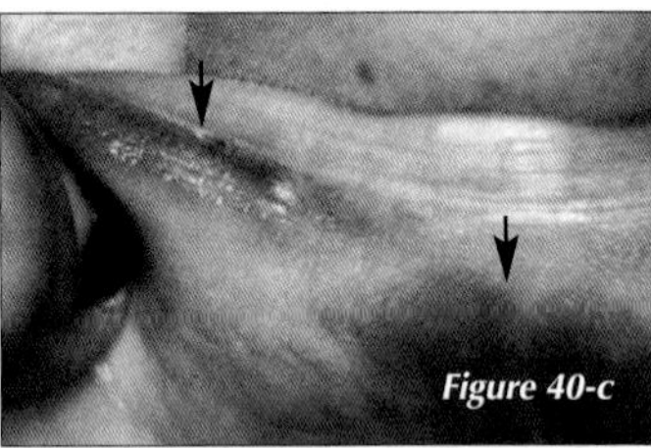

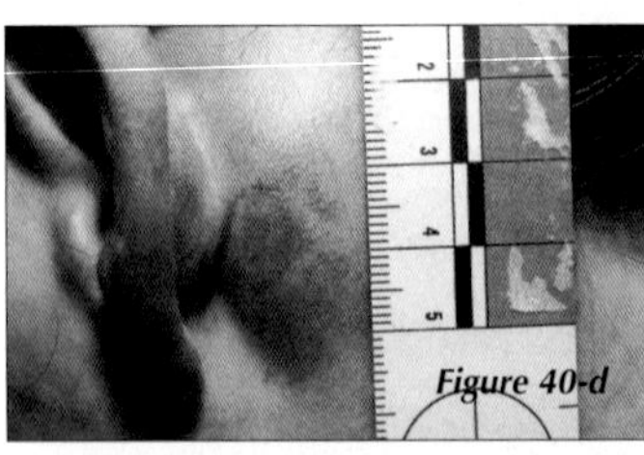

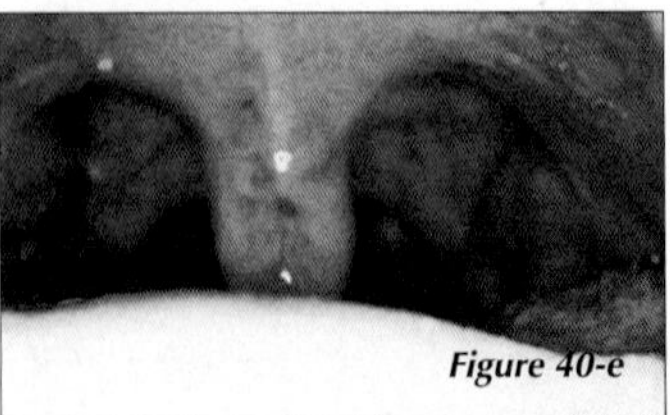

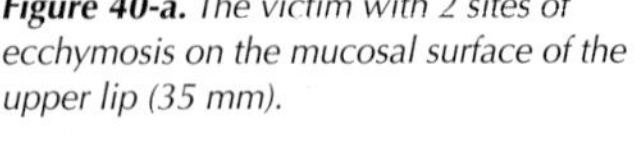

Figure 40-a. *The victim with 2 sites of ecchymosis on the mucosal surface of the upper lip (35 mm).*

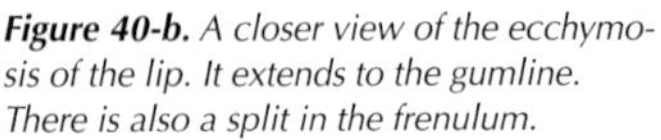

Figure 40-b. *A closer view of the ecchymosis of the lip. It extends to the gumline. There is also a split in the frenulum.*

Figure 40-c. *There is a laceration at the vermillion border of this ecchymotic area of the upper lip.*

Figure 40-d. *A site of ecchymosis behind the earlobe consistent with a history of forced penile penetration of the mouth. This may be called a "clapping" injury (35 mm).*

Figure 40-e. *There are petechiae on the uvula.*

This case was accepted by the district attorney.

Nonassault Variants

Skin-Related Findings

Irritation of the Medial Thighs

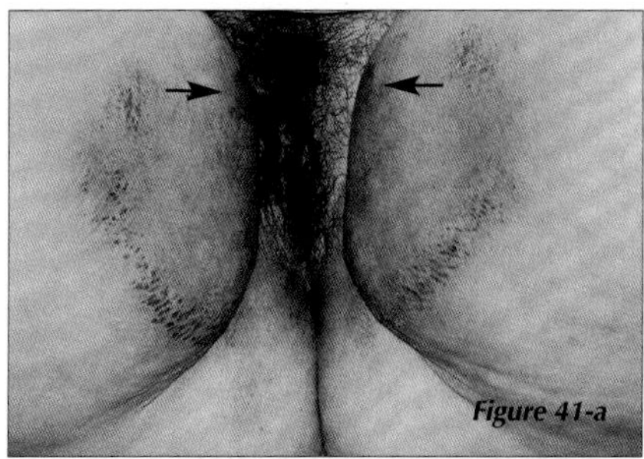

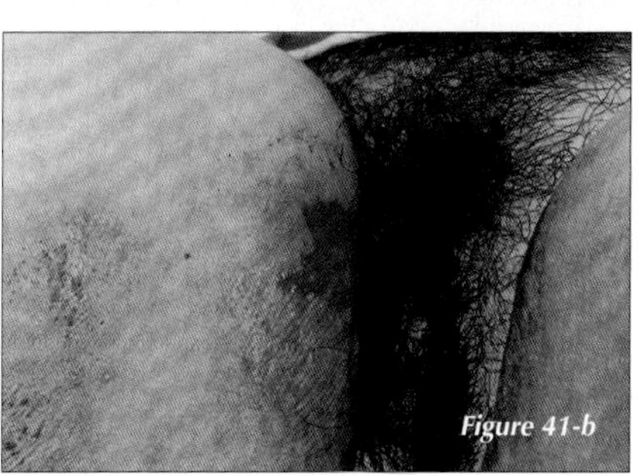

Case Study 41

This is a 300 pound Caucasian female.

Figure 41-a. *There is erythema and hyperpigmentation of the medial thighs extending to the buttocks. There is healing of the breakdown around the perimeter of the erythema. At the arrows, there are oozing abrasions and skin breakdown (35 mm).*

Figure 41-b. *A closer view of the area of open breakdown (35 mm).*

Folliculitis

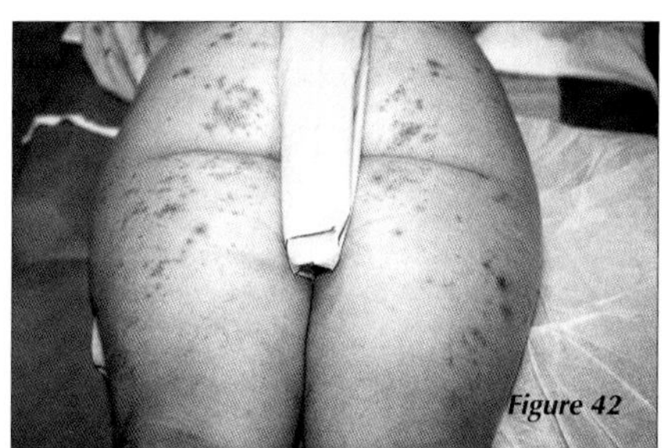

Case Study 42

This is a 43-year-old female.

Figure 42. *She has had a history of folliculitis for over one year from an unknown cause. She was referred to a dermatologist for further examination (35 mm).*

Labial and Vaginal Findings

Lichenification

Case Study 43

Figure 43. *This 18-year-old has lichenification. Note the lack of pubic hair. She does not shave (35 mm).*

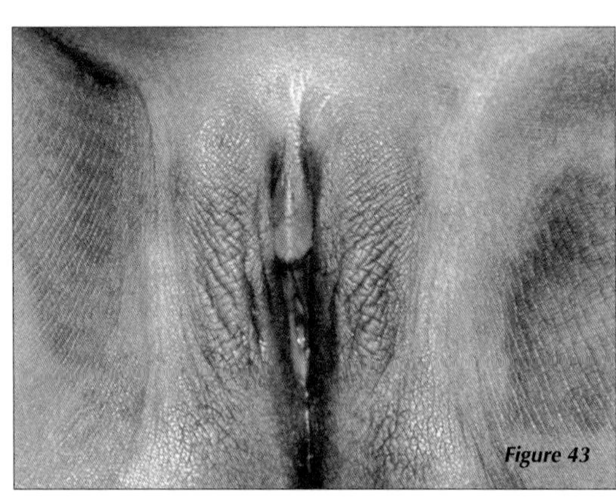
Figure 43

Vulvectomy

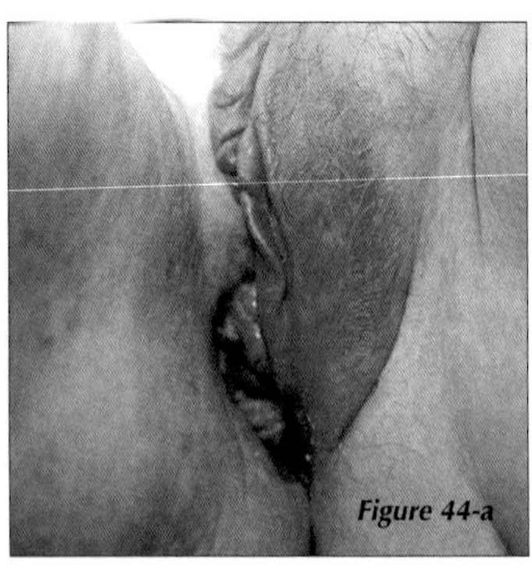
Figure 44-a

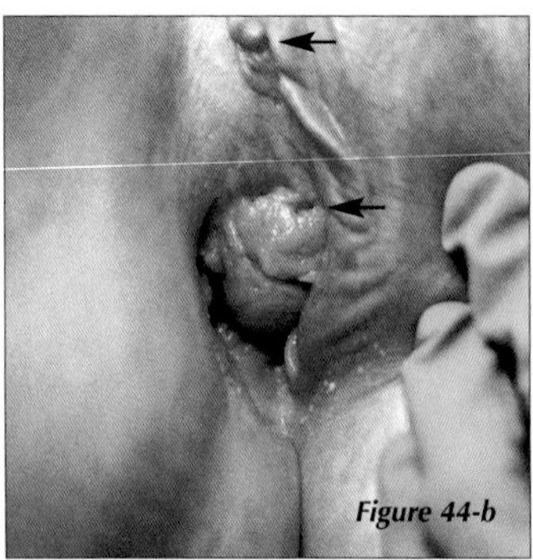
Figure 44-b

Case Study 44

This 40-year-old had vulvar cancer, and the right labium majus and labium minus were surgically removed. She remains sexually active. She is not taking estrogen.

Figure 44-a. *The labium majus and minus on the left are erythematous, as are 2 sites on the medial right thigh. There is thinning of the pubic hair (35 mm).*

Figure 44-b. *The vaginal orifice is visible with the labium majus pulled to the side. The clitoris and urethral opening are visible (35 mm).*

Episiotomy

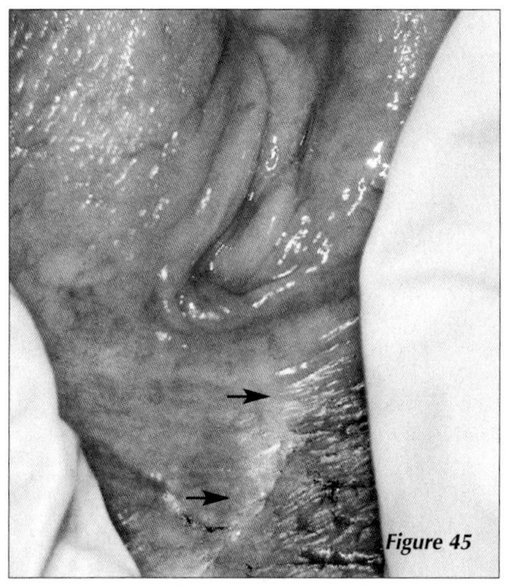
Figure 45

Case Study 45

This 40-year-old female (gravida 2, para 2) has had 2 vaginal deliveries, both with term infants.

Figure 45. *There is a medio-lateral episiotomy that is not easily visible. This photograph was taken 1 hour after consensual penile-vaginal intercourse. There is erythema of the left medial labium, posterior hymen and posterior fourchette.*

Perineum and Perianal Findings

Skin Irritation

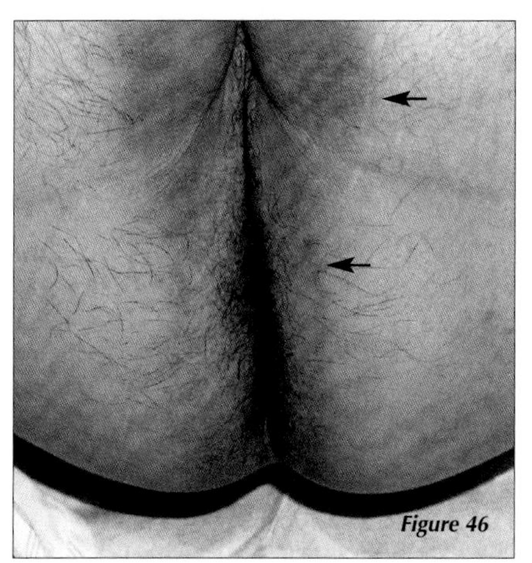
Figure 46

Case Study 46

This 30-year-old heterosexual male has hyperpigmentation and skin thickening. He wears cotton briefs. This photograph was taken during the fall in a tropical climate.

Figure 46. *The hyperpigmentation and skin thickening on the medial thighs and buttocks may be due to rubbing and moisture (35 mm).*

Techniques

Genital Examination

Case Study 47

These 3 photographs demonstrate examination techniques. Although the shape of the hymen is not as significant in adults as it is in children, it is noteworthy to see how different techniques can alter the appearance of the anatomy.

Figure 47-a. *With labial separation, the hymen appears closed, and the posterior fourchette is uninjured.*

Figure 47-b. *With labial separation, the hymen begins to open and appears annular.*

Figure 47-c. *Using labial traction, the hymen now appears crescentic.*

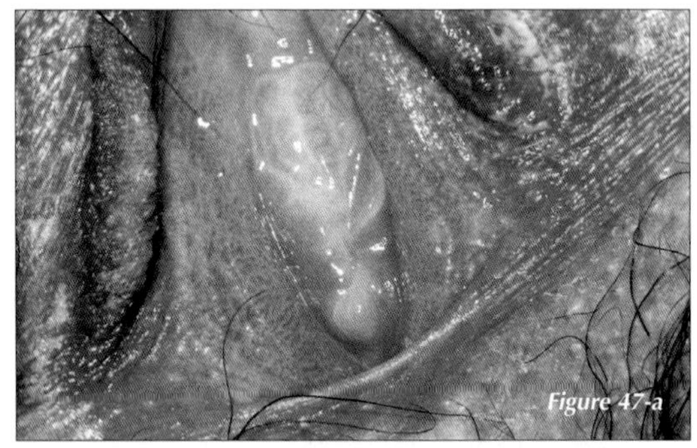

Figure 47-a

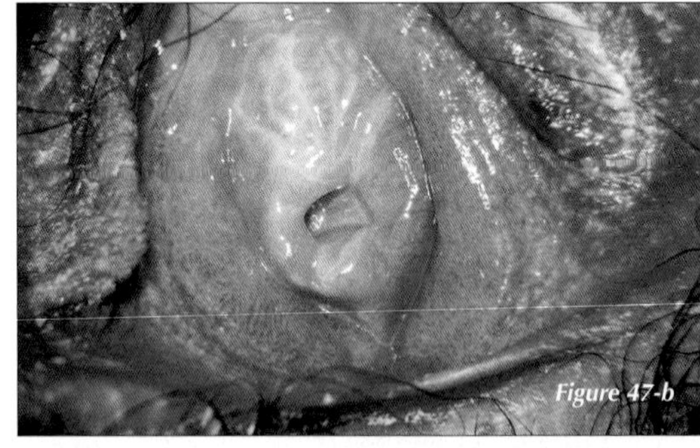

Figure 47-b

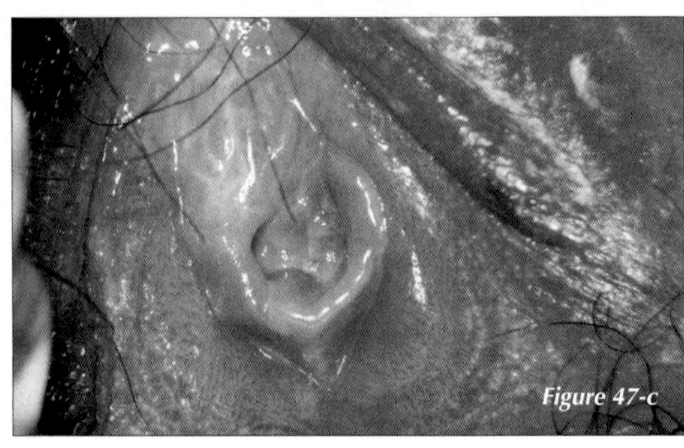

Figure 47-c

Normal Findings

Vestibule

Vestibular Papillations

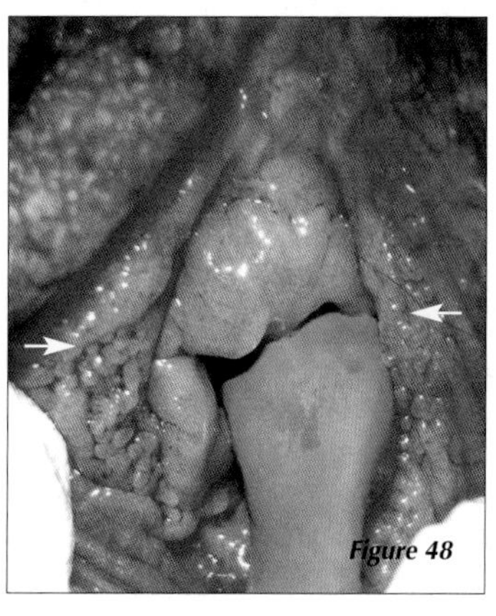

Case Study 48

This 27-year-old Caucasian female was unable to recall whether her mother took diethylstilbestrol nor whether she had a difficult pregnancy.

Figure 48. *There are vestibular papillations visible from 2 to 9 o'clock around the hymen. These papillations are seen most commonly in the vestibule in female offspring whose mothers took diethylstilbestrol during pregnancy.*

Open Bartholin Duct

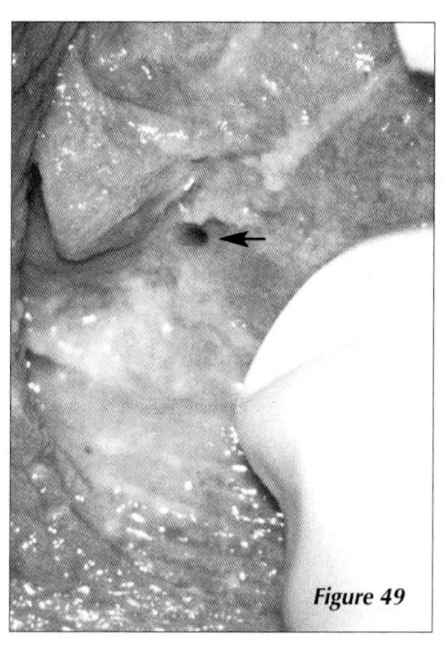

Case Study 49

A 27-year-old Caucasian gravida 0 female.

Figure 49. *The open Bartholin duct is visible. Bartholin glands secrete mucus.*

Periurethral Perihymenal Bands

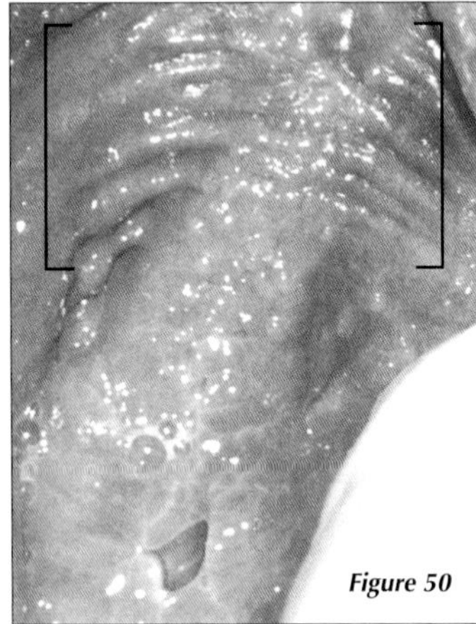

Figure 50

Case Study 50

A sexually active 18-year-old Caucasian gravida 0.

Figure 50. *There are periurethral bands bilaterally.*

Hymens Related to Sexual Experience, Pregnancy, and Number of Vaginal Deliveries

Never Been Pregnant

Case Study 51

This 39-year-old female has been sexually active for 20 years but never pregnant.

Figure 51. *The normally thick hymen has folds or clefts at 4 and 8 o'clock. These need to be more closely examined.*

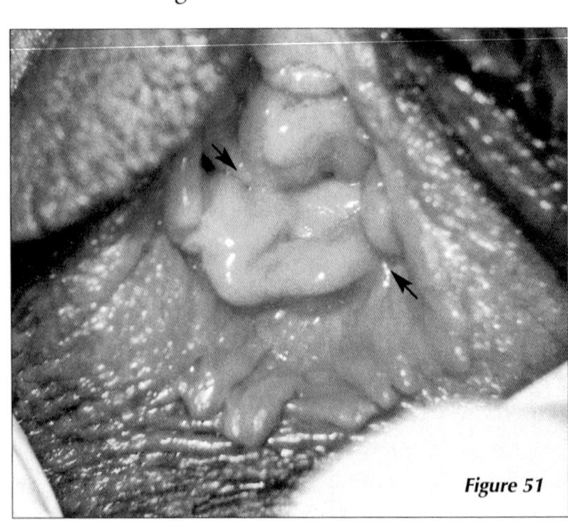

Figure 51

One Vaginal Delivery

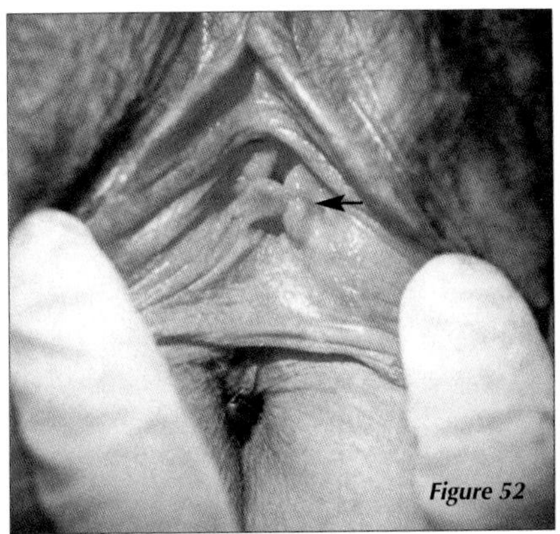
Figure 52

Case Study 52

This 40-year-old obese female (gravida 1) has been sexually active and married for 20 years.

Figure 52. *The left lateral rim of the hymen is visible with a fold or cleft at 3 o'clock. There is a caruncula at 7 to 8 o'clock and a section of hymen visible from 9 to 11 o'clock. A more magnified view using a swab to explore the hymenal rim would be helpful.*

Vaginal Wall

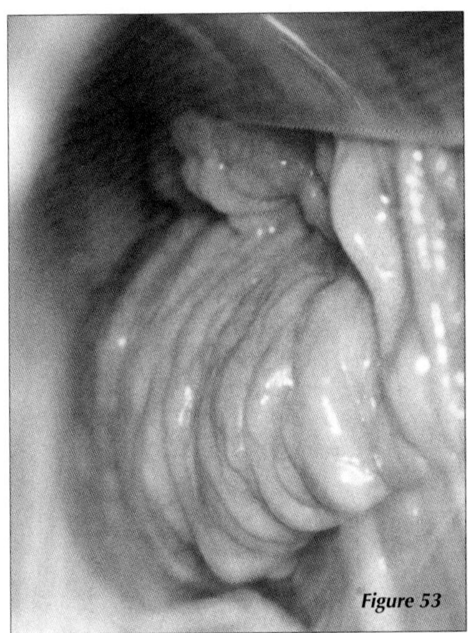
Figure 53

Case Study 53

This 20-year-old has normal rugae on the left vaginal wall.

Figure 53. *The rugae are seen here through the side of the vaginal speculum. The most exterior tissue is the hymen.*

Cervix

Normal Findings

Case Study 54

This 23-year-old (gravida 0) has a normal cervix.

__Figure 54.__ The cervix is rose-colored and shiny, with a slit-like os.

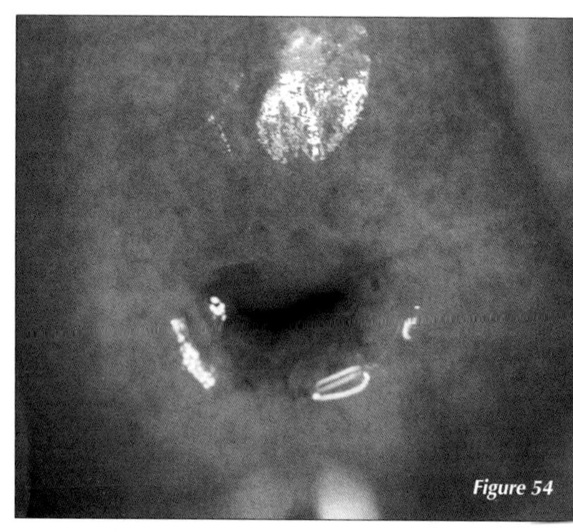

Figure 54

Intrauterine Device String

Case Study 55

This is a 25-year-old sexually active female with an intrauterine device (IUD).

__Figure 55.__ The IUD string in the cervical os has caused no apparent irritation to the cervix. The erythema right at the os may be ectropion. The tissue at 3 and 9 o'clock is the vaginal wall between the blades of the vaginal speculum.

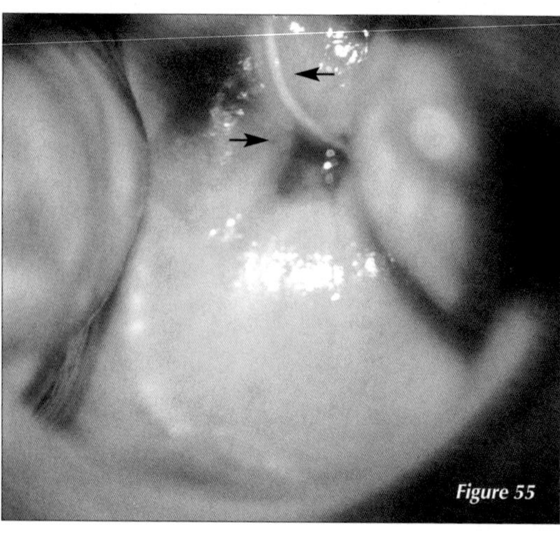

Figure 55

Middle-Aged Adult Sexual Assault: 40-64 Years Old

History of Sexual Assault

Characteristics of the Perpetrator

Stranger

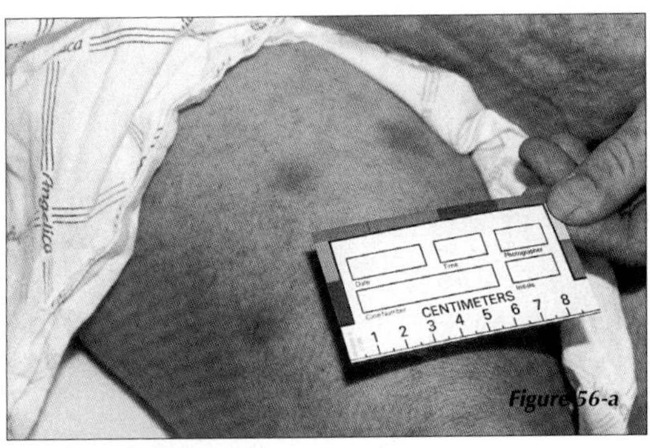

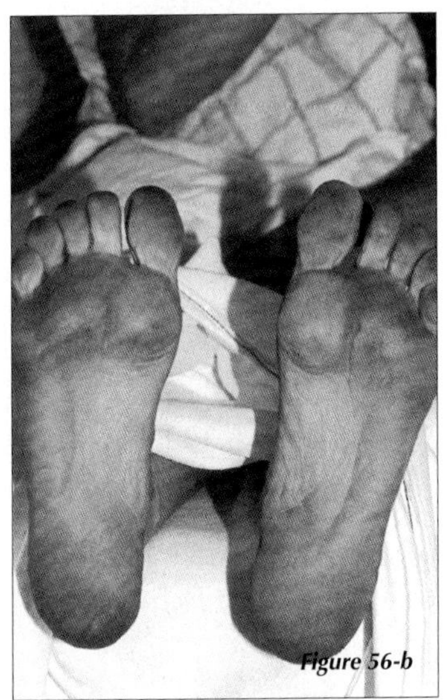

Case Study 56

This 47-year-old female (gravida 1, para 1) was assaulted by 2 strangers. She was picked up by the perpetrators, who then stopped in an empty lot and pushed her out of the car. At knifepoint, they took turns assaulting her, including forced fellatio, forced cunnilingus, and 15 incidents each of penetration of her vagina with penis and fingers. Her anus was penetrated by fingers 6 times and by a penis 15 times. She stated, "They couldn't get it very hard or couldn't come, so they kept trying. I was so scared I went along with it." When they were done, they pushed her back in the car and let her off where they picked her up. She was examined 6 hours after the assault.

Figure 56-a. *There are 3 fingertip-sized ecchymoses on the anterior thigh (35 mm).*

Figure 56-b. *The patient's dirty feet are consistent with the history of being barefoot outdoors.*

Case Study 56
(continued)

Figure 56-c. *The pink hymen is free of acute injury and erythema which might be expected with 15 incidents of forced vaginal penetration. The hymen is visible from 2 to 10 o'clock.*

Figure 56-d. *The posterior fourchette is free of injury.*

The case was inactivated because it was unsubstantiated and the perpetrators were not identified.

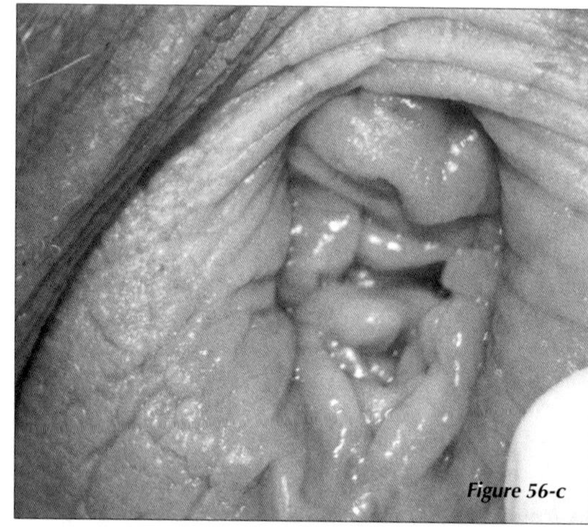

Figure 56-c

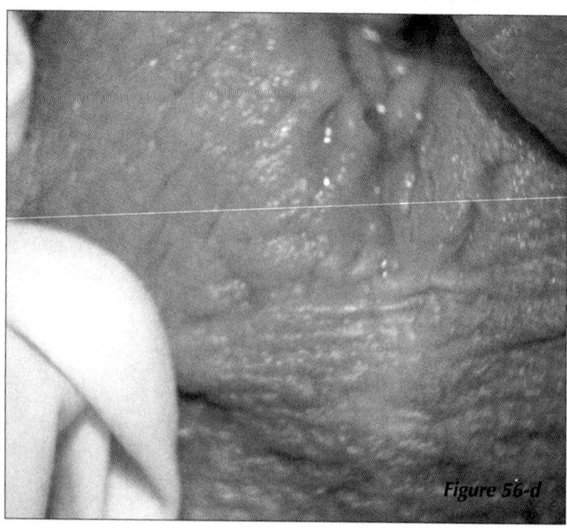

Figure 56-d

NONASSAULT VARIANTS

Nabothian Cyst

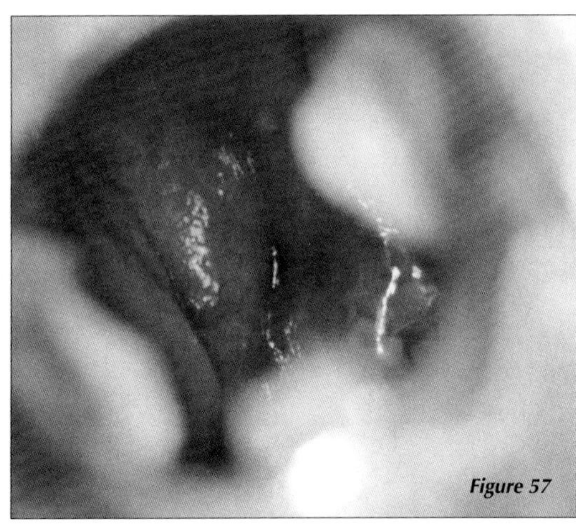

Case Study 57

This 45-year-old female (gravida 0) has had a nabothian cyst for several years. It is examined annually during her pap smears.

Figure 57. *The nabothian cyst.*

Breasts

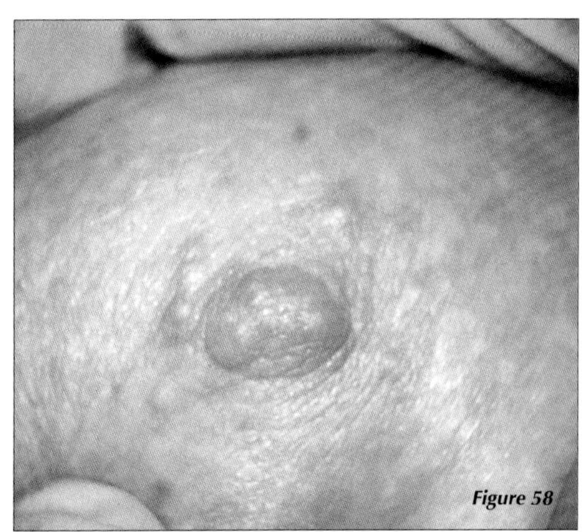

Case Study 58

This 51-year-old is a sober alcoholic. She is on an estrogen-progesterone combination.

Figure 58. *The nipple. The color of the areola has lightened with aging and now blends into the surrounding breast tissue.*

Genital

Case Study 59

This 58-year-old female is a recovering alcohol abuser and a smoker. She is now a Tanner stage 3, having lost much of her pubic hair which is common with aging when exogeneous estrogen is not taken.

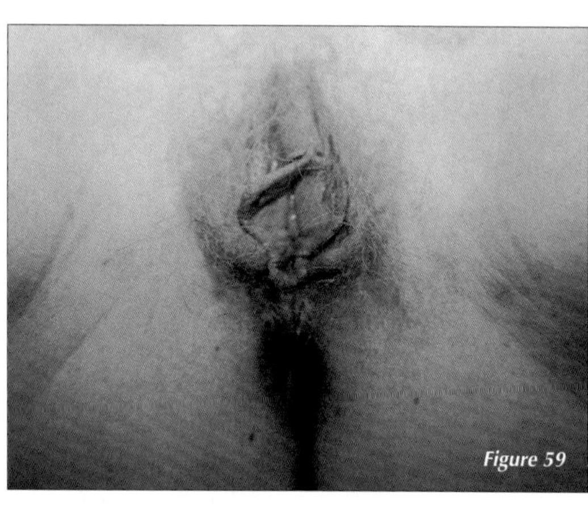

Figure 59. *The pubic hair that remains is sparse.*

Case Study 60

This 50-year-old obese multiparous Hispanic female has been postmenarchal for 3 years and is on no estrogen.

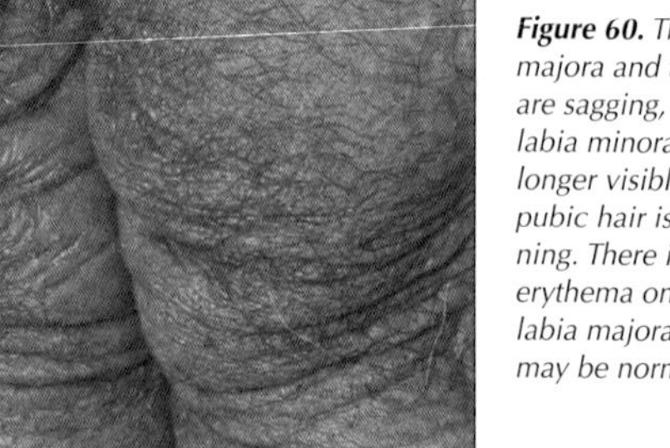

Figure 60. *The labia majora and thighs are sagging, and the labia minora are no longer visible. The pubic hair is thinning. There is erythema on the labia majora, which may be normal.*

Elderly Sexual Assault: 65 and Older

History of Sexual Assault

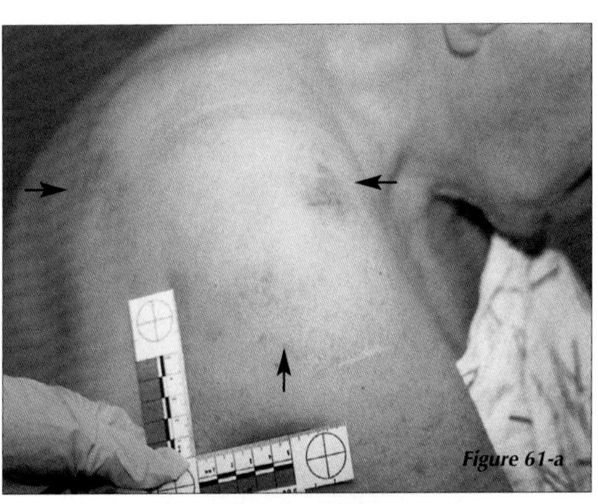

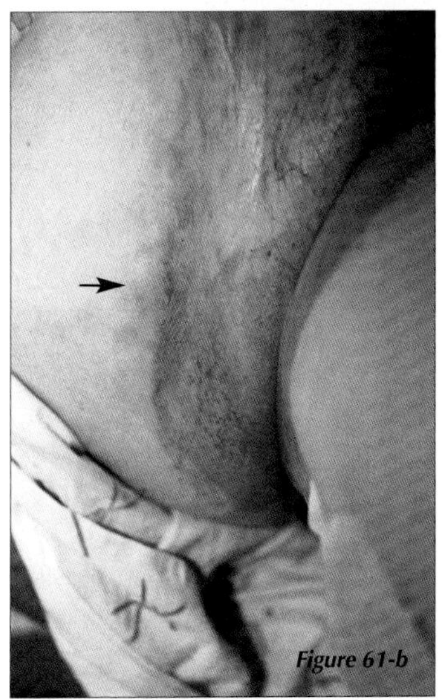

Case Study 61

This 74-year-old female (gravida 6, para 6) is taking no estrogens. She went outside to empty the trash in the evening. Two men (one Caucasian, one Hispanic with a tattoo on his arm) pushed her back inside her house. They pushed her to the floor, kicked her in the abdomen, and hit her above the right eye. She lost consciousness. When she awoke, it was 7 o'clock in the morning and she was naked from the waist down. She arrived for her examination 20 hours after the assault. She was alert and answered direct questions but was hesitant to give details.

Figure 61-a. *The ecchymoses of the right arm, shoulder, and back (35 mm).*

Figure 61-b. *The photograph shows the genital area, obscured by the obese medial thighs. The left leg is extended out, and the right leg is flexed up. The maceration on the inner thighs is related to moisture and obesity (35 mm).*

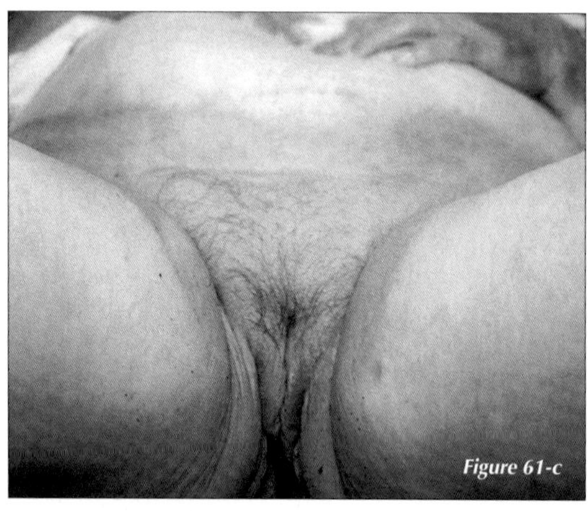

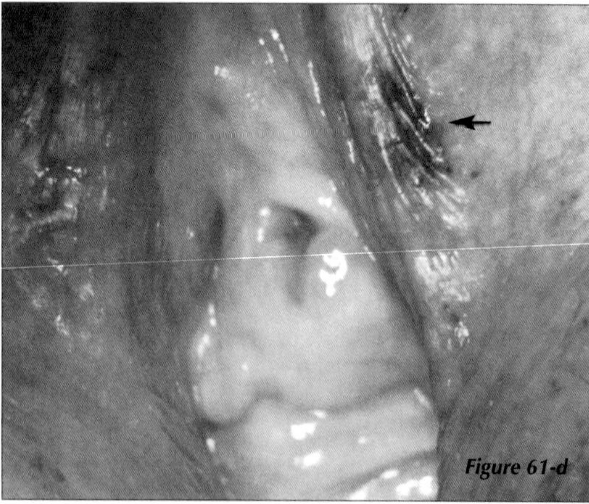

Case Study 61 *(continued)*

Figure 61-c. *There is maceration on the abdomen and inner thighs. Pubic hair is sparse, consistent with the victim's age (35 mm).*

Figure 61-d. *The periurethral area is pink with no acute injury. There is a black lesion on the left labium minus. The color and borders of this lesion are irregular.*

The victim was referred to gynecology for follow-up.

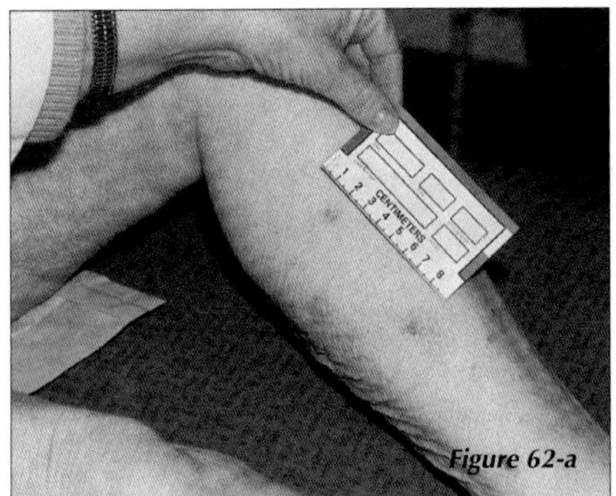

Figure 62-a

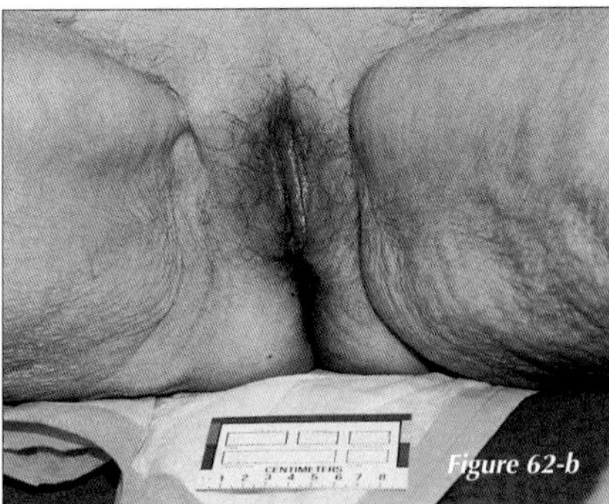

Figure 62-b

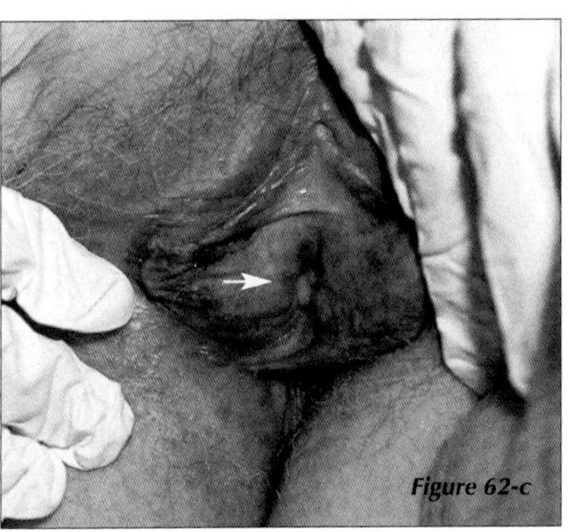

Figure 62-c

Case Study 62

This 79-year-old postmenopausal female (gravida 7, para 5) suffers from diverticulitis and constipation. She is able to stand and transfer but does not ambulate. She is incontinent and wears a diaper. Her diarrhea comes and goes. She lives in a skilled nursing facility and claimed that a male Middle-Eastern medication nurse gave her medication that made her go to sleep. When she woke up, she was naked from the waist down. She was unable to state what he did to her. She was examined in an emergency room 12 hours after she awoke. There was no photographic magnification available at the examination site.

Figure 62-a. *Ecchymosis is visible on the left leg (35 mm).*

Figure 62-b. *The sparse pubic hair and sagging of subcutaneous tissue is consistent with the patient's age. The labia majora and minora are erythematous (35 mm).*

Figure 62-c. *Erythema is present on the right labium majus extending down to the medial thigh. It is also present on the right labium minus (35 mm).*

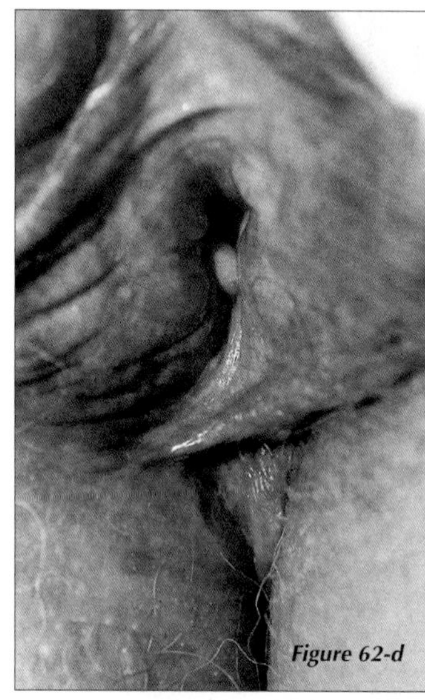

Figure 62-d

Case Study 62
(continued)

Figure 62-d. *There is a hymenal tag protruding from the vaginal orifice. Further separation would allow for more complete evaluation of the vaginal introitus (35 mm).*

Figure 62-e. *The anus is erythematous. Anal tags are visible (35 mm).*

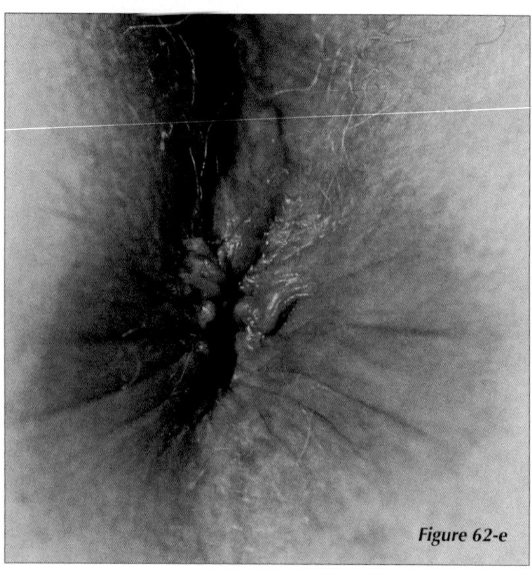

Figure 62-e

Case Study 63

This 94-year-old healthy white female lives in her own home. An unknown man came to the door wanting to use the telephone. She said she would make his call for him, but he pushed in through the door. He penetrated her vagina with his fingers and attempted to penetrate her vagina with his penis while she was on her back. He then put her on her abdomen and put his fingers in her anus and attempted to put his penis in her anus. He became frustrated and did not ejaculate. The victim was examined 2 hours after the assault.

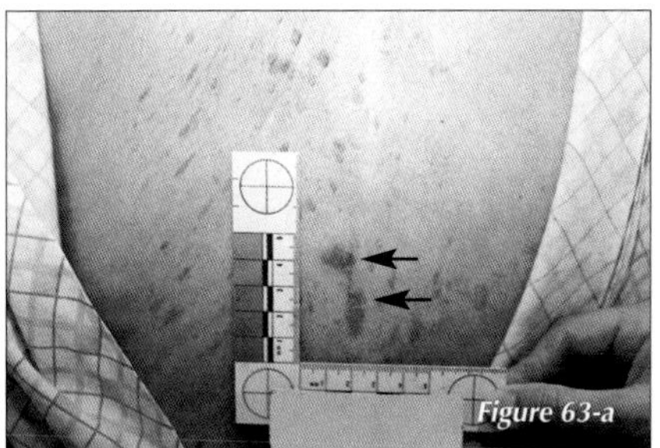

Figure 63-a. *The abrasions on the mid-back are consistent with the victim's story (35 mm).*

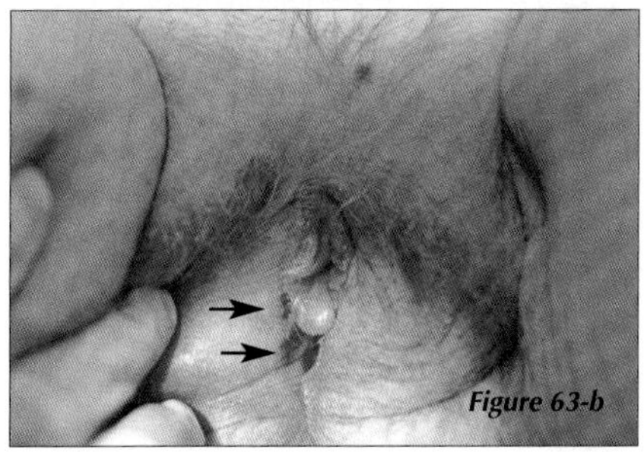

Figure 63-b. *There are lacerations on the right labium minus (35 mm).*

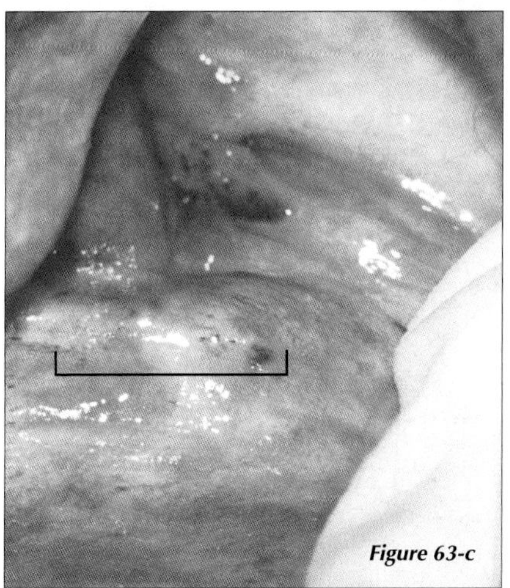

Figure 63-c. *There are abrasions on the posterior fourchette. There is white vaginal discharge present.*

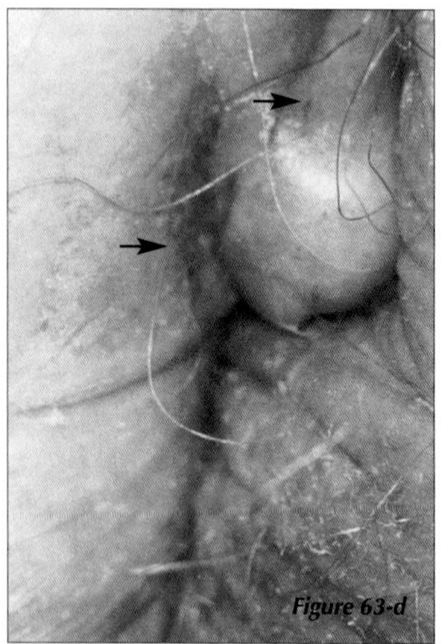

Figure 63-d

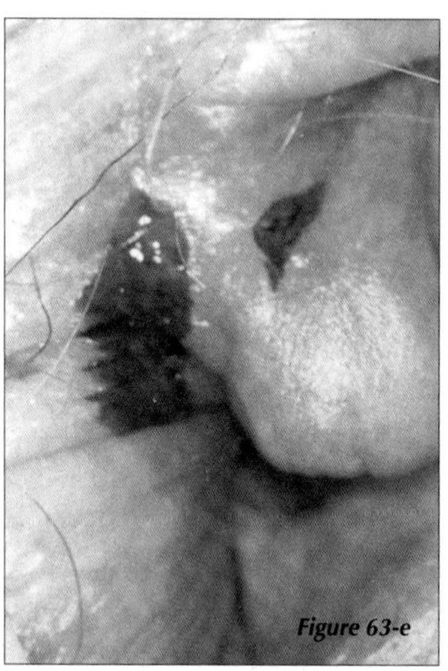

Figure 63-e

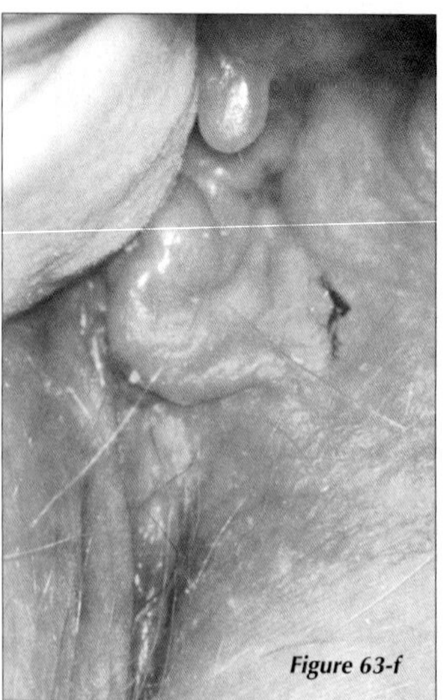

Figure 63-f

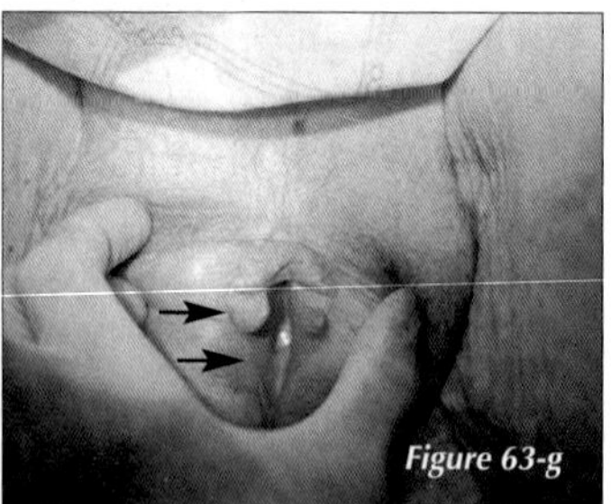

Figure 63-g

Case Study 63 *(continued)*

Figure 63-d. *There is a laceration lateral to the edematous right labium minus.*

Figure 63-e. *The dye uptake of the labial and hymenal lacerations.*

Figure 63-f. *This laceration of the perineum is oozing blood.*

Figure 63-g. *The labium minus laceration is resolved (35 mm).*

Nonassault Variants

Friable Fourchette

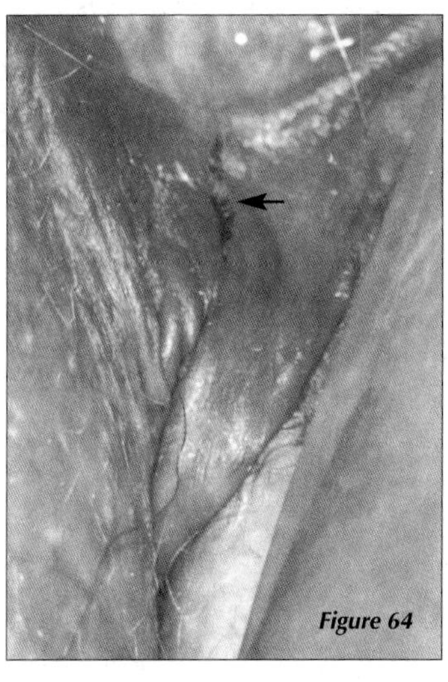

Case Study 64

This 94-year-old female has no ongoing vaginal infection and is not diabetic. She does not take estrogens.

Aged skin is less elastic and therefore less resilient to the separation technique and vaginal speculum exam.

Figure 64. *This posterior fourchette laceration occurred during the speculum examination.*

Rectal Polyp

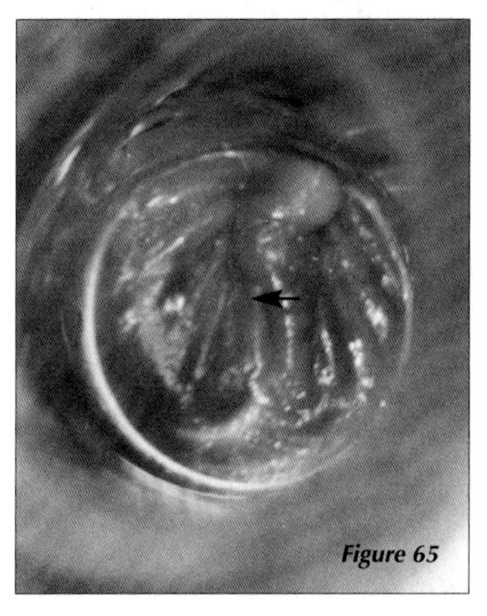

Case Study 65

This 65-year-old female was seen for a report of sexual assault. She denies forced or consensual anal intercourse.

Figure 65. *A rectal polyp is seen through the anoscope. She has no symptoms with this polyp, but she did with the previous one that started to bleed.*

A polyp was removed previously because of bleeding. She was referred for diagnosis and treatment.

NORMAL FINDINGS
Perianal Laxity

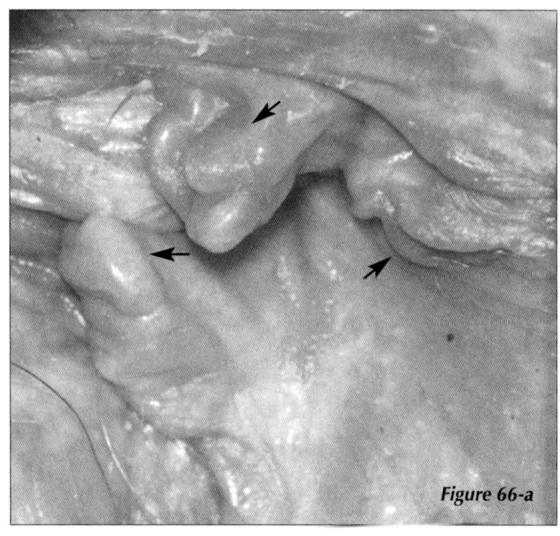
Figure 66-a

Case Study 66

This 88-year-old female states that she is "very healthy for her age." She explains that she has no constipation because of her diet, which includes 2 apples a day, and her daily walk of about 5 blocks.

Figure 66-a. *There are perianal tags superior and lateral to the anus. The anus is beneath the sagging perineal tissue.*

Figure 66-b. *Using separation, the anus is revealed within the redundant perianal tissue.*

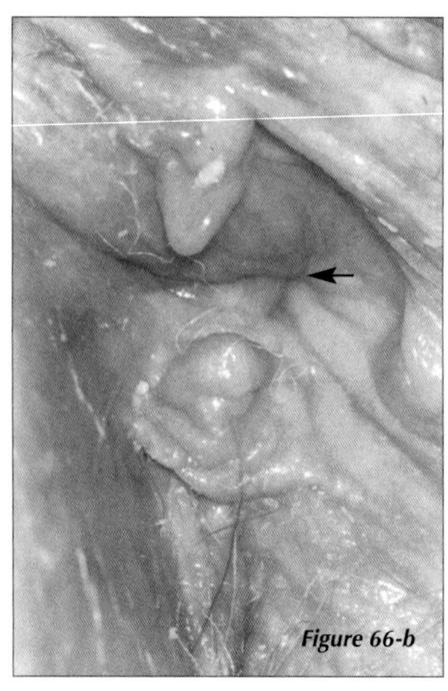
Figure 66-b

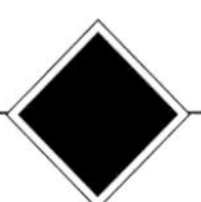

Index

A

B

C

D

E

F

G

H

J

K

L

M

N

S

T

U

V

W

Y

Z

Additional Titles Offered by G.W. Medical Publishing, Inc.

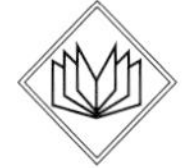

G.W. Medical Publishing, Inc.

Leader of Child Maltreatment and Abuse Publications

77 Westport Plaza Suite 366 • St. Louis, MO 63146

Phone: 1-800-600-0330 • 314-542-4213 • **Fax:** 314-542-4239

www.gwmedical.com

TABLE OF CONTENTS

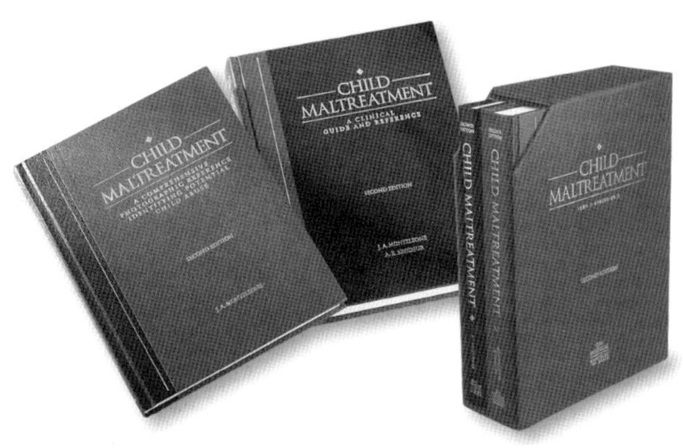

TABLE OF CONTENTS

CHILD MALTREATMENT

TRAINING MODULE AND VISUALS

3 Volume Training Module and Visuals

Angelo P. Giardino, MD, PhD, Editor
James A. Monteleone, MD, Editor
ISBN 1-878060-29-5

$469.95

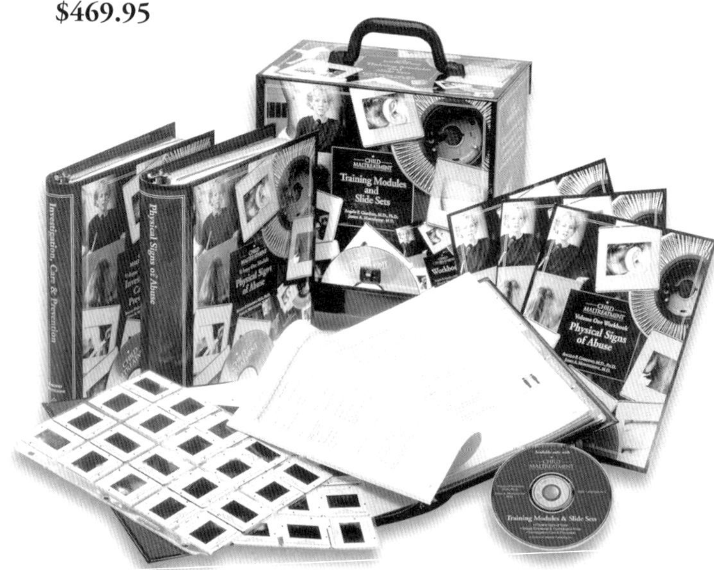

Written by 33 leading experts in various areas of child maltreatment, this training module includes: 392 full-color slides or CD-Rom; 3 instructor's modules, each averaging 225 pages with 36 individual lesson exercises accompanying each section; 15 participant workbooks; and 16 transparency acetate overheads.

This training module package of 3 binders will benefit anyone who trains or teaches others how to *identify, interpret,* and *report* occurrences of child abuse—*law enforcement, medical professionals, social workers, attorneys, teachers, and others.* The presentation of each section flows in an easy-to-follow sequence and is all-inclusive.

Volume One

Physical Signs of Abuse uses color photographs and radiographs to help course participants learn how to distinguish abusive from nonabusive injuries.

Volume Two

Sexual, Emotional & Psychological Abuse enables course participants to identify sexual abuse, delineates which children are at high risk for abuse and neglect, and addresses various psychological disorders.

Volume Three

Investigation, Care & Prevention teaches the steps to take when abuse or neglect is discovered, details the agencies and procedures involved, and helps participants realize strategies for preventing abuse.

The official companion textbook of the 3-volume Training Module is *Child Maltreatment: A Clinical Guide, 2nd ed.*, ISBN 1-878060-22-8. Containing 28 chapters (698 pages) and 242 images, it is a comprehensive encyclopedia of child abuse.

> *"The specialists at the Emergency Medical Services for Children National Resource Center were most impressed with the Child Maltreatment Slide Set. They found this teaching tool to be comprehensive, graphic, and therefore, highly effective."*
>
> **Rebecca Zeltinger, MLS Librarian**
> **National Resource Center**
> **Washington, DC**

TABLE OF CONTENTS

RECOGNITION OF CHILD ABUSE FOR THE MANDATED REPORTER

Written by experts from multiple disciplines, *Recognition of Child Abuse for the Mandated Reporter* incorporates proven approaches for distinguishing possible abuse from conditions that mimic abuse, conducting necessary interviews and examinations, documenting findings and preparing reports, making appropriate referrals, and joining with other caring professionals to prevent child maltreatment. This resource serves as a textbook for students in *medicine, nursing, social services,* and *law enforcement* as they prepare a career involving work with children.

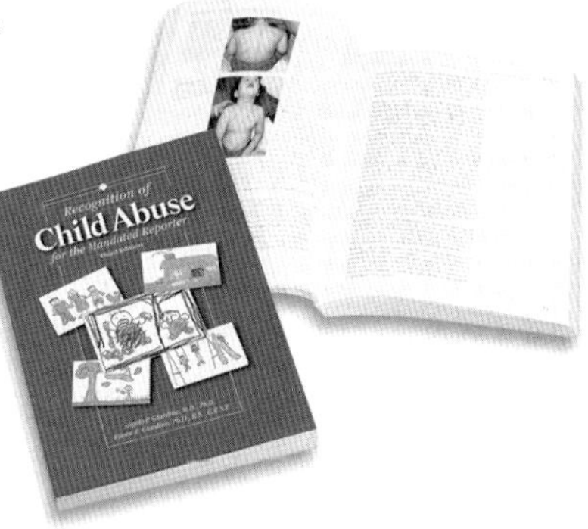

Third Edition

Angelo P. Giardino, MD, PhD
Eileen R. Giardino, PhD, RN, CRNP
466 pages, 80 images, 21 contributors
ISBN 1-878060-52-X

$46.95

TABLE OF CONTENTS

A PARENT'S & TEACHER'S HANDBOOK ON IDENTIFYING AND PREVENTING

CHILD ABUSE

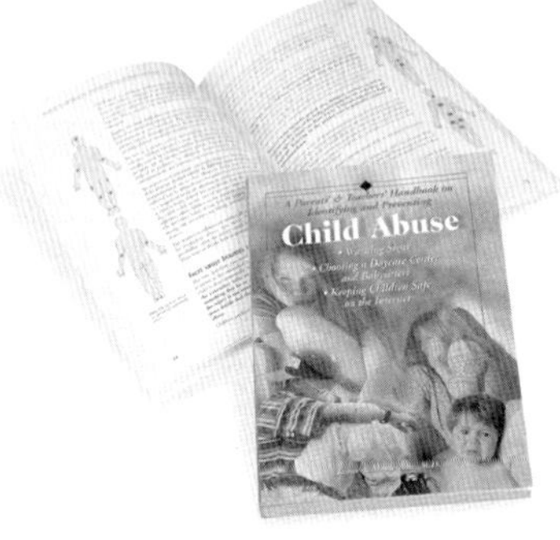

James A. Monteleone, MD
256 pages, 88 photos, 14 illustrations, 18 contributors
ISBN 1-878060-27-9

$19.95

For every parent who has ever felt helpless to protect a child from abusive individuals, this invaluable resource book offers empowerment. In plainspoken language with an easy-to-follow format, ***A Parent's & Teacher's Handbook on Identifying and Preventing Child Abuse*** explains what is and is not abuse, and describes in detail the physical and behavioral indicators of physical, sexual, and psychological abuse. It offers practical strategies on bringing up the subject of personal body safety with children and outlines clear-cut steps to take when a child discloses that he or a friend has been abused.

Drawing on the advice of real families who have dealt with abuse, the handbook describes how the legal and social systems process a child abuse case, giving parents a confidence born of knowing "what happens now."

TABLE OF CONTENTS

NURSING APPROACH

TO THE EVALUATION OF CHILD MALTREATMENT

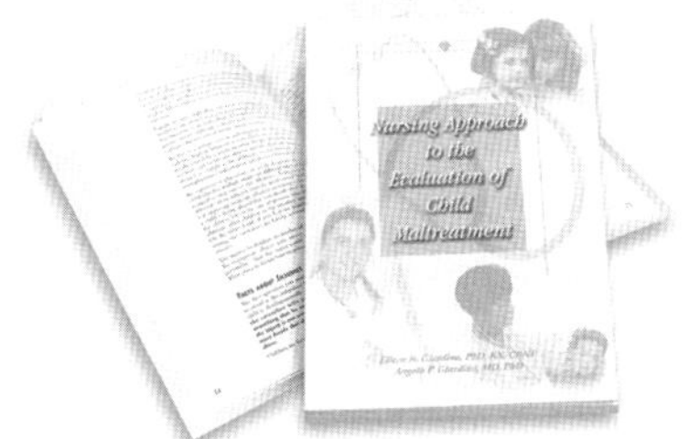

Eileen R. Giardino,
PhD, RN, CRNP
Angelo P. Giardino,
MD, PhD, FAAP
500 pages, 180 images,
20 contributors
ISBN 1-878060-51-1

$49.95

Nurses and nurse practitioners are critical members of child abuse treatment teams. ***Nursing Approach to the Evaluation of Child Maltreatment*** provides the information nurses need to identify, interpret, and report the signs of maltreatment.

Presented in 17 chapters comprising 3 major sections, the areas of physical abuse, sexual abuse, and neglect are extensively addressed. Each chapter is structured to give a general overview of the topic area followed by a detailed treatment plan relevant to the specific types of abuse. In addition, each chapter includes easy-to-use checklists, examination hints, and flow charts for ready access to important information.

TABLE OF CONTENTS

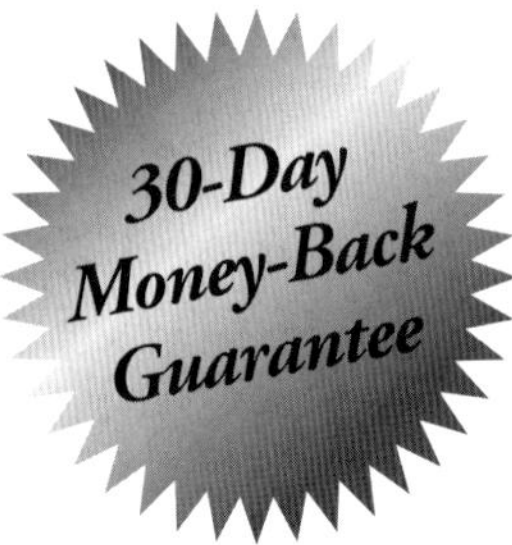

Get the best tools to fight child abuse. Four easy ways to order.

TO ORDER,

complete and mail to:

G.W. Medical Publishing, Inc.
77 Westport Plaza, Suite 366
St. Louis, MO 63146

Call toll-free:
1-800-600-0330
8:30 am – 4:30 pm CST

Fax:
314-542-4239

E-mail:
orders@gwmedical.com

On-line:
www.gwmedical.com

Terms

Please pay personal orders by check or credit card. Make checks payable to G. W. Medical Publishing, Inc. All international orders must be prepaid in U.S. funds. Inquire on shipping costs. Please allow 2-4 weeks for shipping. Call 001-314-542-4213 for international orders.

All orders are billed for postage, handling, and state sales tax where appropriate. All prices subject to change without notice. If using a purchase order, please attach it to this form. **30-Day Money-Back Guarantee:** If you are not 100% satisfied, simply return the book(s) within 30 days in the original shipping carton, by a traceable source. Your money will be promptly refunded without question less a 15% restocking fee.

Four ways to order

1. **Phone:** 1-800-600-0330 Please have your credit card ready when you call.
2. **Fax:** 314-542-4239 Fax this completed form with your company purchase order or credit card information.
3. **Mail:** G.W. Medical Publishing Inc. 77 Westport Plaza, Suite 366 St. Louis, MO 63146
4. **E-Mail:** orders@gwmedical.com

   Web site: www.gwmedical.com

Yes, I'd like to order

Qty	Title/Description	ISBN	Unit	Shipping
	Child Maltreatment Training Module and Visuals Select (1) one: ☐ CD-ROM ☐ 35 mm slide format ☐ Both (additional $125.00)	1-878060-29-5	$469.95	$14.00
	Child Maltreatment Two-Volume Set Second Edition	1-878060-26-0	$229.95	$11.15
	Child Abuse Quick-Reference	1-878060-28-7	$44.95	$6.75
	Recognition of Child Abuse for the Mandated Reporter Third Edition	1-878060-52-X	$46.95	$6.75
	A Parent's & Teacher's Handbook on Identifying and Preventing Child Abuse	1-878060-27-9	$19.95	$6.75
	Sexual Assault Victimization Across the Life Span Two-Volume Set	1-878060-62-7	$229.95	$11.50
	Sexual Assault Quick-Reference	1-878060-38-4	$49.95	$6.75
	Nursing Approach to the Evaluation of Child Maltreatment	1-878060-51-1	$46.95	$6.75

Visit our Web site at www.gwmedical.com to review forthcoming titles.

Please send my books to

Name Title

Company / Organization

Address

City / State / Zip

Phone ( ) Fax ( )

E-Mail Address

I'd like to pay by

Credit Card ❑ Visa ❑ MasterCard

Cardholder's Name

Card Number Exp. Date

Signature of Cardholder

❑ Check Enclosed in U.S. funds (Make payable to G.W. Medical Publishing, Inc.)

❑ Purchase Order No. (This order form must be attached to your company P.O.) Net 10 days after receipt of book(s)

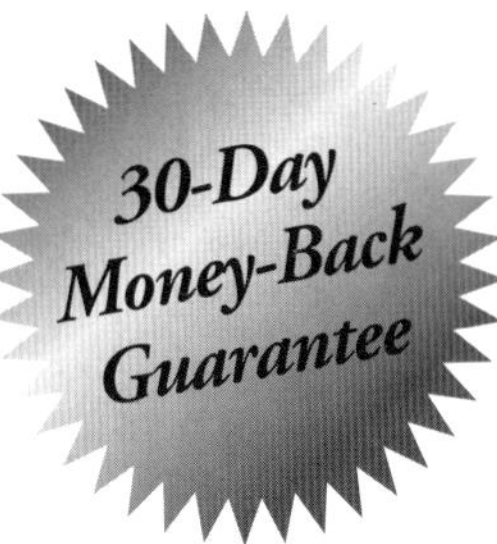

Get the best tools to fight child abuse. Four easy ways to order.

TO ORDER,

complete and mail to:

G.W. Medical Publishing, Inc.
77 Westport Plaza, Suite 366
St. Louis, MO 63146

Call toll-free:
1-800-600-0330
8:30 am – 4:30 pm CST

Fax:
314-542-4239

E-mail:
orders@gwmedical.com

On-line:
www.gwmedical.com

Terms

Please pay personal orders by check or credit card. Make checks payable to G. W. Medical Publishing, Inc. All international orders must be prepaid in U.S. funds. Inquire on shipping costs. Please allow 2-4 weeks for shipping. Call 001-314-542-4213 for international orders.

All orders are billed for postage, handling, and state sales tax where appropriate. All prices subject to change without notice. If using a purchase order, please attach it to this form. **30-Day Money-Back Guarantee:** If you are not 100% satisfied, simply return the book(s) within 30 days in the original shipping carton, by a traceable source. Your money will be promptly refunded without question less a 15% restocking fee.

Four ways to order

1. **Phone:** 1-800-600-0330 Please have your credit card ready when you call.
2. **Fax:** 314-542-4239 Fax this completed form with your company purchase order or credit card information.
3. **Mail:** G.W. Medical Publishing Inc. 77 Westport Plaza, Suite 366 St. Louis, MO 63146
4. **E-Mail:** orders@gwmedical.com

   Web site: www.gwmedical.com

I'd like to order

Title/Description	ISBN	Unit	Shipping
Child Maltreatment Training Module and Visuals Select (1) one: ☐ CD-ROM ☐ 35 mm slide format ☐ Both (additional $125.00)	1-878060-29-5	$469.95	$14.00
Child Maltreatment Two-Volume Set Second Edition	1-878060-26-0	$229.95	$11.15
Child Abuse Quick-Reference	1-878060-28-7	$44.95	$6.75
Recognition of Child Abuse for the Mandated Reporter Third Edition	1-878060-52-X	$46.95	$6.75
A Parent's & Teacher's Handbook on Identifying and Preventing Child Abuse	1-878060-27-9	$19.95	$6.75
Sexual Assault Victimization Across the Life Span Two-Volume Set	1-878060-62-7	$229.95	$11.50
Sexual Assault Quick-Reference	1-878060-38-4	$49.95	$6.75
Nursing Approach to the Evaluation of Child Maltreatment	1-878060-51-1	$46.95	$6.75

our Web site at *www.gwmedical.com* to review forthcoming titles.

ase send my books to

ne Title

npany / Organization

ress

/ State / Zip

ne ( ) Fax ( )

ail Address

ike to pay by

it Card ❑ Visa ❑ MasterCard

holder's Name

Number Exp. Date

ature of Cardholder

eck Enclosed in U.S. funds (Make payable to G.W. Medical Publishing, Inc.)

rchase Order No. (This order form must be attached to your company P.O.)
t 10 days after receipt of book(s)